KIDNEY CANCER

I. INTRODUCTION

1. MOLECULAR GENETICS
OF KIDNEY CANCER

MICHAEL ZIMMER AND OTHON ILIOPOULOS

From The Massachusetts General Hospital Cancer Center and MGH Familial Renal Cancer Clinic, Harvard Medical School, Boston, MA.

INTRODUCTION

Tumorigenesis is a multistep process of genetic and epigenetic changes that occur in an orderly fashion. The order of these changes may navigate through different steps in cancers arising from different organs/tissues. It is likely though that the final outcome is the sequential deregulation of a few key pathways of normal cell growth, namely: inactivation of tumor suppressor genes; activation of oncogenes; evasion of apoptotic cell program; and ultimately induction of angiogenesis and metastasis.[1] Entry points to these genetic alterations were discovered by cloning genes disrupted by tumor-associated chromosomal translocations, harbored in cancer-associated homozygous deletions or underlying familial cancer syndromes.

Thus, identification and cloning of familial cancer susceptibility genes (p53, Rb, VHL, BRCA1/2, PTEN) has implications beyond the familial syndrome they underline. Elucidation of their biochemical function provides entry points into molecular pathways that deregulate normal growth and differentiation. Ultimately they may lead to the identification of critical molecular targets for drug development. In the short term, they may increase our understanding of the full clinical spectrum of familial cancer syndromes and facilitate our ability to develop rational surveillance and genetic counseling programs.

Address for Correspondence: Othon Iliopoulos, Massachusetts General Hospital Cancer Center, 55 Fruit Street, GRJ-904, Boston, MA 02114.

R.A. Figlin (ed.). KIDNEY CANCER. Copyright © 2003. Kluwer Academic Publishers. Boston. All rights reserved.

In this chapter, we will describe primarily Familial Renal Carcinoma syndromes and the genetic events that underlie them. For each familial syndrome, the Online Mendelian Inheritance in Man (OMIM) reference number will be included. The reader is encouraged to visit OMIM (http://www.ncbi.nlm.nih.gov/Omim/) for more detailed description of affected families.

Primary renal epithelial tumors are histologically heterogeneous. The majority of sporadic tumors consists of clear cell carcinoma (75%) and papillary carcinoma (15%), with chromophobe (5%) and oncocytomas (5%) encountered much less frequently.[2] Syndromes of familial renal neoplasms mostly predispose to tumors of specific histology; in the following pages will be discussed according to this classification.

A. FAMILIAL CLEAR CELL RCC

A1. Von Hippel-Lindau Disease (OMIM 193300)

Von Hippel-Lindau (VHL) is a disease of familial predisposition to cancer transmitted in an autosomal dominant fashion. Its incidence is estimated to be 1:36,000 births.[3] Melmon and Rosen described clinical criteria for diagnosis of VHL disease.[4] Cloning of the VHL susceptibility gene[5] has already broadened our understanding of VHL disease clinical spectrum and it may lead to revision of the "classic" clinical criteria.

Clinical Manifestations

Renal cell carcinoma (RCC) and hemangioblastomas (HB) of the central nervous system (CNS) equally contribute to morbidity and mortality of VHL disease. HB usually occur earlier than RCC. The penetrance of the disease is almost complete by the age of 66.

CNS hemangioblastomas, including those in the retina, are the earliest and most characteristic lesion of VHL disease, developing in 60–80% of the patients.[6] They are non-metastatic lesions consisting of stromal cells of neuroectodermal origin and a rich plexus of capillary vessels. They have both solid and cystic component with a variable ratio between the two.[7] VHL-associated hemangioblastomas occur typically in the cerebellum (75%), the spinal cord (20%) and the brain stem (5%). The lesions are multiple and appear in a synchronous or metachronous fashion.[8] In contrast to VHL-associated HB, sporadic HBs tend to occur supra-tentorially, they are usually single and do not reoccur after surgical excision.[9] Simultaneous presence of two spinal HBs is almost pathognomonic of VHL disease. Symptoms occur because of the space occupying nature of HBs and range from simple headaches, to focal neurologic deficits or a clinical presentation of increased intracranial pressure. The main modality for treating HB is surgical excision or stereotactic radiosurgery. The latter is primarily indicated for small (<2 cm) lesions with minimal cystic component that are not located in the brainstem or the spinal cord.

Retinal hemangioblastomas may arise in the periphery of the retina or close to the retinal papilla. The most difficult tumors to treat are encountered within the optic nerve. Retinal HB may be asymptomatic or cause retinal detachement and blindness. With the exception of these within the optic nerve, retinal HBs are treated with laser beam surgery.[10]

VHL patients may develop hundreds of bilateral renal cysts of variable size, deriving from the proximal or distal renal tubules. Renal cysts are usually asymptomatic and there is virtually no report of renal insufficiency attributed solely to VHL-associated cysts.[11] 60–80% of VHL patients develop multiple, bilateral, synchronous or metachronous renal carcinomas, deriving from the cysts or the solid renal parenchyma.[6,12] VHL-associated RCC is exclusively the clear cell type. Cloning of the VHL gene allowed for early diagnosis, identification of family members at risk and institution of surveillance programs. In patients followed by regular imaging of the kidneys RCC are mostly detected as localized, non-metastatic disease and can be treated surgically. Nevertheless, RCCs remain a challenge for VHL patients because they develop multicentrically and metachronously. Repeated surgeries may lead to renal insufficiency; it is now established that the standard of care for VHL-associated RCC is nephron-sparing surgery that can minimize damage of the healthy renal parenchyma.[13] Since the pattern of RCC growth may be variable, small asymptomatic tumors may initially be observed until they reach a size of 3 cm.[14] However, isolated reports of VHL patients with only a primary tumor less than 3 cm and metastatic disease do exist. Molecular markers and imaging techniques reliably predicting RCC and HB activity in VHL patients are urgently needed. Our recent understanding of the functions of the VHL protein may open new areas of target-specific, non-surgical treatment of RCC and HB (see below: functions of pVHL).

VHL-associated pheochromocytomas (PHEO) are usually non-metastatic, multifocal, and bilateral.[15] They tend to cluster in certain, but not all, VHL families and therefore their occurrence provides the basis for clinical subclassification of VHL disease. Specific VHL mutations predispose to PHEO occurrence (see below: VHL mutations). A large study examined the frequency of familial PHEO in 82 consecutive patients presenting with clinical diagnosis of pheochromocytoma: 19% of these patients had germline mutations in the VHL gene while 4% had MEN2 disease. Screeening of family members at risk detected PHEO in 46% of the cases.[16] Diagnosis of PHEO is based on measurement of serum and urine levels of metanephrines and normetanephrines[17] and imaging studies. Abdominal MRI and metaiodobenzylguanidine (MIBG) scintigraphy have 95% imaging sensitivity for pheochromocytoma. Most recently 18-Fluoro-DOPA positron emission tomography (PET) was reported to approach 100% sensitivity in diagnosis of adrenal as well as extra-adrenal PHEO.[15]

Less frequently, VHL patients may develop pancreatic cysts, papillary cystadenomas of the pancreas and pancreatic islet cell tumors.[18,19] Cysts and cystadenomas require treatment when they become symptomatic due to compression of local structures such as the common bile duct. Papillary cystadenomas are non-invading tumors. Islet cell tumors are usually non-functional, but peptide secreting tumors have been described in VHL patients and symptoms depend on the nature of the

Table 1. Criteria for Referal to VHL Clinic (Massachusetts General Hospital).

(1) Any blood relative of an individual diagnosed with VHL disease.
(2) Individuals with one VHL associated lesion★
AND a positive family history (FH) of VHL associated-lesion(s)
(3) Any individual with TWO VHL-associated lesions
(4) Individual with any of the following
Hemangioblastoma (HB) diagnosed at a <30 yo patient
>2 CNS hemangioblastomas (any age of diagnosis)
1 HB + (RCC or PHEO or pancreatic neuroendocrine tumor)
Clear cell Renal Carcinoma (RCC) diagnosed at a <40 yo patient
Bilateral and/or multiple clear cell RCC
Clear cell RCC with a positive FH
Pheochromocytoma (PHEO) diagnosed at a <40 yo patient
Bilateral and/or multiple PHEO
PHEO with a positive FH
>1 Pancreatic Serous Cystadenoma
>1 Pancreatic neuroendocrine tumor
Multiple pancreatic cysts + any VHL associated lesion
Endolymphatic sac tumor (ELST)
Epidiydmal papillary cystadenoma

★ **VHL associated lesions:** hemangioblastoma (HB), clear cell renal carcinoma (RCC), pheochromocytoma (PHE), endolymphatic sac tumor (ELST), epididymal papillary cystadenoma, pancreatic serous cystadenomas, pancreatic neuroendocrine tumors.

secreted peptide. VHL patients are not at high risk for developing mucinous cystadenomas or pancreatic adenocarcinoma.[18] Papillary cystadenomas may also develop in the middle ear (endolymphatic sac tumors) and the organs of mesonephric origin (epididymis in males and adnexal strucutures in females).[20,21]

The clinical indications used in the Massachusetts General Hospital VHL Clinic for evaluating patients for VHL disease are listed in Table 1.

VHL-Associated Mutations

The VHL gene maps to ch. 3p25.[22–24] The gene was cloned in 1993;[5] it consists of there exons and generates at least two mRNA species, one encompassing all exons and one missing exon 2.[5] VHL is expressed in all adult and embryonic tissues examined so far. VHL homologues have been identified in mouse, rat, Drosophila, and C. elegans, but not in S. cerevisiae.[25–28] Genetic studies in Drosophila and C.elegans are in progress and may shed light on critical functions of the protein encoded by the VHL gene (pVHL).

VHL is mutated in almost 100% of the patients presenting with clinical manifestations of VHL disease.[29] Types of mutations include large germline deletions, small intragenic deletions, nonsense mutations and missense mutations. The latter are clustered over the 3′ end of exon 1 and the 5′ of exon 3. All missense mutations map downstream of codon 54. All VHL-associated tumors harbor loss of heterozygosity (LOH) in the VHL locus resulting in loss of the wild-type allele.[30,31] This pattern supports the notion that VHL is a tumor suppressor gene and that inactivation of both alleles is necessary for tumor formation (Knudson's "two-hit" hypothesis). In keeping with this model, VHL is inactivated in 80% of sporadic clear cell renal carcinomas, the majority of sporadic hemangioblastomas and sporadic islet cell tumors of the pancreas.[32–35] RCC of only clear type (conventional) histology harbor VHL mutations. Papillary, chromophobe or oncocytoma have wild-type VHL. Breast, prostate, colon and other non VHL-associated prevalent tumors harbor no mutations in the VHL gene.

VHL disease is phenotypically heterogeneous.[36–38] Type 1 patients develop HB and RCC but not PHEO. Type 2 patients are at risk for PHEO and are subdivided in three subtypes. Type 2A, in addition to PHEO, are at low and type 2B at high risk for RCC. Type 3C patients present as familial PHEO without development of RCC or HB. Germline mutations predisposing to Type 1 disease consist of large or small deletions or nonsense mutations. Only 44% of Type 1 mutations are missense. Based on studies of the crystal strucuture of the protein (see below) Type 1 missense mutations predict total unfolding and inactivation of the protein. In contrast, the overwhelming majority of Type 2 mutations are missense mutations affecting domains of protein-protein interaction but respecting the overall structure of the protein. It is therefore likely that Type 2 mutations retain some protein functions. This information may prove useful for tailoring surveillance programs for each patient's individual risks.

Physiology of VHL−/− Cells

Studies on human renal carcinoma cell lines first indicated that the VHL gene product (pVHL) is involved in the hypoxia signal transduction pathway and that this property of VHL is linked to its ability to mediate tumor suppression. 786-O human renal carcinoma cells lack wild-type pVHL and they grow as tumors when injected into the flank of nude mice. Stable expression of wild-type pVHL in these (and other similarly VHL−/− cell lines) leads to tumor suppression in the mouse xenograft assay, providing functional evidence that pVHL acts as a tumor suppressor gene.[39,40,41,42]

Cells in general sense and respond to hypoxic stimuli (1% ambient oxygen tension) by overexpressing a family of proteins known as hypoxia inducible genes.[43] This family includes growth factors and angiogeneic peptides (such as PDGF, TGF-a, TGF-b, VEGF), enzymes of the intermediate metabolism and molecules involved in remodeling of the extracellular matrix (such as metalloproteinases, plasminogen activator inhibitor-I). Expression of hypoxia inducible proteins remains low under conditions of normoxia. Cells lacking wild-type VHL function (VHL−/− cells) inappropriately overexpress hypoxia inducible proteins.[40,44] This inappropriate overexpression not only may explain the hypervascular nature of VHL-associated tumors (RCC, HB) but it may also provide an explanation for the molecular events leading to transformation of the normal renal epithelium. It is conceivable that constitutive overexpression of proto-oncogenes such as PDGF-B or growth factors such as TGF-a significantly contribute to the malignant phenotype of the VHL−/− cells.

VHL appears to protect cells from environmental "stress" stimuli. Gorospe et al. subjected VHL−/− and isogenic VHL+/+ cells in minimal glucose containing medium culture and noticed that VHL−/− but not pVHL expressing cells died by apoptosis.[45] Similarly, pVHL was reported to protect from UV-mediated apoptosis.[46]

Expression of pVHL may be necessary for serum withdrawal-mediated exit from the cell cycle under specific culture conditions.[47] Pause et al. reported that VHL−/− cells fail to stabilize p27 and do not arrest at G0 stage when serum starved. The mechanism of this phenomenon is not clear. There is no evidence that p27 is directly degraded by pVHL. It is conceivable that the cell cycle arrest is an epiphenomenonon due to titration of growth factors in the conditioned medium: for example VHL−/− cells overexpress TGF-a, which in turn may stimulate cell cycle progression through EGF-receptor activation.

There is evidence that VHL−/− cells exhibit a less differentiated phenotype. VHL−/− cells fail to assemble and deposit a mature extracellular fibronectin matrix. The molecular mechanism for this is not known but it could be attributed to the function of pVHL as E3 substrate receptor: it is conceivable that pVHL is required for degradation of missfolded fibronectin while it resides in the ER, prior to their secretion.[48] Fibronectin may, as part of the extracellular matrix, contribute to regulation of growth and differentiation. Davidowitz et al showed that when VHL+/+ cells are cultured on collagen I they undergo growth arrest at high density and acquire morphological and molecular features of differentiation.[49] In contrast, VHL−/− cells fail to arrest and continue to grow without any evidence of differentiation. Growth of cells in multicellular spheroids is another method to mimic some aspects of cell-to-extracellular matrix interactions and subsequent differentiation. When cultured in spheroids VHL−/− cells form cohesive structures with little extracellular fibronectin deposition.[50] In contrast VHL+/+ cells form tubular structures with salient futures of differentiation, such as polarity of epithelial cells.[50] Rat pluripotential neural progenitor cells may be induced to differentiate into cells with neuronal or glial features. Undifferentiated progenitor cells appear to express low levels of immunohistochemically detectable pVHL.[51] Differentiation into neuronal, but not glial, phenotype correlates with pVHL induction.

Molecular Functions of pVHL

VHL encodes at least two biologically active isoforms. A 213 amino acid phosphoprotein is encoded by the VHL putative ORF (VHL30, 28–30 kD apparent MW).[25,39] A second isoform is produced in cells by internal translation of mRNA initiated at Methionine 54 (VHL19, 19 kD MW).[52,53] All cell lines with wild-type VHL examined so far express both isoforms. No detection of an isoform corresponding to the alternatively spliced mRNA has been reported so far. The pattern of germline mutations indicate that inactivation of both isoforms is necessary for tumor development. Both isoforms undergo nucleocytoplasmic shuttling, in a transcription dependent manner, but the physiologic stimuli regulating this shuttling are not yet known.[54]

Identification and cloning of intracellular proteins stably interacting with pVHL shed light in its biochemical functions. An intracellular multiprotein complex comprises of pVHL, ElonginC, Elongin B, Cullin-2 and the RING-finger protein Rbx-1. The crystal structure of pVHL has been resolved.[55] VHL protein folds into beta and alpha domains. The alpha domain mediates binding of pVHL to Elongin C. The latter bridges pVHL with the N-terminal domain of Cullin-2. A highly conserved domain of Cullin-2 (termed cullin homology doamian-CHD) binds to Rbx-1, which in turn is predicted to recruit a ubiquitin conjugase into the complex. This multiprotein complex is structurally homologuous to yeast SCF complexes (named so after their subunits Skp1, Cdc53 and F-box substrate receptors) and mediates E3-dependent ubuquitination of substrate proteins. Substrate specificity is regulated at the receptor level and pVHL serves as the substrate receptor of the SCF[VHL] complex. Tumor-associated mutation are predicted to either unfold and inactivate pVHL or to disrupt critical protein-protein interactions.[55] Missense mutations in the alpha domain disrupt pVHL-Elongin C interaction and therefore prevent entrance of pVHL into the complex. Missense mutations in the beta domain are predicted to disrupt between pVHL and the putative substrate. In any case, total or partial loss-of-VHL function would lead to inhibition of ubiquitination and therefore constitutive stabilization of the putative substrate.

The proteins identified as the first substrates of pVHL were the Hypoxia Inducible Factors 1a and 2a (HIF 1a/2a).[56] Hypoxia Inducible Factor (HIF) is a heterodimeric transcription factor and a critical mediator of a cellular response to hypoxia.[57] It consists of the hypoxia-regulated alpha subunits 1a, 2a or 3a and the constitutively expressed beta subunits 1b (ARNT), 2b and 3b. When cells sense a normal ambient oxygen tension (21%) the alpha regulatory subunit is ubiquitinated and rapidly destroyed through the proteasome. Hypoxia (1% ambient oxygen tension) stabilizes the alpha subunit, which in turn enters the nucleus, heterodimerizes with a beta subunit, binds to canonical DNA sequences termed Hypoxia Response Elements (HRE), and mediates transcriptional activation of a growing family of hypoxia responsive genes.[58] Stability of HIF alpha subunit is therefore critical regulator of HIF activity. pVHL containing complexes are at least one of the E3 ubiquitin ligases mediating ubiquitination and destruction of HIF1a/2a. VHL protein directly binds to the Oxygen Dependent Degradation (ODD) domain of HIF and mediates its ubiquitination.[59] In a recent series of elegant papers it was shown that this interaction depends on hydroxylation of Proline 564 embedded within the ODD domain.[60,61] The mammalian, C.elegans, and Drosophila prolyl-hydroxylases modifying Proline 564 have been identified and cloned.[62] Hypoxia directly inhibits intracellular prolyl-hydroxylases and consequently disrupts HIF-pVHL interaction, leading to HIF 1a/2a stability and activation of hypoxia inducible genes. Similarly, loss of pVHL function leads to constitutive activation of HIF (Figure 1).

HIF may be a critical factor in tumor development. Almost all solid tumors require angiogenesis for establishment, growth and, potentially, metastasis. HIF is a critical factor for response to tumor-associated hypoxia and angiogenesis. Solid tumors, but not surrounding normal tissue, overexpress HIF. When mouse embryonic stem

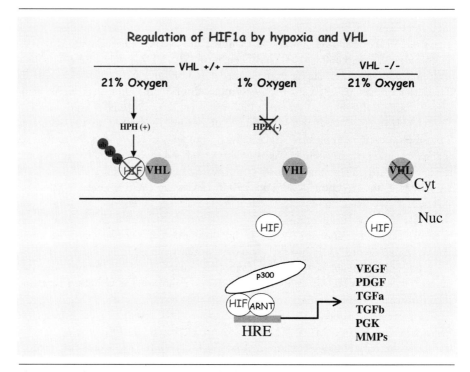

Figure 1. Under normoxic conditions pVHL binds and inactivates HIF, through ubiquitination and proteasomal degradation. When cells are exposed to hypoxia HIF is not modified by HPH and it is detached from pVHL. Stabilized HIF enters the nucleus, heterodimerizes with its constitutively expressed beta subunit and binds DNA at hypoxia response element sites (HRE). VHL−/− cells express HIF constitutively (VHL = Von Hippel-Lindau disease protein. Ub = ubiquitin, HIF = Hypoxia inducible factor subunit 1a or 2a. Cyt = cytoplasm, Nuc = nucleus. ARNT = Arylhydrocarbon Nuclear Translocator/HIF2b).

cells (ES) are injected in nude mice they form teratocarcinomas. HIF−/− ES cells are characterized by marked reduction in tumor formation when subjected in this assay. Peptide-mediated disruption of the interaction of HIF with the transcriptional co-activator p300 led to tumor suppression. In agreement with these findings HIF2a (but not HIF1a) overexpression in VHL+/+ human RCC lines led to tumor formation in the mouse xenograft assay.[63,64] The critical question remains whether HIF inactivation is sufficient for tumor suppression. If this is the case, the therapeutic potential of specific HIF inhibitors in treatment of VHL-associated lesions and perhaps solid tumors generally, is obvious.

Other proteins have been proposed as substrates of pVHL, including activated PKCzeta,[65] and deubuquitinating enzymes.[66] The identity of these molecules as bonafide substrates, and the evaluation of their importance in the generation of VHL-associated lesions, is an area of current research.

A2. Tuberous Sclerosis Complex

Clinical Manifestations

Tuberous sclerosis complex (TSC) is a genetically heterogeneous disease. Two major loci have been linked to the disease and the corresponding genes have been cloned. TSC1 gene (OMIM 191100) maps to ch.9q34[67] and TSC2 (OMIM 191092) to Ch.16p13.3.[68] There is no difference in the clinical manifestations of TSC disease resulting from mutations in either gene, although there are indications that TSC1 mutations underlie clinically milder, and therefore often under-diagnosed, disease.[69]

Major and minor disgnostic criteria for clinical diagnosis of TSC have been compiled and recently revised.[70,71] TSC patients develop predominantly non-malignant, hamartomatous lesions in the CNS (including the retina), kidneys, skin, lungs, and heart (Table 1).

Cortical tubers, calcified subependymal nodules, and subependymal giant cell astrocytomas are CNS lesions characteristic for TSC and constitute part of the major diagnostic criteria.[70] They have characteristic radiologic appearance on brain MRI and cause epilepsy, partial seizures (60% TSC patients), or learning disabilities. Giant cell astrocytomas may obstruct normal cerebrospinal fluid flow and cause symptoms and signs of increased intracranial pressure. Single or miltiple retinal hamartomas occur in approximately 50% of TSC patients and are often asymptomatic.[72] The typical lesion is called mulberry tumor; a grey / yellowish lesion with characteristic surface similar to a mulberry. Flat, discolored retinal hamartomas also occur. Retinal detachement may occur, although this problem is not as frequent as in VHL patients.

The most common kidney lesions in patients with TSC are benign angiomyolipomas. They occur in 70–80% of adults and are possibly the most common TSC lesion. They are usually multiple and bilateral. They grow with age and become symptomatic later in life, causing discomfort, pain, and hematuria—often resulting from hemorrhage within the tumor.[73] Malignant angiomyolipomas, although much less frequent than the hamartomatous ones, do occur.[74] Radiologic differentiation between the two entities is of paramount importance since malignant angiomyolipomas need to be treated surgically. An additional diagnostic dilemma for the physician who follows the TSC patient is the occurence of clear cell renal carcinoma. Lastly, TSC patients may develop oncocytoma. MRI is the method of choice for differential diagnosis between the various kidney tumors, although CT gives very characteristic lesions in case of angiomyolipomas. Multiple and bilateral renal cysts displaying atypical and hyperplastic epithelium are common in TSC patients. The TSC2 gene is adjacent to PKD1 gene. Large germline deletions accompanying both genes have been reported to result in a clinical picture of polycystic kidney disease with features of TSC as angiomyolipomas, termed the "continuous TSC/PKD syndrome".[75]

Skin lesions resulting from TSC include hypomelanotic macules, shagreen patches, and facial angiofibromas.[76] All three, along with the presence of non-traumaticungual or peri-ungual fibromas, constitute major clinical criteria for the presence of the

Table 2. Diagnostic criteria for TSC.

Major features
Facial angiofibromas or forehead plaque
Nontraumatic ungual or periungua fibroma
Hypomelanotic macules (three or more)
Shagreen patch (connective tissue nevus)
Multiple retinal nodular hamartomas
Cortical tuber(1)
Subependymal nodule
Subependymal giant cell astrocytoma
Cardiac rhabdomyoma, single or multiple
Lymphangiomyomatosis (2)
Renal angiomyolipoma (2)

Minor Features
Multiple, randomly distributed pits in dental enamel
Hamartomatous rectal polyps★
Bone cysts
Cerebral white matter radial migration lines(1)
Gingival fibromas
Nonrenal hamartoma★
Retinal achromic patch
Confetti skin lesions
Multiple renal cysts★

Definite TSC: Two major features OR one major + one minor
Probable TSC: One major + one minor feature
Suspect TSC: One major feature OR two or more minor

★ Histological confirmation is suggested.
(1) When cortical tuber and radial migration lines occur together, they should
be counted as one than two features of TSC.
(2) When lymphangiomyomatosis and angiomyolipoma are present, other features of TSC should also be present before a definitive diagnosis is made.
Table 2 is adapted from Roach ES et al "TSC Consensu Conference; revised clinical diagnostic criteria. Journal Child Neuro 1999;14(3): 624–628.

disease. Cardiac rhabdomyomas, single or multiple may occur. Onset of the lesions
clusters early in life or around puberty. Childhood rhabdomyomas tend to regress
spontaneously but the ones around puberty persist and may cause arrythmias. Lung
function is also affected in patients with TSC. Female more often than male patients
may develop lymphangiomyomatosis that may lead to spontaneous pneumothorax
and/or respiratory insufficiency.[77] Other lung lesions include micronodular hyper-
plasia and lung tumors.

Lesions of TSC can be classified as major or minor, depending on their specificity for TSC. Clinical diagnostic criteria comprise a combination of major and/or
minor features as listed in Table 2.

Mutations

The TSC2 gene consists of 42 exons and encodes a 5.5 kb mRNA.[67] The gene is
expressed in all adult human tissue examined so far. Alternative splicing generates
distinct mRNA products. The regulation and biologic significance of these prod-

ucts is not known. Rat,[78] mouse[79] and Drosophila[80,81] homologues of TSC2 have been cloned. The TSC1 gene consists of 23 exons and encodes an 8.6 kb mRNA.

TSC germline mutations can be traced to the parents in approximately one third of all TSC patients.[82] The rest constitute de novo mutations. Evidence exists that a small percentage of "de novo" mutations can be attributed to parent mosaicism.[83,84] Germline TSC2 mutations involve large and small intragenic deletions, nonsense mutations resulting in a truncated protein, and missense mutations to a lesser extent. In the case of contiguous TSC/PKD1 synrdrome, large germline deletions inactivate both genes.[85] The majority of characterized TSC1 mutations are predicted to result in a truncated protein.[69]

Patients with *de novo* TSC mutations are more likely to harbor a germline mutation in the TSC2 gene.[82] In contrast, TSC1 mutations are encountered with higher frequency in familial cases, where the mutation can be traced to one of the parents. It is possible, though, that these differences are due to ascertainment bias: TSC2 mutations result in a more severe disease phenotype, especially mental retardation, compared to that from *TSC1* mutations.[86,87] It is therefore possible that TSC2 mutation carriers might have a reduced reproductive fitness.

Functions of TSC1 and TSC2 Proteins

Genetic and biochemical evidence indicate that TSC2 and TSC1 are tumor suppressor genes. TSC2 gene encodes for a 1,807 amino acid protein that migrates with an apparent molecular weight of approximately 200 kD, named tuberin.[67] TSC1 gene encodes for a 1,164 amino acid protein (130 kD), hamartin, wich binds in vivo and in vitro to tuberin.[88]

Angiomyolipomas, rhabdomyomas and astrocytomas display LOH in the TSC2 or TSC1 locus.[89,90,91] Sporadic counterparts of TSC-associated tumors, in particular renal angiomyolipomas and pulmonary lymphagiomas display LOH in the TSC2 or TSC1 locus.[92,93] Reintroduction of wild type but not mutant tuberin in TSC2−/− cell lines inhibits their growth in vitro and suppresses tumor formation in the nude mouse xenograft assay.[94] These genetic and biological data indicate that TSC1/2 are tumor suppressor genes and that inactivation of both alleles is necessary for tumor formation. It contrast to this model, which holds true for most of the TSC-associated hamartomas, cortical tubers may not display LOH. Recent detailed analysis for molecular events inactivating TSC1/2 provided strong evidence that in several cortical tubers the second allele was not inactivated by LOH.[95] It is therefore possible that a mechanism other than loss of the wild type allele is involved in generation of cortical tubers.

Mice with homozygous inactivation of TSC2 gene die from liver hypoplasia at embryonic day 9.5–12.5. Heterozygous TSC2+/− mice develop multiple and bilateral renal cystadenomas, liver hemangiomas and lung adenomas.[96,97] TSC1+/− heterozygous mice develop a similar pattern of neoplasms,[98] indicating that TSC1/TSC2 proteins have markedly overlapping functions and act in the same signal transduction pathway.

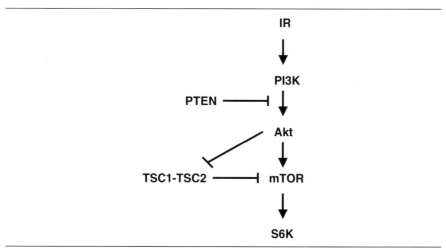

Figure 2. Activation of the PI3K/Akt pathway by loss-of-TSC1/2.
(IR = insulin receptor, PI3K = phosphatidylinositol-3 kinase, TOR = target of rapamycin)

Recent biochemical and genetic experiments place tuberin and hamartin in signaling pathways regulating cell growth. Inactivation of the Drosophila homologues of TSC1 and TSC2 cause inappropriate cell growth of the mutant cells.[80,81] Growth comparison of TSC−/− to TSC+/+ cells, in this genetic model of human disease, shows that TSC−/− cells display a reduced G1 (premitotic) phase. Enhanced growth of TSC−/− cells is accompanied by increased levels of Cyclin A and Cyclin E, leading to increased cell size and proliferation. Reintroduction of both wild type drosophila TSC1 and TSC2, but not each one separately, restores a normal growth profile.[81]

Cell growth and proliferation is controlled by complex mechanisms involving growth factors, growth factor receptors, signaling through adhesion molecules and environmental nutrients. Activation of cell surface receptor tyrosine kinases (RTK) stimulates cell growth, proliferation and possibly cell migration. Lateral branching of a given signal at various steps of RTK signal transduction gives rise to multiple cellular functions controlled by these pathways. Insulin/IGF receptor transmits signaling through activation of IRS-1 and phosphatiolylinostol-3-kinase (PI3K). Activation of PI3K leads (among other signaling events) to phosphorylation and activation of Akt, which in turn activates, via phosphorylation, target of rapamycin (TOR). TOR links growth signaling to protein translation by phosphorylating and activating S6 kinases (S6K). S6K activation leads to increased translation of proteins promoting cell growth and proliferation such as c-myc and Cyclin D1.

A recent series of reports elegantly places the TSC1/TSC2 heterodimer in this signaling pathway.[99–101] The TSC1/TSC2 heterodimeric complex binds directly to and therby inhibits TOR, exerting a negative regulatory influence on cell growth (Figure 2). Activation of PI-3K leads to in vivo phosporylation of S939 and T1462 of TSC2 through Akt/PBK.[102] Phosphorylated TSC2 no longer binds to its heterodimeric partner TSC1 and becomes unstable. Genetic experiments in Drosophila and biochemical experiments in mammalian TSC1 or TSC2−/− cells indicate that loss of TSC protein results in constitutitvely active TOR. Consequently, mutational inactivation of TSC1/TSC2 leads to constitutive activation of TOR-S6K pathway, predisposing cells to uncontrolled growth. A direct clinical importance of these observations is that rapamycin may be a drug of choice for TSC1/2 tumors that are characterized by constitutive TOR upergulation.

Prior to these experiments, our understanding of TSC1/TSC2 function derived from observations that theTSC2 C-terminus has great homology to the catalytic domain of the human GTPase activating protein 3 (GAP3). The Ras superfamily of proteins consists of GTP-binding proteins, present in an "on" state when bound to GTP and switched to an "off" state upon hydrolysis of GTP to GDP. GAP's are proteins that stimulate the intrinsic activity of GTPases and therefore negatively regulate the Ras/Ras-like protein GTP complexes.[103] Immunoprecipitates of endogenous tuberin specifically stimulate the GTPase activity of the Ras related protein Rap1a but not Rap2, H-Ras, Rho or Rac.[104] Cellular fractionation experiments show that TSC2 purifies with the membrane fraction and immunofluorescent studies indicate that TSC2 and Rap1a co-localize to the Golgi apparatus. In addition, tuberin co-immunoprecipitates with Rabaptin, a GAP protein that modulates the activity of Rab5-GTP, a critical component of the endocytic pathway. These findings need to be re-examined in the context of TSC1/TSC2 complex acting downstream of PI3K-Akt.

A3. Constitutional Translocations Involving Chromosome 3p

Families with inherited clear cell RCC harboring germline balanced translocations have been described. These translocations involve the short or long arm of chromosome 3 and, although the cytogenetic analysis establishes their causative association with the occurrence of bilateral multifocal RCC, the mechanism responsible for it has remained in intense debate within the scientific community. We will desribe the traslocations and refer to the competent theories attempting to elucidate the mechanism(s) of carcinogenesis.

The translocations occur between chromosome 3 and either ch. 6, 2, or 8 and appear as follows:

1) t(3;6)(q13;q25)[105] and t(3;6)(q12;q15)
2) t(2;3)(q35;q21)[106,107]
3) t(2;3)(q33;q21)[108] and
4) t(3;8)(p14;q34)[109]

The first explanation put forward by several groups was based on the observation that the derivative chromosome bearing the short arm of ch. 3 (der3) appears lost in cytogenetic studies of the tumors themselves, resulting in one available copy of ch3p within the tumor cell. The VHL tumor suppressor gene encoded by the remaining 3p24 was reported to be mutated in several studies.[109-111] These findings support the view whereby multistep tumorigenesis is inititated by loss of the wild VHL copy (in the der3 chromosome) followed by subsequent mutation of the remaining wild-type allele.[112] Biological experiments addressing the ability of wild type pVHL to suppress tumorigenicity in this seeting could validate the importance of this observation but have not been reported so far due to lack of cell lines derived from translocation-associated tumors.

An alternative explanation predicts that genes spanning the translocations are disrupted and consequently deregulated leading to tumor formation. Efforts to clone these genes led to the identification of several candidates potentially involved in renal tumor formation and provided credence to the hypothesis. Nevertheless, biological confirmation of the involvement of these candidate genes in tumorigenesis remains incomplete and the available indirect evidence for their importance is controversial.

Breaks in ch. 3p14 region disrupt the FHIT (Fragile HIstidine Triad) gene that encodes for an Ap3A hydrolase.[113] Reintroduction of the FHIT gene in FHIT−/− cell lines suppressed tumor formation in the mouse xenograft assay but so did the Ap3A hydrolase deficient mutant.[114] Aberrant transcripts or intragenic deletions were observed in tumors and tumor-derived cell lines but also did so in non-malignant cells. In contrast, antibodies directed against FHIT detected reduced or absent protein in RCC specimens.[115] Mice with germline deletion of the FHIT gene have an increased incidence of carcinogen-induced tumors.[116]

The ch. 8q24 region encompasses the gene TRC8, which is disrupted by the translocations involving this area.[117] The Drosophila TRC8 homologue has similarities with patched gene (PTCH), a growth restrictive gene involved in sonic hedgecog signaling. Mutations of human PTCH lead to the development of basal cell nevus syndrome, an autosomal dominant disease characterized by the presence of multiple basal cell carcinomas.[118] It is therefore possible that TRC8 is a growth restriction/tumor suppressor gene. TRC8 mutations have been detected in RCC.[117]

The 2q33 area and the 3q21 area encode for the genes Deleted In Renal Cancer 1 (DIRC1) and DIRC2 correspondingly. DIRC1's function is unknown.[119] DIRC2 is a member of the major facilitator superfamily (MFS) of transporters, a family of transmembrane proteins facilitating transport of organic anions and cations across cell membrane.[120] Bodmer et al postulated that potential disruption of such a transporter allows for the accumulation of environmental toxins promoting genome instability and therefore predisposing for the "second event" of VHL mutation, as observed in translocation-associated RCC.[120] DIRC2 disruption was noted in early RCC lesions not harboring der3 loss or VHL mutations, supporting the possibility this is an earlier event. It is notable that the second DIRC2 allele was not mutated in translocation-associated or sporadic RCC. Once again, the various models proposed as explanation of 3p translocation-associated RCC require further experimental testing.

A4. Supernumerary Nipple Syndrome

An association between polymastia and renal carcinoma has been reported,[121] indicating that developmental abnormalities of the urothelial tract may predispose to RCC and extrnumerary nipples. Subsequently, a Hungarian family has been described with renal carcinoma and supernumerary nipples.[122] No genetic analysis of this pedigree is available at this point.

A5. Non-VHL. Non-HPRCC Familial RCC

Teh et al reported on the occurrence of clear cell RCC in family members at two consecutive generations.[123] Renal tumors were single and the disease occured between the ages of 50–70. It is not clear if classic germline mutations predispose to this syndrome or polymorphisms on certain genes, coupled with environmental exposure, led to increased susceptibility to RCC.

B. FAMILIAL PAPILLARY RCC

Papillary carcinoma comprises approximately 10% of the sporadic RCC tumors.[2] Classification of a tumor as papillary requires that at least 75% papillary component of the tumor. Histologically, the tumors appear as a fingerlike projection consisting of a fibrovascular core covered by a single or multiple layers of malignant epithelial cells. The presence of fibrovascular core distinguishes the papillary from pseudo-papillary lesions, since the latter lacks this component. Histologically and clinically papillary cancers are subdivided in type 1 and type 2.[2,124] Type 1 neoplasms are characterized by a single or double layer of malignant epithelial cells with eosinophilic or basophilic cytoplasm. In type 2 tumors the epithelial cells are eosinophilic and arrayed in a pseudostratified multilayer. There is evidence that type 1 tumors have a better clinical prognosis than type 2. Familial predisposition to either type 1 or type 2 tumors exists.

Sporadic papillary RCCs are characterized by trisomy of ch. 7, 16, 17 and loss of Y chromosome.

B1. Hereditary Papillary Carcinoma Type 1 (OMIM 1447000)

Family members with HPRCC 1 develop multiple and bilateral papillary type 1 RCC at a much younger age than those with sporadic papillary RCC and the disease is inherited in an autosomal dominant fashion. Zbar et al estimated the frequency of HPRCC to be 1 in 1 million.[112] Linkage analysis mapped the gene responsible for HPRCC 1 to ch. 7q31–q34[125] and Schmidt et al reported activating germline mutations in the MET protooncogene that resides in this area. The mutations segregated with the disease in approximately 80% of the cases.[125] As in sporadic tumors, HPRCC manifests trisomy of ch. 7. The duplicated ch. 7 also harbors a mutation of the MET oncogene.[126]

MET protooncogene maps to Ch.7q31 and consists of 21 exons.[127] It is expressed in hematopoetic, endothelial, and neuronal cells as well as in several adult tissues including the kidney. MET can be rendered oncogenic by either gene amplification or by mutations resulting in constitutive activation of the encoded protein. MET encodes for a 1,390 amino acid precursor protein, which cleaved into alpha and beta chains. The chains are linked by a disulfide bond and form the tyrosine kinase transmembrane c-met receptor.[128]

Hepatocyte growth factor/scatter factor (HGF/SF) is the ligand of c-met receptor.[129] The receptor comprises of an extracellular 50 kD alpha chain linked to a 150 kD transmembrane beta chain. The intracellular part of the receptor has a catalytic domain and a C-terminal "multi-docking domain". Ligand induced dimerization activates the receptor through transphosphorylation at Tyr 1234 and 1235 of the catalytic domain.[130] This initial step leads to autophosphorylation of the receptor at Tyr1349 and 1356 of the "docking" domain, rendering this site competent for interactions with SH2 domain containing proteins.[131] C-met activation results in activation of the PI3K, Grb2/Sos/Ras, Src and PLCgamma pathways. HPRCC-associated mutations map to the catalytic site of the receptor and are predicted to promote phosphorylation of the critical tyrosines.[125] This has been tested experimentally by Schmidt et al, who introduced HPRC1-associated mutant MET in NIH 3T3 cells. The mutant receptor was constitutively phosphorylated and transformed the 3T3 cells.[132]

C-met receptor activation in epithelial cells results in increased proliferation[1] increased motility[2] increased metastatic potential and[3] polarization[4] and tubule formation. Structure-function analysis of the receptor indicates that dissociable downstream pathways are responsible for this phenotype. Ras pathway appears necessary and sufficient for proliferation. Activation of PI3 kinase only appears responsible for increased motility. Activation of both pathways is necessary for acquisition of invasive and metastatic phenotype.[133]

Of particular interest for renal carcinogenesis is the observation that c-met and VHL signaling pathways interact. Stimulation of VHL−/− cells with HGF/SF promotes scattering, secretion of metaloproteinases and inhibition of tissue inhibitor of metaloproteinases. Stable reintroduction of pVHL in these cells markedly decreases these effects of HGF/SF.[134] The molecular mechanism of this interaction is under investigation.

B2. Hereditary Papillary Renal Cell Cancer 2 (HPRCC 2)

This entity is distinct from HPRCC 1. Several families have been identified with RCC of type 2 paillary histology. These families have no mutations in the MET protoncogene and do not have trisomy of ch. 7. So far there is no information regarding the genetic events underlying this familial cancer syndrome.

B3. HPRCC with Familial Cutaneous and Uterine Leiomyomatosis (OMIM 150800)

Launonen et al[135] reported a family whose several members developed uterine leiomyomas, uterine leiomyosarcoma and cutaneous leiomyomas. These are tumors deriving from the smooth muscle cells of the corresponding organs. Four members of this family developed metastatic papillary RCC type 2 (OMIM 605839). The syndrome was inherited in an autosomal dominant fashion with variable penetrance and the tumors appeared around the second or third decade of life. Linkage analysis mapped the gene responsible for the syndrome to ch. 1q42.3–45.[135,136]

A large consortium cloned the gene associated with the disease and showed it is the mitochondrial enzyme fumarate hydratase (FH). Germ line mutations consist of large deletions, small intragenic deletions, nonsense mutations resulting in protein truncation, and missense mutations in conserved amino acids.[137] These mutations predict the destruction of the enzymatic activity of the protein. Genetic analysis indicated that FH is a tumor suppressor gene obeying the Knudson "two-hit" model. Cutaneous, uterine or renal tumors display LOH in the FH locus. Accordingly, lymphoblastoid cell lines from affected individuals had marked reduction in enzymatic FH activity and tumors harboring LOH had no FH activity at all.

The mechanism by which loss of fumarase activity leads to tumor formation can only be postulated at this time. FH is a Krebs cycle enzyme catalyzing the hydration of fularate to malate and thus promoting the Krebs cycle. It is tempting to hypothesize that mitochondrial accumulation of fumarate inhibits the activity of the preceding succinate dehydrogenase enzyme in the Krebs cycle.[138] Germline mutations in B, C, and D subunits of succinate dehydrogenase lead to increased mitochondrial production of reactive oxygen species and cause familial paraganglioma.[139–141] It is therefore possible that fumarate accumulation leads to increased ROS and proliferative advantage of certain cells.[138] This is a hypothesis awaiting confirmation.

B4. HPRCC Associated with Papillary Thyroid Cancer

Families with papillary RCC and papillary thyroid carcinoma have been described.[142] Linkage analysis indicates that the syndrome does not segregate with markers flanking the MET gene and no germline mutations in MET exons that are hotspots for HPRCC1 were detected. Whether or not the genetic events underlying this syndrome are similar to the ones leading to HPRCC1 is unknown.

C. FAMILIAL ONCOCYTOMA
C1. Birt-Hogg-Dube (BHD) Syndrome (OMIM 135150)

Birt, Hogg and Dube first described an inherited dermatologic condition characterized by the development of multiple fibrofolliculomas, trichodiscomas, and acrochordons in individuals older than 25 years.[143]

Fibrofolliculomas and trichodiscomas are benign hamartomatous tumors of the skin originating from structural elements of the hair follicle. Fibrofolliculomas contain predominantly epithelial cells, trichodiscomas have a predominant fibrous component.[144] Clinically they are almost indistinguishable and present as multiple yellowish or skin-colored papules of the face (including oral mucosa), neck, scalp and upper trunk. Acrochordons have a "skin tag" more than "papular" appearance but are most likely histologic variants of fibrofolliculomas and trichodiscomas. Deforming lipomas and collagenomas are less characteristic but they have been recently described in BHD patients.

Members of families affected with BHD syndrome may develop multiple and bilateral renal neoplasms.[145,146] These have been reported to be of various histologies. In 17 affected individuals of a Swedish pedigree two cases of renal cancer were diagnosed: one tumor had mixed clear cell and papillary elements and the second was a chromophobe RCC.[147] Toro et al reported on examining 152 patients from 49 families. Two of these kindreds had renal oncocytomas and the third papillary carcinoma.[145] In a recent review of a large cohort of BHD families the predominant histology of renal tumors was chromophobe RCC [Zbar, 2002 #2085].

In addition to skin and renal lesions BHD patients have lung cysts and suffer from spontaneous pneumothorax [Zbar, 2002 #2085]. Colonic polyps have been initially reported as part of the syndrome but comparison of affected individuals with unaffected controls from the same families provided no evidence that either colonic polyps or colon cancer is associated with BHD [Zbar, 2002 #2085].

Linkage analyses performed independently by the groups of Drs. Berton Zbar and Bin Teh mapped the gene associated with the syndrome to ch. 17p11.2.[147,148] Cloning of the gene is expected in the near fututre.

C2. Familial Renal Oncocytoma

Sporadic and familial oncocytomas of the kidney are mostly non-metastatic benign tumors. Microscopically, they consist of foci of epithelial cells with densely eosinophilic cytoplasm. Electron microscopy studies show a characteristic abundance of mitochondria that "fill" the cytoplasm.[2]

Several case reports describe patients with bilateral, multiple renal oncocytomas. The term "renal oncocytomatosis" was used to describe extreme forms of this clinical presentation. It is not known if the presence of bilateral and numerous lesions indicates familial predisposition.

A clear report of familiar predisposition to oncocytoma was provided by Weinrich et al, who described 5 nuclear families with multiple members affected with renal oncocytomas.[149] On subsequent clinical reevaluation they noted that 3 of these 5 families manifested skin lesions compatible with BHD syndrome (see above). It is therefore likely that several of the previously reported familial renal oncocytomas represent cases of BHD syndrome, although non-BHD associated renal oncocytoma likely exists.

Cytogenetic analysis of sporadic tumors classifies oncocytomas as those characterized by either loss of chromosome 1p or those harboring one of the reported somatic reciprocal translocations: t(9;11) involving 11q13, t(9;11)(p23;q23), t(5;11)(q35;13), and t(1;12)(p36;q13).[150]

REFERENCES

1. Hanahan, D, and RA Weinberg. 2000. The Hallmarks of Cancer. Cell **100**:57–70.
2. Reuter, VE, and JC Presti. 2000. Contemporary approach to the classification of renal epithelial tumors. Seminars in Oncology **27**:124–137.
3. Maher, ER, JRW Yates, R Harries, C Benjamin, R Harris, AT Moore, and MA Ferguson-Smith. 1990. Clinical features and natural history of von Hippel-Lindau Disease. Quarterly Journal of Medicine **77**:1151–1163.

4. Melmon, K, and S Rosen. 1964. Lindau's disease. Am J Med **36**:595–617.
5. Latif, F, K Tory, J Gnarra, M Yao, F-M Duh, ML Orcutt, T Stackhouse, I Kuzmin, W Modi, L Geil, L Schmidt, F Zhou, H Li, MH Wei, F Chen, G Glenn, P Choyke, MM Walther, Y Weng, D-SR Duan, M Dean, D Glavac, FM Richards, PA Crossey, MA Ferguson-Smith, DL Pasiler, I Chumakov, D Cohen, AC Chinault, ER Maher, WM Linehan, B Zbar, and MI Lerman. 1993. Identification of the von Hippel-Lindau Disease Tumor Suppressor Gene. Science **260**:1317–1320.
6. Lamiell, J, F Salazar, and Y Hsia. 1989. von Hippel-Lindau disease affecting 43 members of a single kindred. Medicine **68**:1–29.
7. Wizigmann-Voos, S, and KH Plate. 1996. Pathology, genetics and cell biology of hemangioblastomas. Histol Histopathol **11**:1049–1061.
8. Richard, S, C Campello, L Taillandier, F Parker, and F Resche. 1998. Hemangioblastoma of the central nervous system in von Hippel-Lindau disease. J Intern Med **243**:547–553.
9. Sharma, RR, IP Cast, and C O'Brien. 1995. Supratentorial haemangioblastoma not associated with Von Hippel Lindau complex or polycythaemia: case report and literature review. Br J Neurosurg **9**:81–84.
10. Wittebol-Post, D, FJ Hes, and CJM Lips. 1998. The eye in von Hippel-Lindau disease. Long term follow up of screening and treatment recommendations. J Intern Med **243**:555–561.
11. Neumann, HPH, and B Zbar. 1997. Renal cysts, renal cancer and Von Hippel-Lindau disease. Kidney Int **51**:16–26.
12. Maher, EWA, and A Moore. 1995. Clinical and molecular genetics of von Hippel-Lindau disease. Ophthalmic Genetics **16**:79–84.
13. McClellan, MW, P Choyke, G Weiss, C Manolatos, J Long, R Reiter, RB Alexander, and WM Linehan. 1995. Parenchymal sparing surgery in patients with hereditary renal cell carcinoma. J Urol **153**:913–916.
14. Zbar, B, W Kaelin, E Maher, and S Richard. 1999. Third International Meeting on von Hippel-Lindau disease. Cancer Res **59**:2251–2253.
15. Neumann, PH, S Hoegerle, T Manz, K Brenner, and O Iliopoulos. 2002. How many pathways to pheochromocytoma? Seminars in Nephrology **22**:89–99.
16. Neumann, HPH, DP Berger, G Sigmund, U Blum, D Schmidt, RJ Parmer, B Volk, and G Kirste. 1993. Pheochromocytomas, multiple endocrine neoplasia type 2, and von Hippel-Landau Disease. N Engl J Med **329**:1531–1538.
17. Eisenhofer, G, JW Lenders, WM Linehan, MM Walther, DS Goldstein, and HR Keiser. 1999. Plasma normetanephrine and metanephrine for detecting pheochromocytoma in von Hippel-Lindau disease and multiple endocrine neoplasia type 2. N Engl J Med **340**:1872–1879.
18. Choyke, PL, GM Glenn, MM Walther, NJ Patronas, WM Linehan, and B Zbar. 1995. von Hippel-Lindau disease: genetic, clinical and imaging features. Radiology **194**:629–642.
19. Neumann, HP, E Dinkel, H Brambs, B Wimmer, H Friedburg, B Volk, G Sigmund, P Riegler, K Haag, and SP ••. 1991. Pancreatic lesions in the von Hippel-Lindau syndrome. Gastrenterology **101**:465–471.
20. Humphrey, JS, RD Klausner, and WM Linehan. 1996. Von Hippel-Lindau syndrome: hereditary cancer arising from inherited mutations of the VHL tumor suppressor gene. Cancer Treat Res 1996 **88**:13–39.
21. Iliopoulos, O. 2001. VHL Disease: Genetic and Clinical Observations. Genetic Disorders of Endocrine Neoplasia. Basel Karger (Dahia PML, Eng C. eds) **28**:131–166.
22. Seizinger, BR, GA Rouleau, LJ Ozelius, AH Lane, GE Farmer, JM Lamiell, J Haines, JWM Yuen, D Collins, D Majoor-Krakauer, T Bonner, C Mathew, A Rubenstein, J Halperin, A McConkie-Rosell, JS Green, JA Trofatter, BA Ponder, L Eierman, MI Bowmer, R Schimke, B Oostra, N Aronin, DI Smith, H Drabkin, MH Waziri, WJ Hobbs, RL Martuza, PM Conneally, YE Hsia, and JF Gusella. 1988. Von Hippel-Lindau disease maps to the region of chromosome 3 associated with renal cell carcinoma. Nature **332**:268–269.
23. Crossey, P, E Maher, M Jones, F Richards, F Latif, M Phipps, M Lush, K Foster, K Tory, J Green, B Oostra, J Yates, W Linehan, N Affara, M Lerman, B Zbar, Y Nakamura, and M Ferguson-Smith. 1993. Genetic linkage between von Hippel-Lindau disease and three microsatellite polymorphisms refines the localisation of the VHL locus. Human Molecular Genetics **2**:279–282.
24. Maher, E, E Bentley, J Yates, F Latif, M Lerman, B Zbar, N Affara, and M Ferguson-Smith. 1991. Localization of the gene for von Hippel-lindau disease to a small region of chromosome 3p by genetic linkage analysis. Genomics **10**:957–960.
25. Duan, DR, JS Humphrey, DYT Chen, Y Weng, J Sukegawa, S Lee, JR Gnarra, WM Linehan, and RD Klausner. 1995. Characterization of the VHL tumor suppressor gene product: localization,

complex formation, and the effect of natural inactivating mutations. Proc Natl Acad Sci (USA) **92:**6495–6499.

26. Gnarra, J, J Ward, F Porter, J Wagne, D Devor, A Grinberg, M Emmert-Buck, H Westphal, R Klausner, and W Linehan. 1997. Defective placental vasculogenesis causes embryonic lethality in VHL-deficient mice. Proc Natl Acad Sci U S A **94:**9102–9107.

27. Woodward, ER, A Buchberger, SC Clifford, LD Hurst, NA Affara, and ER Maher. 2000. Comparative sequence analysis of the VHL tumor suppressor gene. Genomics **65:**253–265.

28. Adryan, B, H-J Decker, TS Papas, and T Hsu. 2000. Tracheal development and the von Hippel-Lindau tumor suppressor homolog in Drosophila. Oncogene **19:**2803–2811.

29. Stolle, C, G Glenn, B Zbar, J Humphrey, P Choyke, M Walther, S Pack, K Hurley, C Andrey, R Klausner, and W Linehan. 1998. Improved detection of germline mutations in the von Hippel-Lindau disease tumor suppressor gene. Hum Mutat3 **12:**417–423.

30. Prowse, A, A Webster, F Richards, S Richard, S Olschwang, F Resche, N Affara, and E Maher. 1997. Somatic inactivation of the VHL gene in Von Hippel-Lindau disease tumors. American Journal of Human Genetics **60:**765–761.

31. Lubensky, IA, JR Gnarra, P Bertheau, MM Walther, WM Linehan, and Z Zhuang. 1996. Allelic deletions of the VHL gene detected in multiple microscopic clear cell renal lesions in von Hippel-Lindau disease patients. American Journal of Pathology **149:**2089–2094.

32. Gnarra, JR, K Tory, Y Weng, L Schmidt, MH Wei, H Li, F Latif, S Liu, F Chen, F-M Duh, I Lubensky, DR Duan, C Florence, R Pozzatti, MM Walther, NH Bander, HB Grossman, H Brauch, S Pomer, JD Brooks, WB Isaacs, MI Lerman, B Zbar, and WM Linehan. 1994. Mutations of the VHL tumour suppressor gene in renal carcinoma. Nature Genetics **7:**85–90.

33. Shuin, T, K Kondo, S Torigoe, T Kishida, Y Kubota, M Hosaka, Y Nagashima, H Kitamura, F Latif, B Zbar, MI Lerman, and M Yao. 1994. Frequent somatic mutations and loss of heterozygosity of the von Hippel-Lindau tumor suppressor gene in primary human renal cell carcinomas. Cancer Res **54:**2852–2855.

34. Kanno, H, K Kondo, S Ito, I Yamamoto, S Fujii, S Torigoe, N Sakai, M Hosaka, T Shuin, and M Yao. 1994. Somatic mutations of the von Hippel-Lindau Tumor supressor gene in sporadic central nervous systems hemangioblastomas. Cancer Research **54:**4845–4847.

35. Vortmeyer, AO, IA Lubensky, F Fogt, WM Linehan, U Khettry, and Z Zhuang. 1997. Allelic deletion and mutation of the von Hippel-Lindau tumor suppressor gene in pancreatic microcystic adenomas. Am J Pathol **151:**951–956.

36. Chen, F, T Kishida, M Yao, T Hustad, D Glavac, M Dean, JR Gnarra, ML Orcutt, FM Duh, G Glenn, J Green, YE Hsia, J Lamiell, HW Ming, L Schmidt, T Kalman, I Kuzmin, T Stackhouse, F Latif, WM Linehan, M Lerman, and B Zbar. 1995. Germline mutations in the von hippel-lindau disease tumor suppressor gene: correlations with phenotype. Human Mutation **5:**66–75.

37. Crossey, PA, FM Richards, K Foster, JS Green, A Prowse, F Latif, MI Lerman, B Zbar, NA Affara, MA Ferguson-Smith, and ER Maher. 1994. Identification of intragenic mutations in the von Hippel-Lindau disease tumor suppressor gene and correlation with disease phenotype. Hum Mol Gen **3:**1303–1308.

38. Maher, E, A Webster, F Richards, J Green, P Crossey, S Payne, and A Moore. 1996. Phenotypic expression in von Hippel-Lindau disease: Correlations with germline VHL gene mutations. Journal of Medical Genetics **33:**328–332.

39. Iliopoulos, O, A Kibel, S Gray, and WG Kaelin. 1995. Tumor Suppression by the Human von Hippel-Lindau Gene Product. Nature Medicine **1:**822–826.

40. Gnarra, JR, S Zhou, MJ Merrill, J Wagner, A Krumm, E Papavassiliou, EH Oldfield, RD Klausner, and WM Linehan. 1996. Post-transcriptional regulation of vascular endothelial growth factor mRNA by the VHL tumor suppressor gene product. Proc Natl Acad Sci **93:**10589–10594.

41. Knebelmann, B, S Ananth, HT Cohen, and VP Sukhatme. 1998. Transforming growth factor a is a target for the von Hippel-Lindau tumor suppressor protein. Cancer Res **58:**226–231.

42. Ananth, S, B Knebelmann, W Gruning, M Dhanabal, G Walz, IE Stillman, and VP Sukhatme. 1999. Transforming growth factor beta1 is a target for the von Hippel-Lindau tumor suppressor and a critical growth factor for clear cell renal carcinoma. Cancer Res **59:**2210–2216.

43. Semenza, GL. 1999. Perspectives on oxygen sensing. Cell **98:**281–284.

44. Iliopoulos, O, C Jiang, AP Levy, WG Kaelin, and MA Goldberg. 1996. Negative Regulation of Hypoxia-Inducible Genes by the von Hippel-Lindau Protein. Proc Natl Acad Sci **93:**10595–10599.

45. Gorospe, M, JM Egan, B Zbar, M Lerman, L Geil, I Kuzmin, and NJ Holbrook. 1999. Protective function of von Hippel-Lindau protein against impaired protein processing in renal carcinoma cells. Mol Cell Biol **19:**1289–1300.

46. Schoenfeld, AR, T PArris, A Eisenberger, EJ Davidowitz, M De Leon, F Talasazan, P Devarajan, and RD Burk. 2000. The von Hippel Lindau tumor suppressor gene protects cells from UV-mediated apoptosis. Oncogne **19**:5851–5857.

47. Pause, A, S Lee, KM Lonergan, and RD Klausner. 1998. The von Hippel-Lindau Tumor Suppressor Gene is Required for Cell Cycle Exit Upon Serum Withdrawal. Proc Natl Acad Sci (USA).

48. Ohh, M, RL Yauch, KM Lonergan, JM Whaley, AO Stemmer-Rachamimov, DN Louis, BJ Gavin, N Kley, WG Kaelin, O Iliopoulos, and WG Kaelin. 1998. The von Hippel-Lindau Tumor Suppressor Protein is Required for Proper Assembly of an Extracellular Fibronectin Matrix. Mol Cell **1**:In Press.

49. Davidowitz, EJ, AR Schoenfeld, and RD Burk. 2001. VHL induces renal cell differentiation and growth arrest through integration of cell-cell and cell-extracellular matrix signaling. Mol Cell Biol **21**:865–874.

50. Lieubeau-Teillet, B, J Rak, S Jothy, O Iliopoulos, W Kaelin, and RS Kerbel. 1998. VHL gene mediated growth suppression and induction of differentiation in renal cell carcinoma cell grown as multicellular tumor spheroids. Cancer Research **58**:4957–4962.

51. Kanno, H, F Saljooque, I Yamamoto, S Hattori, M Yao, T Shuin, and H-S U. 2000. Role of the von HIppel-Lindau tumor suppressor protein during neuronal differentiation. Cancer Res **60**:2820–2824.

52. Iliopoulos, O, M Ohh, and W Kaelin. 1998. pVHL19 is a biologically active product of the von Hippel-Lindau gene arising from internal translation initiation. Proc Natl Acad Sci USA **95**: 11661–11666.

53. Schoenfeld, A, E Davidowitz, and R Burk. 1998. A second major native von Hippel-Lindau gene product, initiated from an internal translation start site, functions as a tumor suppressor. Proc Natl Acad Sci U S A **195**:8817–8822.

54. Lee, S, M Neumann, R Stearman, R Stauber, A Pause, G Pavlakis, and R Klausner. 1999. Transcription-Dependent Nuclear-Cytoplasmic Trafficking Is Required for the Function of the von Hippel-Lindau Tumor Suppressor Protein. Mol Cell Biol **19**:1486–1497.

55. Stebbins, CE, WG Kaelin, and NP Pavletich. 1999. Structure of the VHL-ElonginC-ElonginB complex: implications for VHL tumor suppressor function. Science **284**:455–461.

56. Maxwell, PH, RMS Wiesene, GW Chang, SC Clifford, EC Vaux, ME Cockman, CC Wykoff, CW Pugh, ER Maher, and PJ Ratcliffe. 1999. The tumour suppressor protein VHL targets hypoxia-inducible factors for oxygen-dependent proteolysis. Nature **399**:271–275.

57. Semenza, GL. 1998. Hypoxia-inducible factor 1: master regulator of O2 homeostasis. Curr Opin Genet Dev **8**:588–594.

58. Semenza, GL. 1999. Regulation of mammalian O2 homeostasis by hypoxia-inducible factor 1. Annu Rev Cell Dev Biol **15**:581–578.

59. Ohh, M, CW Park, M Ivan, MA Hoffman, TY Kim, LE Huang, N Pavletich, V Chau, and WG Kaelin. 2000. Ubiquitination of hypoxia-inducible factor requires direct binding to the beta-domain of the von Hippel-Lindau protein. Nat Cell Biol **2**:423–427.

60. Jaakkola, P, D Mole, YM Tian, MI Wilson, J Gielbert, LSJ Gaskel, AA Kriegsheim, HF Hebestreit, M Mukherji, CJ Schofield, PH Maxwell, CW Pugh, and PJ Ratcliffe. 2001. Targeting of HIF-alpha to the von Hippel-Lindau Ubiquitylation Complex by O2-Regulated Prolyl Hydroxylation. Science **292**:468–472.

61. Ivan, M, K Kondo, H Yang, W Kim, J Valiando, M Ohh, A Salic, JM Asara, WS Lane, and WG Kaelin. 2001. HIF1a targeted for VHL-mediated destruction by proline hydroxylation: implications for oxygen sensing. Science **292**:464–468.

62. Epstein, ACR, JM Gleadle, and LAEA McNeill. 2001. C. Elegans EGL-9 and mammalian homologs define a family of Dioxygenases that regulate HIF by Prolyl Hydroxylation. Cell **107**:43–54.

63. Maranchie, JK, JR Vasselli, J Riss, JS Bonifacino, WM Linehan, and RD Klausner. 2002. The contribution of VHL substrate binding and HIF1-alpha to the phenotype of VHL loss in renal cell carcinoma. Cancer Cell **1**:247–255.

64. Kondo, K, J Klco, E Nakamura, M Lechpammer, and WG Kaelin. 2002. Inhibition of HIF is necessary for tumor suppression by the von Hippel-Lindau protein. Cancer Cell **1**:237–246.

65. Okuda, H, K Saitoh, S Hirai, K Iwai, Y Takaki, M Baba, N Minato, S Ohno, and T Shuin. 2001. The von Hippel-Lindau tumor suppressor protein mediates ubiquitination of activated atypical protein kinase C. J Biol Chem **276**:43611–43617.

66. Li, Z, X Na, D Wang, SR Schoen, EM Messing, and G Wu. 2002. Ubiquitination of a novel deubiquitinating enzyme requires direct binding to von Hippel-Lindau tumor suppressor protein. J Biol Chem **277**:4656–4662.

67. 1993. European Consostrium on Tuberous Sclerosis: Identification and characterization of the tuberous sclerosis gene on chromosome 16. Cell **75**:1305–1315.
68. 1997. Consortium: Identification of the TSC1 gene on chromosome 9q34. Science **277**:805–808.
69. Niida, Y, N Lawrence-Smith, A Banwell, E Hammer, J Lewis, RL Beauchamp, K Sims, V Ramesh, and L Ozelius. 1999. Analysis of both TSC1 and TSC2 for germline mutations in 126 unrelated patients with tuberous sclerosis. Hum Mutat **14**:412–422.
70. Roach, ES, MR Gomez, and H Northurp. 1988. Tuberous sclerosis complex consensus conference: revised clinical diagnostic criteria. J Child Neurology **13**:624–628.
71. Roach, ES, FJ DiMario, and H Northurp. 1998. Tuberous sclerosis consensus conference: recommendations for diagnostic evaluation. J Child Neurology **14**:401–407.
72. Zimmer-Galler, IE, and DM Robertson. 1995. Long-term observation of retinal lesions in tuberous sclerosis. Am J Ophthalmol **119**:318–324.
73. Ewalt, DH, E Sheffield, SP Sparagana, MR Delgado, and ES Roach. 1998. Renal lesion growth in children with tuberous sclerosis complex. J Urol 1998 Jul;**160(1)**:141–145 **160**:141–145.
74. Al-Saleem, T, LL Wessner, BW Scheithauer, K Patterson, ES Roach, SJ Dreyer, K Fujikawa, J Bjornsson, J Bernstein, and EP Henske. 1998. Malignant tumors of the kidney, brain, and soft tissues in children and young adults with the tuberous sclerosis complex. Cancer **83**:2208–2216.
75. Martignoni, G, F Bonetti, M Pea, R Tardanico, M Brunelli, and JN Eble. 2002. Renal disease in adults with TSC2/PKD1 contiguous gene syndrome. Am J Surg Pathol **26**:198–205.
76. Siegel, DH, and R Howard. 2002. Molecular advances in genetic skin diseases. Curr Opin Pediatr **14**:419–425.
77. Pacheco-Rodriguez, G, AS Kristof, LA Stevens, Y Zhang, D Crooks, and J Moss. 2002. Giles F. Filley Lecture: Genetics and gene expression in lymphangioleiomyomatosis. Chest **121**:56S–60S.
78. Yeung, RS, G-H Xiao, F Jin, W-C Lee, JR Testa, and AG Knudson. 1994. Predisposition to renal carcinoma in the Eker rat is determined by germ-line mutation of the tuberous sclerosis 2 (TSC2) gene. Proc Nat Acad Sci **91**:11413–11416.
79. Rennebeck, G, EV Kleymenova, R Anderson, RS Yeung, K Artzt, and CL Walker. 1998. Loss of function of the tuberous sclerosis 2 tumor suppressor gene results in embryonic lethality characterized by disrupted neuroepithelial growth and development. Proc Natl Acad Sci USA **95**:15629–15634.
80. Ito, N, and GM Rubin. 1999. Gigas, a Drosophila homolog of tuberous sclerosis gene product-2, regulates the cell cycle. Cell **96**:529–539.
81. Tapon, N, N Ito, BJ Dickson, JE Treisman, and IK Hariharan. 2001. The Drosophila tuberous sclerosis complex gene homologs restrict cell growth and cell proliferation. Cell **105**:345–355.
82. MacCollin, M, and D Kwiatkowski. 2001. Molecular genetic aspects of the phakomatoses: tuberous sclerosis complex and neurofibromatosis 1. Curr Opin Neurol **14**:163–169.
83. Kwiatkowska, J, J Wigowska-Sowinska, D Napierala, R Slomski, and DJ Kwiatkowski. 1999. Mosaicism in tuberous sclerosis as a potential cause of the failure of molecular diagnosis. N Engl J Med **340**:703–707.
84. Rose, VM, KS Au, G Pollom, ES Roach, HR Prashner, and H Northrup. 1999. Germ-line mosaicism in tuberous sclerosis: how common? Am J Hum Genet **64**:986–992.
85. Brook-Carter, PT, B Peral, and C Ward, et al. 1994. Deletion of the TSC2 and PKD1 gene associated with severe infantile polycystic kidney disease-A contiguous gene syndrome. Nat Genet **8**:328–332.
86. Dabora, SL, S Jozwiak, DN Franz, PS Roberts, A Nieto, J Chung, YS Choy, MP Reeve, E Thiele, JC Egelhoff, J Kasprzyk-Obara, D Domanska-Pakiela, and DJ Kwiatkowski. 2001. Mutational analysis in a cohort of 224 tuberous sclerosis patients indicates increased severity of TSC2, compared with TSC1, disease in multiple organs. Am J Hum Genet **68**:64–80.
87. Langkau, N, N Martin, R Brandt, K Zugge, S Quast, G Wiegele, A Jauch, M Rehm, A Kuhl, RM Mack-Vette, B Zimmerhackl, and B Janssen. 2002. TSC1 and TSC2 mutations in tuberous sclerosis, the associated phenotypes and a model to explain observed TSC1/TSC2 frequency ratios. Eur J Pediatr **161**:393–402.
88. Van Slegtenhorst, M, M Nellist, B Nagelkerken, J Cheadle, R Snell, A van den Ouweland, A Reuser, JP Sampson, D Halley, and P Sluijs. 1998. Interaction between hamartin and tuberin, TSC1 and TSC2 gene products. Hum Mol Genet **7**:1053–1057.
89. Green, AJ, M Smith, and JRW Yates. 1994. Loss of heterozygosity on chromosome 16p13.3 in hamartomas from tuberous sclerosis patients. Nature Genet **6**:192–196.
90. Sepp, T, JR Yates, and AJ Green. 1996. Loss of heterozygosity in tuberous sclerosis hamartomas. J Med Genet **33**:962–964.

91. Henske, EP, HP Neumann, BW Scheithauer, EW Herbst, MP Short, and DJ Kwiatkowski. 1995. Loss of heterozygosity in the tuberous sclerosis (TSC2) region of chromosome band 16p13 occurs in sporadic as well as TSC-associated renal angiomyolipomas. Gene Chromosomes Cancer **13**: 295–298.

92. Carsillo, T, A Astrinidis, and EP Henske. 2000. Mutations in the tuberous sclerosis complex gene TSC2 are a cause of sporadic pulmonary lymphangioleiomyomatosis. Proc Natl Acad Sci **97**: 6085–6090.

93. Henske, EP, HP Neumann, BW Scheithauer, EW Herbst, MP Short, and DJ Kwiatkowski. 1995. Loss of heterozygosity in the tuberous sclerosis (TSC2) region of chromosome band 16p13 occurs in sporadic as well as TSC-associated renal angiomyolipomas. Genes Chromosomes Cancer **13**:295–298.

94. Jin, F, R Wienecke, GH Xiao, JC Maize, JE DeClue, and RS Yeung. 1996. Suppression of tumorigenicity by the wild-type tuberous sclerosis 2 (Tsc2) gene and its C-terminal region. Proc Natl Acad Sci **93**:9154–9159.

95. Niida, Y, AO Stemmer-Rachamimov, M Logrip, D Tapon, R Perez, DJ Kwiatkowski, K Sims, M MacCollin, DN Louis, and V Ramesh. 2001. Survey of somatic mutations in tuberous sclerosis complex (TSC) hamartomas suggests different genetic mechanisms for pathogenesis of TSC lesions. Am J Hum Genet **69**:493–503.

96. Kobayashi, T, O Minowa, J Kuno, H Mitani, O Hino, and T Noda. 1999. Renal carcinogenesis, hepatic hemangiomatosis, and embryonic lethality caused by a germ-line Tsc2 mutation in mice. Cancer Res **59**:1206–1211.

97. Onda, H, A Lueck, PW Marks, HB Warren, and DJ Kwiatkowski. 1999. Tsc2(+/−) mice develop tumors in multiple sites that express gelsolin and are influenced by genetic background. J Clin Invest **104**:687–695.

98. Kobayashi, T, O Minowa, Y Sugitani, S Takai, H Mitani, E Kobayashi, T Noda, and O Hino. 2001. A germ-line Tsc1 mutation causes tumor development and embryonic lethality that are similar, but not identical to, those caused by Tsc2 mutation in mice. Proc Natl Acad Sci **98**:8762–8767.

99. Potter, CJ, LG Pedraza, and T Xu. 2002. Akt regulates growth by directly phosphorylating Tsc2. Nat Cell Biol **4**:658–665.

100. Gao, X, Y Zhang, P Arrazola, O Hino, T Kobayashi, RS Yeung, B Ru, and D Pan. 2002. Tsc tumour suppressor proteins antagonize amino-acid-TOR signalling. Nat Cell Biol **4**:699–704.

101. Inoki, K, Y Li, T Zhu, J Wu, and KL Guan. 2002. TSC2 is phosphorylated and inhibited by Akt and suppresses mTOR signalling. Nat Cell Biol **4**:648–657.

102. Manning, BD, AR Tee, MN Logsdon, J Blenis, and LC Cantley. 2002. Identification of the tuberous sclerosis complex-2 tumor suppressor gene product tuberin as a target of the phosphoinositide 3-kinase/akt pathway. Mol Cell **10**:151–162.

103. Luttrell, LM, Y Daaka, and RJ Lefkowitz. 1999. Regulation of tyrosine kinase cascades by G-protein-coupled receptors. Curr Opin Cell Biol **11**:177–183.

104. Wienecke, R, A Koning, and J DeClue. 1995. Identification of tuberin, the tuberous sclerosis 2 product. Tuberin possesses specific Rap1GAP activity. J Biol Chem **270**:16409–16414.

105. Kovacs, G, P Brusa, and W De Riese. 1989. Tissue-specific expression of a constitutional 3;6 translocation: development of multiple bilateral renal-cell carcinomas. Int J Cancer **43**:422–427.

106. Bodmer, D, MJ Eleveld, MJ Ligtenberg, MA Weterman, BA Janssen, DF Smeets, PE de Wit, A van den Berg, E van den Berg, MI Koolen, and A Geurts van Kessel. 1998. An alternative route for multistep tumorigenesis in a novel case of hereditary renal cell cancer and a t(2;3)(q35;q21) chromosome translocation. Am J Hum Genet **62(6)**:1475–1483:1475–1483.

107. Bodmer, D, M Eleveld, M Ligtenberg, M Weterman, A van der Meijden, M Koolen, C Hulsbergen-van der Kaa, SD Smits A, and A Geurts van Kessel. 2002. Cytogenetic and molecular analysis of early stage renal cell carcinomas in a family with a translocation (2;3)(q35;q21). Cancer Genet Cytogenet **134**:6–12.

108. Podolski, J, T Byrski, S Zajaczek, T Druck, DB Zimonjic, NC Popescu, G Kata, A Borowka, J Gronwald, J Lubinski, and RK Huebne. 2001. Characterization of a familial RCC-associated t(2;3)(q33;q21) chromosome translocation. J Hum Genet **46**:685–693.

109. Li, FP, HJ Decker, B Zbar, VP Stanton, G Kovacs, BR Seizinger, H Aburatani, AA Sandberg, S Berg, and S Hosoe, et al. 1993. Clinical and genetic studies of renal cell carcinomas in a family with a constitutional chromosome 3;8 translocation. Ann Intern Med **118**:106–111.

110. Schmidt, L, F Li, RS Brown, S Berg, F Chen, MH Wei, K Tory, MI Lerman, and B Zbar. 1995. Mechanism of Tumorigenesis of Renal Carcinomas Associated with the Constitutional Chromosome 3;8 Translocation. Cancer J Sci Am **1**:191.

111. Eleveld, MJ, D Bodmer, G Merkx, A Siepman, SH Sprenger, MA Weterman, MJ Ligtenberg, J Kamp, W Stapper, JW Jeuken, D Smeets, A Smits, and A Geurts Van Kessel. 2001. Molecular analysis of a familial case of renal cell cancer and a t(3;6)(q12;q15). Genes Chromosomes Cancer **31**:23–32.

112. Zbar, B. 2000. Inherited epithelial tumors of the kidney: old and new disease. Semin Cancer Biol **10**:313–318.

113. Ohta, M, H Inoue, MG Cotticelli, K Kastury, R Baffa, J Palazzo, Z Siprashvili, M Mori, P McCue, and EA Druck T. 1996. The FHIT gene, spanning the chromosome 3p14.2 fragile site and renal carcinoma-associated t(3;8) breakpoint, is abnormalin digestive tract cancers. Cell **84**:587–597.

114. Siprashvili, Z, G Sozzi, LD Barnes, P McCue, AK Robinson, V Eryomin, L Sard, E Tagliabue, A Greco, L Fusetti, G Schwartz, MA Pierotti, CM Croce, and K Huebner. 1997. Replacement of Fhit in cancer cells suppresses tumorigenicity. Proc Natl Acad Sci U S A **94**:13771–13776.

115. Hadaczek, P, Z Siprashvili, M Markiewski, W Domagala, T Druck, PA McCue, Y Pekarsky, M Ohta, K Huebner, and J Lubinski. 1998. Absence or reduction of Fhit expression in most clear cell renal carcinomas. Cancer Res **158**:2946–2951.

116. Fong, LY, V Fidanza, N Zanesi, LF Lock, LD Siracusa, R Mancini, Z Siprashvili, M Ottey, SE Martin, T Druck, P McCue, CM Croce, and K Huebner. 2000. Muir-Torre-like syndrome in Fhit-deficient mice. Proc Natl Acad Sci **97**:4742–4747.

117. Gemmill, RM, JD West, F Boldog, N Tanaka, LJ Robinson, DI Smith, F Li, and HA Drabkin. 1998. The hereditary renal cell carcinoma 3;8 translocation fuses FHIT to a patched-related gene, TRC8. Proc Natl Acad Sci U S A **95**:9572–9577.

118. Bale, AE, and KP Yu. 2001. The hedgehog pathway and basal cell carcinomas. Hum Mol Genet **10**:757–762.

119. Druck, T, J Podolski, T Byrski, L Wyrwicz, S Zajaczek, G Kata, A Borowka, J Lubinski, and K Huebner. 2001. The DIRC1 gene at chromosome 2q33 spans a familial RCC-associated t(2;3)(q33;q21) chromosome translocation. J Hum Genet **46**:583–589.

120. Bodmer, D, M Eleveld, M Kater-Baats, I Janssen, B Janssen, M Weterman, E Schoenmaker, M Nickerson, M Linehan, B Zbar, and AG van Kessel. 2002. Disruption of a novel MFS transporter gene, DIRC2, by a familial renal cell carcinoma-associated t(2;3)(q35;q21). Hum Mol Genet 2002 Mar 15;**11(6)**:641–649; **11**:641–649.

121. Goedert, JJ, EA McKeen, and JF Fraumeni. 1981. Polymastia and renal adenocarcinoma. Ann Intern Med **95**:182–184.

122. Mehes, K. 1996. Familial association of supernumerary nipple with renal cancer. Cancer Genet Cytogenet **86**:129–130.

123. Teh, B, S Giraud, F Sari, S Hii, J Bergerat, LCJ Limacher, and D Nicol. 1997. Familial non-VHL non-papillary clear-cell renal cancer. Lancet **349**:848–849.

124. Zbar, B, and M Lerman. 1998. Inherited carcinomas of the kidney. Advances Cancer Research **75**:163–201.

125. Schmidt, L, F Duh, F Chen, T Kishida, G Glenn, P Choyke, S Scherer, Z Zhuang, I Lubensky, M Dean, R Allikmets, A Chidambaram, U Bergerheim, J Feltis, C Casadevall, A Zamarron, M Bernues, S Richard, C Lips, M Walther, L Tsui, L Geil, M Orcutt, T Stackhouse, and BEA Zbar. 1997. Germline and somatic mutations in the tyrosine kinase domain of the MET proto-oncogene in papillary renal carcinomas. Nature Genetics **16**:68–73.

126. Zhuang, Z, WS Park, S Pack, L Schmidt, AO Vortmeyer, E Pak, T Pham, RJ Weil, S Candidus, IA Lubensky, WM Linehan, B Zbar, and G Weirich. 1998. Trisomy 7-harbouring non-random duplication of the mutant MET allele in hereditary papillary renal carcinomas. Nat Genet 1998 Sep;**20(1)**:66–69; **20**:66–69.

127. Duh, FM, SW Scherer, LC Tsui, MI Lerman, B Zbar, and L Schmidt. 1997. Gene structure of the human MET proto-oncogene. Oncogene **15**:1583–1586.

128. Bardelli, A, C Ponzetto, and PM Comoglio. 1994. Identification of functional domains in the hepatocyte growth factor and its receptor by molecular engineering. J Biotechnol **37**:109–122.

129. Bottaro, DP, JS Rubin, DL Faletto, AM Chan, TE Kmiecik, GF Vande Woude, and SA Aaronson. 1991. Identification of the hepatocyte growth factor receptor as the c-met proto-oncogene product. Science **251**:802–804.

130. Ponzetto, C, A Bardelli, Z Zhen, F Maina, P dalla Zonca, S Giordano, A Graziani, G Panayotou, and PM Comoglio. 1994. A multifunctional docking site mediates signaling and transformation by the hepatocyte growth factor/scatter factor receptor family. Cell **77**:261–271.

131. Naldini, L, E Vigna, R Ferracini, P Longati, L Gandino, M Prat, and PM Comoglio. 1991. The tyrosine kinase encoded by the MET proto-oncogene is activated by autophosphorylation. Mol Cell Biol **4**:1793–1803.

132. Nakaigawa, N, G Weirich, L Schmidt, and B Zbar. 2000. Tumorigenesis mediated by MET mutant M1268T is inhibited by dominant-negative Src. Oncogene **19:**2996–3002.
133. Giordano, S, Z Zhen, E Medico, G Gaudino, F Galimi, and PM Comoglio. 1993. Transfer of motogenic and invasive response to scatter factor/hepatocyte growth factor by transfection of human MET protooncogene. Proc Natl Acad Sci **90:**649–653.
134. Koochekpour, S, M Jeffers, PH Wang, C Gong, GA Taylor, LM Roessler, R Stearman, JR Vasselli, WG Stetler-Stevenson, WG Kaelin, WM Linehan, RD Klausner, JR Gnarra, and GF Vande Woude. 1999. The von Hippel-Lindau tumor suppressor gene inhibits hepatocyte growth factor/scatter factor-induced invasion and branching morphogenesis in renal carcinoma cells. Mol Cell Biol **19:**5902–5912.
135. Launonen, V, O Vierimaa, M Kiuru, J Isola, S Roth, E Pukkala, P Sistonen, R Herva, and LA Aaltonen. 2001. Inherited susceptibility to uterine leiomyomas and renal cell cancer. Proc Natl Acad Sci **98:**3387–3392.
136. Alam, NA, S Bevan, and MEA Churchman. 2001. Localization of a gene (MCUL1) for multiple cutaneous leiomyomata and uterine fibroids to chromosome 1q42.3–q43. Am J Hum Genet **68:**1264–1269.
137. Consortium, TML. 2002. Germline mutations in FH predispose to dominantly inherited uterine fibroids, skin leiomyomata and papillary renal cell cancer. Nat Genet **30:**306–310.
138. Rustin, P. 2002. Mitochondria, from cell death to proliferation. Nat Genet **30:**352–353.
139. Baysal, BE, RE Ferrell, JE Willett-Brozick, EC Lawrence, D Myssiorek, A Bosch, A van der Mey, PE Taschner, WS Rubinstein, EN Myers, CW Richard, CJ Cornelisse, P Devilee, and B Devlin. 2000. Mutations in SDHD, a mitochondrial complex II gene, in hereditary paraganglioma. Science **287:**848–851.
140. Astuti, D, F Douglas, TW Lennard, IA Aligianis, ER Woodward, DG Evans, C Eng, F Latif, and ER Maher. 2001. Germline SDHD mutation in familial phaeochromocytoma. Lancet **357:** 1181–1182.
141. Niemann, S, and U Müller. 2000. Mutations in *SDHC* cause autosomal dominant paraganglioma, type 3. Nature Genet **26:**268–270.
142. Malchoff, CD, M Sarfarazi, B Tendler, F Forouhar, G Whalen, V Joshi, A Arnold, and DM Malchoff. 2000. Papillary thyroid carcinoma associated with papillary renal neoplasia: genetic linkage analysis of a distinct heritable tumor syndrome. J Clin Endocrinol Metab **85:**1758–1764.
143. Birt, AR, GR Hogg, and WJ Dube. 1977. Hereditary multiple fibrofolliculomas with trichodiscomas and acrochordons. Arch Dermatol **113:**1674–1677.
144. Scalvenzi, M, G Argenziano, E Sammarco, and M Delfino. 1998. Hereditary multiple fibrofolliculomas, trichodiscomas and acrochordons: syndrome of Birt-Hogg-Dube. J Eur Acad Dermatol Venereol **11:**45–47.
145. Toro, JR, G Glenn, P Duray, T Darling, G Weirich, B Zbar, M Linehan, and ML Turner. 1999. Birt-Hogg-Dube syndrome: a novel marker of kidney neoplasia. Arch Dermatol **135:**1195–1202.
146. Roth, JS, AD Rabinowitz, M Benson, and ME Grossman. 1993. Bilateral renal cell carcinoma in the Birt-Hogg-Dube syndrome. J Am Acad Dermatol **29:**1055–1056.
147. Khoo, SK, M Bradley, FK Wong, MA Hedblad, M Nordenskjold, and BT Teh. 2001. Birt-Hogg-Dube syndrome: mapping of a novel hereditary neoplasia gene to chromosome 17p12–q11.2. Oncogene **20:**5239–5242.
148. Schmidt, LS, MB Warren, ML Nickerson, G Weirich, V Matrosova, JR Toro, ML Turner, P Duray, M Merino, S Hewitt, CP Pavlovich, G Glenn, CR Greenberg, WM Linehan, and B Zbar. 2001. Birt-Hogg-Dube syndrome, a genodermatosis associated with spontaneous pneumothorax and kidney neoplasia, maps to chromosome 17p11.2. Am J Hum Genet **69:**876–882.
149. Weirich, G, G Glenn, RK Junke, M Merino, S Storkel, I Lubensky, P Choyke, S Pack, M Amin, MM Walther, WM Lineha, and B Zbar. 1998. Familial renal oncocytoma: clinicopathological study of 5 families. J Urol **160:**335–340.
150. Leroy, X, E Leteurtre, PH Mahe, B Gosselin, B Delobel, and MF Croquette. 2002. Renal oncocytoma with a novel chromosomal rearrangement, der(13)t(13;16)(p11;p11), associated with a renal cell carcinoma. J Clin Pathol **55:**157–158.

2. MECHANISMS OF IMMUNE DYSFUNCTION IN RENAL CELL CARCINOMA

ITHAAR H. DERWEESH, M.D.[1,3], CHARLES S. TANNENBAUM, PhD.[1], PATRICIA A. RAYMAN[1], M.S., AND JAMES H. FINKE, PhD.[1,2,3]

[1]*Department of Immunology, Lerner Research Institute*

[2]*Experimental Therapeutics*

[3]*Glickman Urological Institute, Cleveland Clinic Foundation, Cleveland, Ohio*

INTRODUCTION

The immunologic control of carcinogenesis was first demonstrated by Gross in 1943,[1] who made the observation that inbred mice could be immunized against tumor transplants from syngeneic animals. In 1970, the concept of "immune surveillance" was developed by Burnet,[2] who proposed that cancers express unique antigens that would allow their detection by the host's immune system. Subsequent discovery of T cell subsets, TCR complex, antigen presentation, MHC restriction and molecular approaches to identify antigens have contributed to our understanding of T cell immunity to tumors.

Development of an effectual immune response against neoplastic cells requires activation of T cells following recognition of tumor-associated antigens expressed on the appropriate antigen presenting cells.[3,4] This cell-mediated immune response involves activation of cytotoxic CD8+ T cells as well as CD4+ T cells. CD8+ T cells recognize antigenic peptides presented by major histocompatibility complex (MHC) Class I molecules whereas CD4+ T cells recognize antigenic peptides presented by MHC Class II molecules along with the appropriate costimulatory molecules.[4]

Activation of type 1 CD4+ cells leads to production of cytokines such as interleukin-2 (IL-2) that provides a critical signal for clonal expansion of antigen-activated lymphocytes.[5] IL-2 signaling also upregulates expression of effector molecules

Address for Correspondence: James Finke, Department of Immunology, NB3, Cleveland Clinic Foundation, 9500 Euclid Avenue, Cleveland, Ohio 44195. E-mail: finkej@ccf.org (granzyme B and pore-forming protein) required for the cytolytic function of CD8+ T cells. Another critical cytokine is gamma-interferon (IFNγ), produced by both type 1 (Th1) helper CD4+ and a subset of CD8+ T cells, that further promotes the development of a cellular response by enhancing MHC and costimulatory molecule expression as well as by activating macrophages.[5] Activation of T-cell immunity is dependent on normal intracellular signaling through the T-cell receptor and subsequent downstream induction of a variety of transcriptional factors that regulate gene expression of cytokines, chemokines, and receptors involved in T cell responses.[6,7]

Renal cell carcinoma has been an archetypal system by which host-tumor immune interactions have been characterized, described and exploited. A role for immunological modulation in the natural history of renal cell carcinoma was first suggested by indirect observations. Nephrectomy for metastatic renal cell carcinoma occasionally resulted in metastatic tumor regression,[8] and nephrectomy in combination with resection of solitary metastasis, particularly in the lung has been associated with long-term survival.[9] Furthermore, the development of metastatic disease 10 years or longer after resection of an apparently localized cancer indicates that the cancer had metastasized prior to nephrectomy but that the metastatic foci had been contained by the immune system.

In 1980, Rosenberg and co-workers reported that lymphoid cells could be generated in vitro that were cytotoxic against a broad range of murine and human tumor targets.[10] Subsequently IL-2 was shown to stimulate growth of T cells with antitumor reactivity and mediate regression of cancer in experimental animal models and selected patients with advanced cancers.[11] In 1994, Rosenberg and coworkers updated their experience with high-dose bolus IL-2 in 149 patients with metastatic renal cell carcinoma, reporting a 7% complete regression and 13% partial regression, with durable responses in the complete regression group.[12] On the basis of this and similar data (demonstrating a 14% overall response rate—5% CR, 9% PR),[13] high-dose bolus IL-2 achieved Food and Drug Administration approval in high performance status patients who had undergone nephrectomy.

Recently, an emerging strategy for immune modulation of advanced RCC is allogeneic peripheral blood stem cell transplantation. This strategy relies on an allogeneic T cell graft versus tumor effect. Donor T cell populations targeting allogeneic antigens expressed on the patient's malignant cells are thought to be the driving force of the graft-versus-tumor effect. This strategy has proven to be successful in treating a variety of hematologic malignancies,[14] and preliminary results have been generated in the treatment of metastatic renal cell carcinoma that has been refractory to other immunomodulatory approaches. The first series demonstrated a 53% regression rate (10 out of 19 patients), with a 37% partial response rate (7 of 19 patients) and a 15% complete response (3 of 19 patients).[15]

Indeed, substantial progress has been made on identifying tumor-associated antigens that are recognized by autologous T cells in RCC patients (Table 1).[16] Moreover, T cells isolated and expanded in vitro from a number of different tumor types including RCC have been shown to either secrete cytokines like IFNγ in response to autologous tumor or to mediate tumor specific cytotoxicity.[17]

Table 1. Tumor-associated antigens for RCC.

Antigen	% RCC Expressing	Reference
Carboxyl Esterase	75%	Ronsin et al, 1999[158]
Gp75 (TRP-1)	11%	Neumann et al, 1998[16]
RAGE-1	21%	Neumann et al, 1998[16]
PRAME	40%	Neumann et al, 1998[16]
Her2/neu	40–45%	Brossart et al, 1998;[159] Zhang et al, 1997[160]
MAGE-1	0–22%	Neumann et al, 1998;[16] Traversari et al, 1992[161]
MAGE-3	76%	Neumann et al, 1998[16]

An emerging body of literature indicates that the tumor may evade immune system-mediate destruction by distinct mechanisms, many of which are directed towards altering the function of T cells.[18–20] Potential mechanisms include: Reduced expression of antigen presenting machinery by tumor cells and the induction of anergy, and later a more global T cell hyporesponsiveness, type 2 bias, and TR cell deletion (apoptosis). Any one or more of these mechanisms may thus present a barrier to the development of an effective anti-tumor immune response. This chapter reviews the evidence for immune dysfunction in T cells from patients with RCC and the mechanisms that may contribute to it.

IMMUNE DYSFUNCTION IN T CELLS FROM PATIENTS WITH RENAL CELL CARCINOMA

At the tumor, there is typically a significant infiltrate of mononuclear cells composed primarily of T lymphocytes and variable numbers of macrophages with minimal presence of NK, B cells, or granulocytes.[21] The T-cell infiltrate is composed of both CD4+ and CD8+ subsets and following in vitro expansion with IL-2, T cell lines (CD4+ and CD8+) and clones that preferentially respond to autologous RCC can be detected in a subset of patients.[17,22,23] Despite this infiltrate, however, there is little evidence demonstrating the presence of a type 1 immune response in the tumor bed. Only a low percentage of infiltrating lymphocytes express mRNA for either IL-2 or IFNγ, two cytokines critical for the development of an immune response.[24,25] Similar findings have been reported for other tumor types.[26] There is also very little expression of the high affinity IL-2 receptor (5%) on tumor infiltrating lymphocytes (TILs) that is usually up-regulated on activated T cells.[18] However, most of TIL express CD45RO, which is a marker of primed T cells, and show minimal CD45RA that is expressed on naïve lymphocytes. The predominance of CD45RO+ T cells within in the tumor versus peripheral blood is likely due to a selective migration of the CD45RO+ cells into tissue rather than a predominance of functionally activated T cells in the tumor environment.[18,27]

TIL are also known to be functionally impaired when isolated from the tumor and stimulated in vitro. TIL from different tumor types including RCC are defective in their ability to proliferate to a variety of stimuli[18,19,28] Exogenous IL-2 added to the cultures was not very effective in initiating cell cycle progression since most TIL appear to be arrested in G0.[29] The cytolytic activity of TIL from RCC tumors is also impaired. This may be due in part to reduced expression of granzyme B mRNA in approximately half of the TIL since granzyme B plays a significant role in the cytotoxic process.[30] The functional deficits in TIL appear to be selective because IL-2Rα expression and cytokine production (IL-2 and IFNγ) following in vitro activation is normal.[18] Immune dysfunction can also be seen in vivo in patients with advanced disease. Delayed type hypersensitivity of some RCC patients is impaired since they fail to respond to common recall antigens: PPD, mumps, and Candida.[31] Additionally, the response rate to PPD skin testing with stage I RCC was higher than that of patients with stage IV disease.[32]

DEFECTIVE ANTIGEN PRESENTATION MAY CONTRIBUTE TO THE ABSENCE OF A POTENT IMMUNE RESPONSE TO RCC

Recently, the molecular basis of recognition of tumor antigens by cytotoxic T cells (CTL) has become better elucidated. CTL directed against autologous RCC have been generated, including MHC-restricted CD8+ lines.[17,23,33,34] However, before CTL recognition of discrete RCC tumor antigens can result in effective antitumor activity in vivo, there must first be efficient processing of antigenic peptides and presentation in a MHC class I-restricted manner by the tumor cells or dedicated antigen presenting cells (APCs) to the appropriate effector T cells in a MHC class II-restricted manner.

Tumors and other epithelial cells have the potential to present foreign antigen on their surface to T cells; however, these peptides must first be processed and loaded into the MHC class I binding cleft. Class I molecules assemble in the endoplasmic reticulum (ER) with peptides generated from cytosolic proteins by the cytosolic proteases[35] and by multicatalytic proteosomal subunits such as low-molecular weight proteins 2 (LMP2), LMP7 and LMP10.[36] These peptide fragments then associate with the ATP dependent peptide transport associated with antigen processing (TAP) and are translocated to the ER where they are loaded onto MHC class I molecules prior to expression on the cell surface.[37] Downregulation of components of antigen processing and presenting machinery, which may attenuate the antitumor response by providing neoplastic cells with a mechanism for escaping CTL-mediated recognition and destruction, has been identified in RCC as well as tumors of the lung, liver, prostate, colon, cervix, skin and breast.[38] The defects include reduced or absent expression of MHC class I heavy and light chains, diminished levels of TAP proteins, as well as deficient expression of LMP proteosomal complexes.[39] With respect to RCC, reduction of mRNA and protein levels of these molecules appears more pronounced in RCC cells that have acquired metastatic potential, suggesting that the process of malignant transformation may include progressive loss of these functionally important molecules.[39] In addition, by increasing the levels of TAP in RCC, either through cytokine treatment with IFNγ[38] or by transfection with TAP-1 cDNA,[40] higher expression of MHC class I-molecules on the tumor cell surface and enhanced tumor specific, class I-restricted CTL recognition can be achieved.[37,38]

Dendritic cells (DC), considered to be the most potent antigen-presenting cells, represent 1% of the population of mononuclear cells in the peripheral blood and have been described in almost every tissue except the brain and cornea.[41,42] They are the most potent stimulators of T-cell proliferation and activation in mixed leukocyte reactions (MLR). Immature DCs from peripheral blood express HLA-DR, costimulatory molecules B7.1 (CD80), B7.2 (CD86) and CD40. Peripheral blood and tissue DCs take up antigens by endocytosis and phagocytosis,[43] and subsequently migrate to the draining lymph nodes where they mature to fully competent antigen-presenting cells expressing CD83, the most specific marker for mature DCs.[44,45] The state of complete maturation correlates with high-level expression of costimulatory molecules B7.1 (CD80), B7.2 (CD86), adhesion molecule ICAM-1(CD54) and antigen-presenting complexes (HLA-DR, CD1a). DCs participate in tumor immunity by migrating into tumors, where they acquire antigen, undergo activation, and migrate to lymph nodes to initiate a T-lymphocyte response against tumor-associated antigens.

Maturation, differentiation, state of activation and distribution of DCs in tumors seem to be closely controlled and regulated by a variety of microenvironmental signals including cytokines and other surface molecule expression on neighboring cells.[46] The milieu of cytokines might induce development of intratumoral immune tolerance.[47] Interleukin-10, produced by some tumors and lymphocytes, might down regulate the expression of MHC class II and B7.2 and thus reduce the state of activation and the capacity of antigen presentation.[48]

Earlier studies described the correlation of DC presence in primary tumors with progression of disease and patient survival.[49,50] Tumor infiltrating DCs (TiDCs) found in colorectal carcinomas were immunologically incompetent by the demonstration of reduced expression of the costimulatory molecule B7.2 (CD86) as well as a failure of upregulating this molecule in cultures with IL-4 and GM-CSF. TiDCs isolated and cultured from RCC tumors showed similar results.[51] A recent study described small but significant subpopulations of TiDCs in human RCC, with low numbers of TiDCs expressing maturation markers CD83.[52] Furthermore, intratumoral DCs are weak stimulators of T-cell proliferation in MLR and show low cytokine production.[52] Thus, escape of tumor cells from the immune response may result from a defective differentiation or function of professional antigen-presenting cells (APC), i.e., dendritic cells (DC). This hypothesis was tested by Menetrier et al.,[53] who demonstrated that RCC cell lines were found to release soluble factors that inhibit the differentiation of CD34+ cells into DC and trigger their commitment towards monocytic cells with a potent phagocytic capacity but lacking APC function. Antibodies against IL-6 and granulocyte colony-stimulating factor (GM-CSF) attenuated the inhibitory effects of RCC cell lines, and recombinant IL-6 and/or GM-CSF was found to inhibit differentiation of DC similarly to RCC.

T CELL ANERGY

Anergy is a state in which T cells are alive but incapable of producing IL-2 and expanding in response to specific antigenic stimulation.[54,55] The functional alterations of anergic T cells are also associated with select signaling defects. This includes a reduction in the activation of the kinases ZAP-70, RAS and ERK and as well as impaired activation of the transcription factors, AP-1 and NFAT.[56] The anergizing signal also appears to activate the kinase, fyn as well as increase intracellular calcium and cyclic AMP. In turn, cAMP upregulates cyclin-dependent kinase inhibitor p27kip1 that may ultimately block cell cycle progression.[56]

The development of T cell anergy appears to be an early event in tumor progression.[57] While T cell anergy has been well described in animal models and in vitro,[54,55] it is not known whether the unresponsiveness that is observed in cancer patient T cells represents anergy. Antigen specific T cells have been detected within melanoma lesions after vaccination. Immunization was apparent in most lesions as evident by IFNγ mRNA expression that appeared to correlate with high antigen expression by tumors (gp100).[58] However, IFNγ expression was not associated with a significant inflammatory response or T cell accumulation.[58,59] While IFNγ was expressed in tumor there was an absence of IL-2 mRNA, a cytokine critical for T cell proliferation and that is absent in anergic cells.[58] Furthermore, detection of these antigen-reactive T cells in the tumor did not correlate with clinical responses. The presence of tumor antigen-specific T cells in the tumor and blood in the absence of clinical responses, in many cases, demonstrates the need for additional functional analysis of these effector cells. Although these studies show that tumor specific T cells can infiltrate tumors following immunotherapy, it is not clear whether these cells are typically functional, in an anergic state or undergoing apoptosis. Studies are underway to examine the functional status of tumor antigen specific T cells in RCC patients. Whether these cells will exhibit potent anti-tumor activity or will be tolerant is an important question to address.

Possible Mechanisms of T Cell Anergy

There are several mechanisms that may play a role in the induction of T cell anergy in cancer patients (Table 2).

Defective Dendritic Cell (DC) Signaling of T Cells

The lack of co-stimulation or CD40 ligation appears to be responsible for anergy induction in murine tumor models.[60] In these models, antigen-presenting cells (APC) can induce T cell tolerance to self-antigens due to the inability to activate APC via CD40. Tolerance of tumor specific CD4+ T cells can be reversed by in vivo ligation of CD40.[61] With some tumors it may be possible to overcome anergy.

Table 2. Possible Mechanisms of Anergy in Cancer Patient T cells.

- Defective Dendritic Cell stimulation of T cells:
  — No costimulation (Boussiotis et al, 1996)[60]
  — No CD40 ligation; tolerance reversible with in vivo ligation of CD40 (Sotomayor et al, 1999)[61]
- Persistent antigenic stimulation of T cells by tumor (Welsh, 2001)[63]
- IL-10 (Wittke et al, 1999)[64]

Recent studies in transgenic mice show that expression of a tolerizing antigen does not block the in vitro stimulation and recovery of T cells capable of initiating tumor cell destruction.[62] Whether defective APC and CD40 signaling may be important to the induction of T cell anergy in human cancers remains to be evaluated in more detail.

Persistent Antigen Stimulation

Dysfunction of antigen specific T cells has been reported in persistent infections where high doses of virus appear to cause clonal exhaustion.[63] Recent studies utilizing MHC tetramers have revealed a complex process where there is evidence of activation-induced cell death of T cells that recognize the nucleoprotein of LCMV. These cells show signs of impaired cytokine production, become annexin V positive (an early event in apoptosis) and disappear. However, specific T cells to the glycoprotein GP33 become anergized but do not undergo AICD and persist.[63] The fact that T cells recognizing different antigenic epitopes behave differently may be due to the degree of antigen stimulation. It may be that continuous antigenic stimulation by the tumor can contribute to immune dysfunction in the antigen specific T cells of cancer patients, although this possibility has not been explored in depth.

Interleukin 10

(IL-10) is an immunosuppressive cytokine that has been detected in renal cell carcinoma tumors[25] as well as in elevated amounts in the serum of patients with advanced RCC.[64] IL-10 has been described as a cytokine of the type 2 response. It is able to suppress antigen-presenting cells by down-regulation of HLA class I and II molecules on dendritic cells and by induction of anergy of T-lymphocytes through the inhibition of the CD28 co-stimulatory pathway.[65] However, IL-10 only blocks T cells stimulated by low numbers of triggered T-cell receptors, a condition that is dependent on CD28 co-stimulation. IL-10 does not affect T cells that receive a strong T cell receptor signal and are independent of CD28 co-signaling.

T CELL UNRESPONSIVENESS IN CANCER PATIENT T CELLS

A more global immune dysfunction has been observed in animal tumor models and in cancer patients that is typically associated with more advanced tumor burden. Reduced T cell function is characterized by a hyporesponsiveness to challenge with common recall antigens.[31] Furthermore, defective T cell function is most evident in TIL, and is characterized by impaired proliferation and reduced cytotoxic effector function.[17] Within the tumor microenvironment, there is also minimal induction of inflammatory genes such as IFNγ and IL-2 mRNA.[66] In a subset of RCC patients, diminished T cell function has also been observed in peripheral blood T cells, that is mostly associated with the reduced production of type 1 response cytokines, IL-2 and IFNγ.[67,68] Related to the occurrence of global immune dysfunction in T cells for cancer patients are changes in the function and expression of the T cell receptor (TCR), defects in downstream TCR signaling, and attenuation of the lytic activity of T cell lines associated with suppression of NFκB translocation.

Table 3. Mechanisms By Which Tumors Reduce Zeta Chain Levels.

- Hydrogen peroxide production by activated granulocytes and macrophages (Kono et al, 1996; Schmielau and Finn, 2001)[72,77]
- Caspase activity in apoptotic T cells (zeta chain is a substrate for caspase 3) (Gastman et al, 1999; Gastman et al, 2000)[78,79]
- Repeated stimulation through TCR or TNFR can reduce zeta expression (Ochoa and Longo, 1995; Isomaki et al, 2001)[68,82]
- Reduced L-arginine in the tumor microenvironment (Taheri et al, 2001)[83]

Coinciding with the phenomenon of global immune dysfunction in cancer patients there is a demonstrated alteration in the expression and/or function of T cell receptor linked signaling events. The most examined defect in T cell signaling is the reduction in expression of the ζ chain of the TCR complex. The TCR consists of a ligand specific α/β heterodimer noncovalently associated with CD3 and ζ subunits to form an eight chain complex (αβγδε2ζ2). Of these eight chains, the cytoplasmic domain of the ζ chain alone is capable of transducing TCR signaling events.[69] Reduced expression of the ζ chain has been observed by western immunoblot or flow cytometry in T cells from patients with a variety of tumors, including, melanoma, cervical cancer and Hodgkin's disease.[68] The decrease in ζ in T cells of RCC patients has been controversial, with some reports showing variable levels of reduced expression[19,70] and others showing no reduction.[71] Reduction in ζ chain expression has been correlated in some studies with a decrease in either proliferation or type 1 cytokine production.[68] Decreased levels of ζ chain in T cells appear to correlate with disease progression and overall survival in cervical cancer,[72] Hodgkin's disease[73] and oral carcinoma.[74] It may be that ζ chain expression levels in T cells will be useful as a predictor for survival although more studies are needed. However, it is not clear whether it will be useful for monitoring responses to immunotherapy.[75]

Table 3 demonstrates mechanisms by which the reduction in ζ chain levels may occur. Hydrogen peroxide produced by activated granulocytes (in the blood) and macrophages (in the tumor) is known to decrease ζ chain expression in T cells. Degradation can be prevented by the addition of hydrogen peroxide scavengers.[76,77] ζ degradation may also result from caspase activity induced in apoptotic T cells. In vitro experiments demonstrated that induction of apoptosis in T cells coincides with ζ chain degradation that is blocked by the addition of a pan-caspase inhibitor and that ζ can be a substrate for caspase-3.[78,79] Indeed, elevated caspase-3 activity and increased peripheral T cell apoptosis has been demonstrated to coexist with down-regulation of TCR ζ molecules in patients with melanoma[80] and gastric carcinoma.[81] In vitro studies have also shown that repeated stimulation via TCR or by TNF can reduce the expression of ζ in T cells.[68,82] Thus, ζ may be modulated by chronic stimulation. There is also another report suggesting that the decrease in ζ chain expression may, in part, be due to reduced L-arginine levels in the tumor microenvironment.[83]

Table 4. Potential Mechanisms for Tumor-Induced NFκB Defect.

- Hydrogen peroxide inhibition of NFκB Correlated with reduced expression of TH1 cytokines (Malmberg et al, 2001)[93]
- Ganglioside suppressed NFκB activation in T cells (Uzzo et al, 1999)[89,90]

There are also reports of defects in downstream TCR signaling in T cells from cancer patients. This includes reduced tyrosine phosphorylation of multiple substrates, including PLCγ.[84] Assessment of free intracellular calcium concentrations after mitogen stimulation also revealed less mobilization of calcium compared to normal T lymphocytes. Whether these alterations are related to defective ζ chain expression is not known.

The transcription factor, Nuclear factor kappaB (NFκB) regulates the expression of various genes essential for cell function and survival.[85,86] Tumor-induced inhibition of the lytic activity of tumor-specific T lines correlated with suppression of NFκB translocation.[87] Other studies in animal models[88] and renal cancer patients[89] have demonstrated defective activation of the transcription factor NFκB in TIL and peripheral blood derived T cells. The major difficulty is in the nuclear accumulation of the most transactivating NFκB dimer, RelA/p50, following T cell activation. Impaired NFκB activation is observed in T cells from 50% of RCC patients but in less than 5% of NED (no evidence of disease) patients and healthy individuals.[90] Studies from knockout mice defective in NFκB proteins demonstrate that NFκB is a cell survival factor that regulates expression of multiple anti-apoptotic genes including Bfl-1/A1, Bcl-2 and the cellular inhibitors of apoptosis family of genes.[91] There is also data suggesting a role for NFκB in the regulation of the cells involved in type 1 but not type 2 responses.[92] Studies are in progress to determine if the defect in NFκB of patients' T cells is related to increased sensitivity to apoptosis or to the bias for a type 2 response. The inhibition of NFκB activation appears to be mediated by soluble products present in the tumor microenvironment (Table 4). Hydrogen peroxide production presumably by macrophages blocked NFκB activation, primarily in memory T cells, that correlated with reduced expression of type 1 cytokines.[93] Select gangliosides from RCC also inhibit NFκB activation in T cells.[89] Finally, in a transgenic animal model, the induction of tolerance to self-antigens correlated with a lack of activation of NFκB.[94] Our recent findings also suggest that a reduction in NFκB activation, induced by RCC derived gangliosides can sensitize T cells to activation induced cell death.[95]

SHIFT TO A TYPE 2 RATHER THAN A TYPE 1 RESPONSE

Immune responses could be divided into two functional subsets on the basis of the immunoregulatory cytokines that these clones produced.[96,97] Type 1 responses are characterized by production of IL-2 and IFNγ whereas type 2 responses are characterized by the production of IL-4, IL-5, and IL-10. Though initially recognized as a phenomenon of immune regulation in CD4+ T helper (Th) cells and later

CD8+ T lymphocytes, cytokine production that characterizes type 1 and type 2 responses may by also be carried out by non–T-cell leukocytes, such as monocytes/macrophages, natural killer (NK) cells, B cells, mast cells, and eosinophils.[5] Type 1 responses are recognized to stimulate the development of cell-mediated immunity (CMI) whereas type 2 responses were more important for humoral immunity (B-cell development and antibody production). Furthermore, it has been demonstrated that some of these immunoregulatory cytokines possess cross-regulatory properties such that they not only enhance one type cytokine production but also suppressed the other type of response and the cells that produced it. The cross-regulatory properties of type 1 and type 2 cytokines are linked in an inverse relationship that exists between CMI and humoral immunity in response to antigenic stimuli. Thus, some type 1 (IFNγ, IL-12) cytokines downregulate humoral immunity by decreasing the levels of Th2 cells and type 2 cytokines. Conversely, some type 2 (IL-4, IL-10) cytokines downregulate CMI by decreasing the levels of type 1 response cells and the cytokines they elaborate.[5]

It is generally accepted and supported by animal studies that type 1 cytokines promote the development of an anti-tumor cell-mediated immune response. The production of IFNγ is particularly linked to the generation of an effective immune response responsible for rejecting tumors.[98,99] The cytokine IL-2 is required for T cell proliferation and acquisition of cytotoxic effector function characteristic of a type 1 response, whereas the cytokines IL-4 and IL-10 on the other hand promote a type 2 response that is necessary for a humoral immune response.[5] There is evidence in both animal models and in human neoplasms that the tumor microenvironment can shift the balance to a predominately type 2 response. The induction of various immunotherapeutic approaches that favor a shift back to a type 1 response typically results in the development of an effective tumor immune response.[100] This has been best documented in animal studies. To the extent it has been examined in cancer patients, there is evidence that in the peripheral blood, the type 2 response is predominant. This is supported by several observations. In a variety of different tumors, including renal cell carcinoma and pancreatic carcinoma, there is increased production of type 2 as opposed to type 1 cytokines.[101,102] Furthermore, measurement of intracellular levels of cytokines in RCC patients by immunocytometry demonstrates a change from a type 1 to type 2 response with increasing tumor stage.[67] Therefore, in some cancer patients type 2 bias, and under- or low IFN expression by the bulk CD4+ T cell population, may reflect the influence of tumor antigen specific CD4+ T cells. Studies are ongoing to determine whether immunotherapy can induce primarily a type 1 response in the tumor specific T cell populations, and the effect this will have on the clinical response. The mechanisms involved in shifting the cytokine response in cancer patients to a type 2 response are not well delineated. However, several investigations suggest that TGFβ, IL-10, FasL, and gangliosides may be involved in this process (Table 5).

Tumor-derived TGFβ has been demonstrated to drive the balance to a type 2 response by upregulation of the production of IL-10[103] or by a direct effect on tumor infiltrating lymphocytes.[104] IL-10 is known to play a role in down regulat-

Table 5. Mechanisms by which Tumor Microenvironment may produce type 2 hyporesponsiveness.

- TGF-β (Maeda et al, 1996)[103]
  — Drive the balance to type 2 response by unpregulation of IL-10 production.
  — Inhibit TH1-type responses directly by a direct effect on tumor infiltrating lymphocytes (Ortegel et al, 2002)[104]
- IL-10
  — Downregulates the expression of type 1 response cytokines (Bellone et al, 1999)[102]
  — Augment the immunosuppressive activity of TGFβ by enhancing the expression of TGFβ II receptors (Cottrez and Groux, 2001)[105]
- Clearance of antigen-specific IFNγ producing T cells via Fas mediated-apoptosis (Ribas et al, 2000; Muschen et al, 2001)[109,110]
- Gangliosides
  — Downregulate expression of type 1 cytokines (Irani, 1998)[124]
  — Increase production of IL-10 (Kanada, 1999)[125]

---

ing the expression of type 1 cytokines and may also augment the immunosuppressive activity of TGFβ by enhancing the expression of TGFβ II receptors.[105] The role of IL-10 as an inhibitor of type 1 immunity is not entirely clear from the animal studies. However, in a limited number of studies in cancer patients there is correlative data linking IL-10 and TGFβ expression and the presence of a type 2 response in peripheral blood T cells. For example, in pancreatic carcinoma patients, co-expression of TGF-beta and IL-10 in tumor tissue was associated with elevated levels of both cytokines in the sera and with the predominance of a type 2 cytokine expression pattern in response to anti-CD3 antibody.[102] Furthermore, serial sampling of fine-needle aspirates of identical metastases from melanoma patients receiving IL-2-based vaccinations has been performed to assess changes in expression of IL-10, TGFβ and IFNγ mRNA levels by quantitative real-time PCR. Attenuated expression of IL-10 in pretreatment tissues of responding lesions was noted, and IFNγ transcript levels were found to increase after treatment in regressing as compared to non-regressing lesions.[157] A potential role for IL-10 and TGFβ in regulating type 1 cytokine responses is beginning to be addressed in the tumor. These types of studies should provide information on whether the pre-treatment profile of cytokines in the tumor will influence clinical responses to immunotherapy. On the other hand, the contribution of IL-10 to promoting type 2 responses and dampening the development of an effective anti-tumor immune response in animal models is complicated by the observations from multiple groups indicating that IL-10 may also promote anti-tumor immunity under certain conditions. In these studies, IL-10 production by type 2 cells was found to inhibit neovascularization of tumors.[106–108]

It is also possible that the shift to a type 2 response in tumor bearing hosts, in some cases, is due to the clearance of antigen-specific IFNγ producing T cells (Th1 cells). Elimination of Th1 cells was attributable to Fas-receptor mediated clearance in a murine melanoma model.[109] In breast cancer patients, depletion of CD4+ and CD8+ peripheral blood lymphocytes was significantly correlated with Fas Ligand (FasL) expression in the tumors. This might be suggestive for a relationship between FasL expression by breast cancer and systemic immunosuppression.[110]

One proposed mechanism of tumor escape is the release, by tumor cells, of soluble factors into their microenvironment, leading to the suppression of the immune response.[111] Several groups have suggested that gangliosides, a class of biologically active cell surface glycolipids, may function as soluble modulators of the immune response. Upregulated levels of ganglioside expression have also been identified in several human epithelial cancers[112] including neuroblastoma, melanoma, retinoblastoma, and hepatoma as well as RCC.[113] Evidence that gangliosides may be active in the suppression of the antitumor immune response include studies demonstrating that tumor cells synthesize and shed gangliosides into their microenvironment,[111,114–117] coupled with studies showing that gangliosides are highly immunosuppressive in vitro. The mechanisms of ganglioside-induced Immunosuppression are multiple. Gangliosides inhibit multiple steps in the cellular immune response, including, Ag processing and presentation,[118] lymphocyte proliferation,[119,120] inhibition of IL-2-induced T cell proliferation,[121] down-regulation of CD4 expression[122] and the generation of a cytotoxic response.[123] Most recently, it has been shown that exposure of mouse splenocytes to gangliosides results in reduced gene transcription of the type 1 response cytokines IL-2 and IFNγ, while leaving gene transcription of the type 2 response associated cytokines, IL-4 and IL-10, unaffected.[124] Others have reported a ganglioside-induced increase in T cell IL-10 production.[125] Together, these findings suggest that shed tumor gangliosides may shift the balance of the antitumor immune response from a type 1 response toward a type 2 response, possibly leading to a reduction in the cellular antitumor immune response critical for tumor elimination.

TUMOR INDUCTION OF APOPTOSIS IN T CELLS DIMINISHES EFFECTIVE ANTITUMOR IMMUNITY

Recent evidence suggests that cell mediated immunity may be downregulated through apoptotic pathways.[126] Indeed, apoptosis of antigen specific T cells is considered a major mechanism by which T cell responses are shut down after antigenic exposure.[127] Repeated antigen stimulation of T cells is known to increase their sensitivity to apoptosis. There is also growing evidence that apoptotic mechanisms regulate the development of an effective immune response to tumor cells.[95,128] Apoptotic T cells have been reported in several different tumor types, though it is unclear whether the level of apoptosis relates to stage, grade or clinical outcome. Spontaneous apoptosis of a subset of T cells in the peripheral blood of patients with advanced melanoma and gastric cancer has been observed.[80,81] There is also evidence that T cells from cancer patient showed a heightened sensitivity to activation induced cell death (AICD). That is, T cells undergo apoptosis following activation via the T cell receptor complex.[129] Possible mechanisms of apoptosis of T cells in cancer patients include tumor expressed death receptors and their ligands, a death receptor independent pathway involving mitochondrial damage and ganglioside sensitization (Table 6).

The caspases, a family of cysteine proteases, play critical roles in the execution phase of apoptosis and are responsible for many of the biochemical and morpho-

Table 6. Mechanisms of Tumor-Induced T cell Apoptosis.

- Death Receptors/Death Ligands
  - Fas Ligand (Whiteside and Rabinowich, 1998; Uzzo et al, 1999)[149,129]
  - CD27/CD27L (Wischhusen et al, 2002)[153]
  - DR4,DR5/TRAIL (Koyama et al, 2002)[154]
- Death Receptor independent pathway involving mitochondrial damage (Gastman et al, 2000)[79]
  - Ganglioside sensitization through the mitochondrial pathway (Kristal and Brown, 1999; de Maria et al, 1997)[155,156]

---

logical changes associated with apoptosis.[130] Two main pathways of caspase activation have been delineated. Thus, there are at least two major mechanisms by which a caspase cascade may be initiated: (a) one involving capase-8; and (b) the other involving caspase-9 as the most apical caspase. In the first pathway, activation of initiator caspase-8 or caspase-10 is triggered by ligation of death receptors of the TNF family of immune effectors, including Fas, TNFR1, or Death Receptor 3 by their respective ligands (FasL, TNF, TRAIL). Caspase-8 has been identified as the most apical caspase in apoptosis induced by several death receptors, including Fas and TNFR1.[131,132] Fas-associated death domain (FADD)[133] is recruited directly to ligated Fas or indirectly to ligated TNFR1, resulting in recruitment and autoactivation of caspase-8. Active caspase-8 cleaves and activates downstream caspases, initiating the caspase cascade. Caspase 8 activates caspases 3 and 7, and caspase 3 activates caspase 6.[134] Caspases 3 and 6 have specific roles in the nuclear changes accompanying apoptosis, while caspase 7 is responsible for mitochondrial permeability transition and cytoplasmic shrinkage.[134]

Caspase-9 has been proposed as the initiating caspase in a pathway of apoptosis that is death receptor independent.[135,136] The second pathway is essentially controlled by mitochondria. Induction of cell death in response to a variety of apoptotic stimuli is associated with mitochondrial release of cytochrome c, an event that is blocked by antiapoptotic members of the Bcl-2 family and promoted by proapoptotic members, such as Bax and Bak.[137-139] In the cytosol, cytochrome c, together with dATP, forms a complex with APAF-1 that results in activation of caspase-9[135] and the downstream effector caspases caspase-3, -6, and -7.[136,140] Potential mechanisms for the release of cytochrome c include opening of mitochondrial PT pores, the presence of specific channels for cytochrome c release, or mitochondrial swelling and rupture of the outer membrane, but without loss of mitochondrial membrane potential.[141] There is evidence that both pathways, the death receptor as well as the mitochondrial pathway, are involved in T cell induced apoptosis by the tumor or its micro-environment.

Death Receptor Pathway–Fas Ligand

Fas Ligand (FasL) belongs to the tumor necrosis factor (TNF) family of immune effectors which includes TNF, lymphotoxin, CD40 ligand, CD27 ligand, CD 30 ligand and TRAIL (TNF-related apoptosis-inducing ligand).[142] FasL induces apoptosis resulting in the death of cells expressing the FAS receptor (APO-1, CD95). Whereas FasL is predominantly found in activated T cells[143] and natural killer cells,[144] its receptor is expressed in many other cell types.[142] The Fas/FasL system plays a critical role in the regulation of a variety of facets of the immune response. Fas/FasL-mediated apoptosis is involved in the induction of tolerance to autoantigens,[145,146] formation of immune sanctuaries,[146] down-regulation of lymphocyte expansion via-cell-cell interaction, and the reduction of excess active lymphocytes following an immune response.[147,148]

However, tumor cells may take advantage of these mechanisms to escape immune detection and destruction. Malignant cells from an increasing number of solid tumors[149] including RCC[129] have been shown to express FasL and tumor infiltrating lymphocytes are potential targets for these FasL expressing tumor cells.[150] T cells derived from the peripheral blood as well as those infiltrating the tumor have been shown to express Fas receptor.[129,150] These cells are therefore potential targets for apoptosis mediated by FasL expressing tumor. When preactivated allogeneic T cells or the Jurkat T cell line were co-cultured with RCC tumors expressing FasL, they exhibited DNA breaks as measured by TUNEL assay.[129] This lethal interaction was partially blocked by antibodies against FasL, supporting its role in T cell death. Apoptosis of T cells was blocked by 50% when anti-FasL antibody was added to the T cell-tumor cultures.[129] Furthermore, there is clear and consistent evidence for T cell apoptosis in the tumor bed of RCC malignancies. Taken together, these data support the role of tumor-mediated apoptosis as a mechanism of inhibition of an effective T cell response to renal tumors. The blocking antibody experiments suggest that Fas/FasL interaction is involved, however more definitive approaches are required to clearly elucidate the role of FasL in the induction of apoptosis in T cells.

While the Fas/FasL pathway appears to play an important role in the deletion of activated tumor reactive T cells, investigators have not always been able to demonstrate FasL expression by specific tumor types. For example, melanoma-specific T cells are induced to undergo activation induced cell death following MHC class I-restricted recognition of the tumor in a Fas-dependent fashion,[151] notwithstanding the FasL-negativity of the melanoma lines used in the assays.[151,152] Apoptosis of these tumor specific T cells was prevented and normal immune functions maintained by the addition of pan caspase inhibitors to the cultures, suggesting a role for T cell fratricide in this process.

The process of activation induced cell death (AICD) is critical to the downregulation and termination of a completed immune response. Ordinarily, when stimulated T cells are reactivated, they undergo apoptosis so as to prevent overexuberance of the T cell response. However the spontaneous apoptosis of T cells reported in the peripheral blood of some patients may also occur via the Fas pathway.[80,81] This is supported by the observation that the majority of the apoptotic T cells are expressing the Fas receptor.[80] This finding suggests that when T cells are stimulated by tumor antigen, they may undergo cell death rather than cell activation. AICD is likely the result of increased expression of FasL on the T cells. FasL positive T cells coming in contact with one another will trigger the Fas pathway and induce apoptosis. The current data suggest that AICD in this setting involves the Fas pathway.[80] Therefore definitive approaches are required to clearly elucidate the role of FasL in the induction of apoptosis in T cells. Some of the proposed experiments should be able to distinguish apoptosis induced by FasL expression on tumor versus T cell recognition resulting in AICD, and currently our lab is actively engaged in investigations regarding this subject.

Other Death Receptors

Recently, other members of the TNF family have been demonstrated to induce apoptosis in T cells. Tumor membrane-bound CD70 has been noted to mediate T cell apoptosis induced by gliomas.[153] Furthermore, immunohistochemical studies have demonstrated that membrane-bound TRAIL was noted to be constitutively expressed at high levels in localized and further upregulated metastatic gastric carcinoma carcinomas patients, and this upregulation in expression correlated with an increase in apoptosis of tumor infiltrating lymphocytes as detected by TUNEL.[154]

Mitochondrial Pathway

With respect to the receptor independent, mitochondrial controlled apoptotic pathway, Gastman et al.[79] reported that apoptosis of T cells induced by squamous cell carcinoma of the head and neck (SCCHN) was only partly Fas dependent. The involvement of mitochondria in tumor-induced apoptosis of T cells was demonstrated by changes in mitochondrial permeability, by release of cytochrome c to the cytosol, and by the presence of active subunits of caspase-9 in T cells co-cultured with tumor cells. One possible mechanism for initiating apoptosis pathway via the mitochondrial may involve the expression of gangliosides on tumor cells. Gangliosides, specifically GD3 ganglioside, have been demonstrated to generate apoptotic signals in leukemic T cells[155] through the induction of mitochondrial membrane permeability, changes which lead to cytochrome c release and activation of downstream caspases.[156]

To further elucidate the significance of mitochondria in tumor-induced T-cell death, we investigated the effects of various inhibitors of the mitochondrial pathway. Specific antioxidants significantly blocked the DNA degradation induced in T cells by co-cultured tumor cells. These data and others demonstrate that in addition to the Fas-mediated death receptor pathway, a mitochondria-dependent pathway may also be involved in tumor-induced apoptosis of T lymphocytes. Work is proceeding by a number of laboratories, including ours, to further delineate which tumor derived products can induce apoptosis, and the mechanisms by which they act. Understanding how tumors can inhibit the immune response to malignant cells may provide ways in which to prevent these defects and thus promote anti-tumor immunity.

REFERENCES

1. Gross L. Intradermal immunization of G3H mice against a sarcoma that originated in an animal of the same line. Cancer Res. 3:326–333, 1943.
2. Burnet M. Immunologic surveillance. Oxford: Pergamon press, 1970.
3. Altman A, Cogeshall K, and Mustelin T. Molecular events mediating T cell activation. Adv. Immunol. 48:227–360, 1990.
4. Foss FM. Immunologic mechanisms of antitumor activity. Semin. Oncol. 29(3 Suppl 7):5–11, 2002.
5. Lucey DR, Clerici M, and Shearer GM. Type 1 and type 2 cytokine dysregulation in human infectious, neoplastic, and inflammatory diseases. Clin. Microbiol. Rev. 9:532–562, 1996.
6. Ullman KS, Northrop JP, Verweij CL, and Crabtree GR. Transmission of signals from the T lymphocyte antigen receptor to the genes responsible for cell proliferation and immune function: the missing link. Annu. Rev. Immunol. 8:421–452, 1990.
7. Singer AL, and Koretzky GA. Control of T cell function by positive and negative regulators. Science. 296:1639–1640, 2002.
8. Montie JE, Stewart BH, Straffon RA, et al. The role of adjunctive nephrectomy in patients with metastatic renal cell carcinoma. J. Urol. 117:272–275, 1977.
9. Mountain CF, Khalil KG, Hermes KE, and Frazier OH. The contribution of surgery to the management of carcinomatous pulmonary metastases. Cancer 41:833–840, 1978.
10. Yron I, Wood TA, Spiess P, and Rosenberg SA. In vitro growth of murine T cells: V. The isolation and growth of lymphoid cells infiltrating syngeneic solid tumors. J. Immunol. 125:238–245, 1980.
11. Rosenberg SA. Immunotherapy of patients with advanced cancer using interleukin-2 alone or in combination with lymphokine-activated killer cells. In Devita VT, Hellman S, and Rosenberg SA, eds. Important advances in Oncology 1988. Philadelphia, JB. Lippincott. Company. 217–257, 1988.
12. Rosenberg SA, Yang JC, Topalian SL, et al. Treatment of 283 consecutive patients with metastatic melanoma or renal cell cancer using high-dose bolus interleukin-2. JAMA. 271:907–913, 1994.
13. Fyfe G, Fisher RI, Rosenberg SA, Sznol M, Parkinson DR, and Louie AC. Results of treatment of 255 patients with metastatic renal cell carcinoma who received high-dose recombinant interleukin-2 therapy. J. Clin. Oncol. 13:688–696, 1995.
14. Bahceci E, Read EJ, Leitman S, Childs R, Dunbar C, Young NS, and Barrett J. CD34+ cell dose predicts relapse and survival after T-cell-depleted HLA-identical hematopoietic stem cell transplantation (HSCT) for hematological malignancies. Br. J. Haematol. 108:404–414, 2000.
15. Childs R, Chernoff A, Contentin N, Bahceci E, Schrump D, Leitman S, Read EJ, Tisdale J, Dunbar C, Linehan WM, Young NS, and Barrett AJ. Regression of metastatic renal-cell carcinoma after nonmyeloablative allogeneic peripheral-blood stem-cell transplantation. N. Eng. J. Med. 343:750–758, 2000.
16. Neumann E, Engelberg A, Decker J, Storkel S, Jaeger E, Huber C, and Seliger B. Heterogeneous espression of the tumor-associated antigens RAGE, PRAME, and Glycoprotein 75 in human renal cell carcinoma; candidates for T-cell—based immunotherapy. Cancer Res. 58:4090–4095, 1998.
17. Finke JH, Rayman P, Hart L, Alexander JP, Edinger MG, Tubbs RR, et al. Characterization of TIL subsets from human renal cell carcinoma: specific reactivity defined by cytotoxicity IFNγ secretion and proliferation. J. Immunother. 15:91–104, 1994.
18. Alexander P, Kudoh S, Melsop KA, Hamilton TA, Edinger MG, Tubbs RR, Sica D, Tuason L, Klein E, Bukowski RM, et al. T-cell infiltrating renal cell carcinoma display a poor proliferative response even though they can produce IL-2 and express IL2 receptors, Cancer Res. 53:1380–1387, 1993.
19. Tartour E, Latour S, Mathiot C, Thiounn N, Mosseri V, Joyeus I, et al. Variable expression of CD3-γ chain in tumor-infiltrating lymphocytes (TIL) derived from renal-cell carcinoma: relationship with TIL phenotype and function, Int. J. Cancer. 63:205–212, 1995.
20. Finke J, Ferrone S, Frey A, Mufson A, and Ochoa A. Where have all the T cells gone? Mechanisms of immune evasion by tumors. Immunol. Today. 20:158–160, 1999.
21. Finke JH, Tubbs R, Connelly B, Pontes E, and Montie J. Tumor-infiltrating lymphocytes in patients with renal-cell carcinoma. Ann. N. Y. Acad. Sci. 532:387–394, 1988.
22. Belldegrun A, Muul LM, and Rosenberg SA. Interleukin 2 expanded tumor-infiltrating lymphocytes in human renal cell cancer: isolation, characterization, and antitumor activity. Cancer Res. 48:206–214, 1988.
23. Schendel DJ, Oberneder R, Falk CS, Jantzer P, Kressenstein S, Maget B, Hofstetter A, Riethmuller G, and Nossner E. Cellular and molecular analyses of major histocompatibility complex (MHC) restricted and non-MHC-restricted effector cells recognizing renal cell carcinomas: problems and perspectives for immunotherapy. J. Mol. Med. 75:400–413, 1997.

24. Nakagomi H, Pisa P, Pisa EK, Yamamoto Y, Halapi E, Backlin K, Juhlin C, and Kiessling R. Lack of interleukin-2 (IL-2) expression and selective expression of IL-10 mRNA in human renal cell carcinoma. Int. J. Cancer. 63:366–371, 1995.
25. Wang Q, Redovan C, Tubbs R, Olencki T, Klein E, Kudoh S, Finke J, and Bukowski RM. Selective cytokine gene expression in renal cell carcinoma tumor cells and tumor-infiltrating lymphocytes. Int. J. Cancer. 61:780–785, 1995.
26. Pisa P, Halapi E, Pisa EK, Gerdin E, Hising C, Bucht A, Gerdin B, and Kiessling R. Selective expression of interleukin 10, interferon gamma, and granulocyte-macrophage colony-stimulating factor in ovarian cancer biopsies. Proc. Natl. Acad. Sci. USA 89:7708–7712, 1992.
27. Cardi G, Mastrangelo ML, and Beard D. Deletion of T cells with the CD4+ CD45R+ phenotype in lymphocytes that infiltrate subcutaneous metastases of human melanoma. Cancer Res. 49:6562–6565, 1989.
28. Miescher S, Whiteside TL, Moretta L, and von Fliendner V. Clonal and frequency analyses of tumor-infiltrating T lymphocytes from human solid tumors. J. Immunol. 138:4004–4011, 1987.
29. Rayman P, Uzzo RG, Kolenko V, Bloom T, Cathcart MK, Molto L, Novick AC, Bukowski RM, Hamilton T, and Finke JH. Tumor-induced dysfunction in interleukin-2 production and interleukin-2 receptor signaling: a mechanism of immune escape. Cancer J. Sci. Am. 6:S81–S87, 2000.
30. Kudoh S, Redovan C, Rayman P, Edinger M, Tubbs RR, Novick A, Finke JH, and Bukowski RM. Defective granzyme B gene expression and lytic response in T lymphocytes infiltrating human renal cell carcinoma. J. Immunother. 20:479–487, 1997.
31. Klugo RC. Diagnostic and therapeutic immunology of renal cell cancer. Henry Ford Med. J. 27:106–109, 1979.
32. Amano T, Koshida K, Nakajima K, Nato K, and Hisazums H. PPD, PHA and SU-PS skin test in genitourinary malignancies. Acta. Urologica. Japonica. 31:2107–2111, 1985.
33. Bernhard H, Karbach J, Wolfel T, Busch P, Storkel S, Stockle M, Wolfel C, Seliger B, Huber C, Mayer zum Buschenfelde KH, et al. Cellular immune response to human renal-cell carcinomas: definition of a common antigen recognized by HLA-A2-restricted cytotoxic T-lymphocyte (CTL) clones. Int. J. Cancer. 59:837–842, 1994.
34. Finke JH, Rayman P, Edinger M, Tubbs RR, Stganley J, Klein E, and Bukowski R. Characterization of a human renal cell carcinoma specific cytotoxic CD8+ T cell lline. J. Immunother. 11:1–11, 1992.
35. van Endert PM. Genes regulating MHC class I processing of antigen. Curr. Opin. Immunol. 11:82–88, 1999.
36. Seliger B, Maeurer MJ, and Ferrone S. Antigen-processing machinery breakdown and tumor growth. Immunol. Today. 21:455–464, 2000.
37. Seliger B, Hammers S, Hohne A, Zeidler R, Knuth A, Gerharz CD, and Huber C. IFN-gamma-mediated coordinated transcriptional regulation of the human TAP-1 and LMP-2 genes in human renal cell carcinoma. Clin. Cancer. Res. 3:573–578, 1997.
38. Seliger B, Hohne A, Jung D, Kallfelz M, Knuth A, Jaeger E, et al. Expression and function of the peptide transporters in escape variants of human renal cell carcionomas. Exper. Hematol. 25:608–614, 1997.
39. Seliger B, Hohne A, Knuth A, Bernhard H, Meyer T, Tampe R, Momburg F, and Huber C. Analysis of the major histocompatibility class I antigen presentation machinery in normal and malignant renal cells: evidence for deficiencies associated with transformation and progression. Cancer Res. 56:1756–1760, 1996.
40. Kallfelz M, Jung D, Hilmes C, Knuth A, Jaeger E, Huber C, and Seliger B. Induction of immuno-genicity of a human renal-cell carcinoma cell line by TAP1-gene transfer. Int. J. Cancer. 81:125–133, 1999.
41. Steinman RM. The dendritic cell system and its role in immunogenicity. Ann. Rev. Immunol. 9:271–296, 1991.
42. Hart DN. Dendritic cells: unique leukocyte populations which control the primary immune response. Blood. 90:3245–3287, 1997.
43. Scheicher C, Mehlig M, Dienes H, and Reske K. Uptake of microparticle-adsorbed protein antigen by bone marrow-derived dendritic cells results in upregulation of interleukin-1α and interleukin-12 p40/p35 and triggers prolonged, efficient antigen presentation. Eur. J. Immunol. 25:1566–1572, 1995.
44. Larsen CP, Ritchie SC, Hendrix R, Linsley PS, Hathcock KS, Hodes RJ, Lowry RP, and Pearson TC. Regulation of immunostimulatory function and costimulatory molecule (B7.1 and B7.2) expression on murine dendritic cells. J. Immunol. 152:5208–5219, 1994.

45. Zhou L, and Tedder TF. Human blood dendritic cells selectively express CD83, a member of the immunoglobulin superfamily. J. Immunol. 154:3821–3835, 1995.

46. Austyn JM. The dendritic cell system and anti-tumor immunity. In. Vivo. 7:193–201, 1993.

47. Buelens C, Willems F, Delvaux A, Pierard G, Delville JP, Velu T, and Goldman M, Interleukin-10 differentially regulates B7-1 (CD80) and B7-2 (CD86) expression on human peripheral blood dendritic cells. Eur. J. Immunol. 25:2668, 1995.

48. Nomori H. Histiocytes in nasopharyngeal carcinoma in relation to prognosis. Cancer. 57:100, 1986.

49. Nakano T, Oka K, Arai T, Morita S, and Tsuremoto, H. Prognostic significance of Langerhans cell infiltration in radiation therapy for squamous cell carcinoma of the uterine cervix. Arch. Pathol. Lab. Med. 113:507, 1989.

50. Chaux P, Moutet M, Faivre J, Martin F, and Martin, M. Inflammatory cells infiltrating human colorectal carcinomas express HLA class II but not B7-1 and B7-2 costimulatory molecules of the T-cell activation. Lab. Invest. 74:975, 1996.

51. Thurnher M, Radmayr C, Ramoner R, Ebner S, Bock G, Klocker H, Romani N, and Bartsch G. Human renal cell carcinoma tissue contains dendritic cells. Int. J. Cancer. 67:1, 1996.

52. Troy AJ, Summers KL, Davidson PJ, Atkinson CH, and Hart DN. Minimal recruitment and activation of dendritic cells within renal cell carcinoma. Clin. Cancer. Res. 4:585–593, 1998.

53. Menetrier-Caux C, Montmain G, Dieu MC, Bain C, Favrot MC, Caux C, Blay JY. Inhibition of the differentiation of dendritic cells from CD34(+) progenitors by tumor cells: role of interleukin-6 and macrophage colony-stimulating factor. Blood. 92:4778–4791, 1998.

54. Schwartz RH. T cell clonal anergy. Curr. Opin. Immunol. 9:351–357, 1997.

55. Mondino A, Khoruts A, and Jenkins MC. The anatomy of T-cell activation and tolerence. Proc. Natl. Acad. Sci. USA. 93:2245–2252, 1996.

56. Appleman LJ, Tzachani D, Grader-Beck T, van Puijenbroek AAFL, and Boussiotis VA. Helper T cell anergy: from biochemistry to cancer pathophysiology and therapeutics. J. Mol. Med. 78:673–683, 2001.

57. Staveley-O'Carroll K, Sotomayor E, Montgomery J, Borello I, Hwang L, Fein S, Pardoll D, and Levitsky H. Induction of antigen-specific T cell anergy: An early event in the course of tumor progression. Proc. Natl. Acad. Sci. USA. 95:1178–1183, 1998.

58. Kammula US, Lee KH, Riker AI, Wang E, Ohnmacht GA, Rosenberg SA, and Marincola FM. Functional analysis of antigen-specific T lymphocytes by serial measurement of gene expression in peripheral blood mononuclear cells and tumor specimens. J. Immunol. 163:6867–6875, 1999.

59. Nielsen M-B, and Marincola FM. Melanoma vaccines: the paradox of T cell activation without clinical response. Cancer Chemother Pharmacol. 46:S62–S66, 2000.

60. Boussiotis VA, McArthur JG, Gribben JG, and Nadler LM. The role of B7-1/B7-2:CD28/CTLA-4 pathways in the prevention of anergy, induction of production immunity and down-regulation of the immune response. Immunol. Rev. 153:5–26, 1996.

61. Sotomayor EM, Borello I, Tubb E, Rattis F-M, Bien, Lu Z, Fein S, Schoenberger S, and Levitsky HI. Conversion of tumor-specific CD4[+] T-cell tolerance to T-cell priming through in vivo ligation of CD40. Nature Medicine. 5:780–787, 1999.

62. Ohlen C, Kalos M, Hong DJ, Shur, AC, and Greenberg PD. Expression of a tolerizing tumor antigen in peripheral tissue does not preclude recovery of high-affinity CD8[+] T Cells or CTL immunotherapy of tumors expressing the antigen. J. Immunol. 166:2863–2870, 2001.

63. Welsh RM. Assessing CD8 T Cell number and dysfunction in the presence of antigen. J. Exp. Med. 193:19–22, 2001.

64. Wittke F, Hoffmann R, Buer J, Dallmann I, Oevermann K, Sel S, Wandert T, Ganser A, and Atzpodien J. Interleukin 10 (IL-10): an immunosuppressive factor and independent predictor in patients with metastatic renal cell carcinoma. Br. J. Cancer. 79:1182–1184, 1999.

65. Akdis CA, and Blaser K. Mechanisms of interleukin-10-mediated immune suppression. Immunology. 103:131–136, 2001.

66. Olive C, Cheung C, Nicol D, and Falk MC. Expression of cytokine mRNA transcripts in renal cell carcinoma. Immunol. Cell. Biol. 76:357–362, 1998.

67. Onishi T, Onishi Y, Goto H, Tomita M, and Abe K. An assessment of the immunological status of patients with renal cell carcinoma based on the relative abundance of T-helper 1- and -2 cytokine-producing CD4+ cells in peripheral blood. BJU. Int. 87:755–759, 2001.

68. Ochoa AC, and Longo DL. Alteration of signal transduction in T cells from cancer patients. In Important Adv. Oncol., Devita VD, Hellman S, and Rosenberg SA, eds., JB. Lipponcott, Philadelphia. 43–54, 1995.

69. Chan AC, Irving BA, and Weiss A. New insights into T-cell antigen receptor structure and signal transduction. Curr. Opin. Immunol. 4:246–252, 1992.
70. Bukowski RM, Rayman P, Uzzo R, Bloom T, Sandstrom K, Peereboom D, Olencki T, Budd GT, Mclain D, Elson P, Novick A, and Finke JH. Signal transduction abnormalities in T lymphocytes from patients with advanced renal carcinoma: Clinical relevance and effects of cytokine therapy. Clin. Canc. Res. 4:2337–2347, 1998
71. Cardi G, Heaney JA, Schned AR, Phillips DM, Branda MT, and Ernstoff MS. T-cell receptor zeta-chain expression on tumor-infiltrating lymphocytes from renal cell carcinoma. Cancer Res. 57:3517–3519, 1997.
72. Kono K, Ressing ME, Brandt RMP, Melief CJM, Potkul RK, Andersson B, Petersson M, Kast WM, and Kiessling R. Decreased expression of signal-transducing zeta chain in peripheral T cells and natural killer cells in patients with cervical cancer. Clin. Cancer Res. 2:1825–1828, 1996.
73. Frydecka I, Kaczmarek P, Bocko D, Kosmaczewska A, Morilla R, and Catovsky D. Expression of signal-transducing zeta chain in peripheral blood T cels and natural killer cells in patients with Hodgkin's disease in different phases of the disease. Leuk. Lymphoma. 35:545–554, 1999.
74. Reichert TE, Day R, Wagner EM, and Whiteside TL. Absent or low expression of the s chain in T cells at the tumor site correlates with poor surival in patients with oral carcinoma. Cancer Res. 58:5344–5347, 1998.
75. Keilholz U, Weber J, Finke JH, Gabrilovich DI, Kast WM, Disis ML, Kirkwood JM, Scheilbenbogen C, Schlom J, Maino VC, Lyerly HK, Lee PP, Storkus W, Marincola F, Worobec A, and Atkins MB. Immunologic monitoring of cancer vaccine therapy: results of a workshop sponsored by the society for biological therapy. J. Immunother. 25:97–138, 2002.
76. Kono K, Salazar-Onfray F, Petersson M, Hansson J, Masucci G, Wasserman K, Nakazawa T, Anderson P, and Kiessling R. Hydrogen peroxide secreted by tumor-specific T-cell and natural killer cell-mediated cytotoxicity. Eur. J. Immunol. 26:1308–1313, 1996.
77. Schmielau J, and Finn OJ. Activated granulocytes and gralulocyte-derived hydrogen peroxide are the underlying mechanism of suppression of T-Cell Function in Advanced Cancer Patients. Cancer Res. 61:4756–4760, 2001.
78. Gastman BR, Johnson DE, Whiteside TL, and Rabinowich H. Caspase-mediated degradation of T-cell receptor zeta-chain. Cancer Res. 59:1422–1427, 1999.
79. Gastman BR, Johnson DE, Whiteside TL, Rabinowich H. Tumor-induced apoptosis of T lymphocytes: elucidation of intracellular apoptotic events. Blood. 95:2015–2023, 2000.
80. Saito T, Dworacki G, Gooding W, Lotze MT, and Whiteside TL. Spontaneous apoptosis of CD8+ T lymphocytes in peripheral blood of patients with advanced melanoma. Clin. Cancer Res. 6: 1351–1364, 2000.
81. Takahashi A, Kono K, Amemiya H, Iizuka H, Fujii H, and Matsumoto Y. Elevated caspase-3 activity in peripheral blood T cells coexists with increased degree of T-cell apoptosis and downregulation of TCR zeta molecules in patients with gastric cancer. Clin. Cancer Res. 7:74–80, 2001.
82. Isomaki P, Panesar M, Annenkov A, Clark JM, Foxwell BMJ, Chernajjovsky Y, and Cope AP. Prolonged exposure of T cells to TNF down-regulates TCRz and expression of the TCR/CD3 complex at the cell surface. J. Immunol. 166:5495–5507, 2001.
83. Taheri F, Ochoa JB, Faghiri Z, Culotta K, Park H-J, Lan MS, Zea AH, and Ochoa AC. L-arginine regulates the expression of the T-cell receptor z chain (CD3z) in Jurkat Cells. Clin. Cancer Res. 7:765s–958s, 2001.
84. Morford LA, Elliott LH, Carlson SL, Brooks WH, and Roszman TL. T cell receptor-mediated signaling is defective in T cells obtained from patients with primary intracranial tumors. J. Immunol. 159:4415–4425, 1997.
85. Rayet B, and Gelinas C. Aberrant rel/nfkb genes and activity in human cancer. Oncogene. 18:6938–6947, 1999.
86. Ng CS, Novick AC, Tannenbaum CS, Bukowski RM, and Finke JH. Mechanisms of immune evasion by renal cell carcinoma: tumor-induced T-lymphocyte apoptosis and NFkappaB suppression. Urology. 59:9–14, 2002.
87. Gati A, Guerra N, Giron-Michel J, Azzarone B, Angevin E, Moretta A, Chouaib S, and Caignard A. Tumor cells regulate the lytic activity of tumor-specific cytotoxic T lymphocytes by modulating the inhibitory natural killer receptor function. Cancer Res. 61:3240–3244, 2001.
88. Ghosh P, Komschilies KL, Cippitelli M, Longo DL, Subleski J, Ye J, Sica A, Young HA, Wiltrout RH, and Ochoa AC. Gradual loss of T-Helper 1 populations in spleen of mice during progressive tumor growth. J. Nat. Cancer Inst. 87:1478–1483, 1995.

89. Uzzo RG, Rayman P, Klenko V, Clark PE, Cathcart MK, Bloom T, Novick AC, Bukowski RM, Hamilton T, and Finke JH. Renal cell carcinoma-derived gangliosides suppress nuclear factor-κB activation in T cells. J. Clin. Invest. 104:769–776, 1999.
90. Uzzo RG, Clark PE, Rayman P, Bloom T, Rybicki L, Novick AC, Bukowski RM, and Finke JH, Alterations in NFκB activation in T Lymphocytes of Patients with renal cell carcinoma. J. Nat. Cancer Ins. 91:718–721, 1999(b).
91. Hatada EN, Krappmann D, and Scheidereit C. NF-kappaB and the innate immune response. Curr. Opin. Immunol. 12:52–58, 2000.
92. Aronica MA, Mora A, Mitchell DB, Finn PW, Johnson JE, Sheller JR, and Boothby MR. Preferential role for NF-κB/Rel signaling in the type 1 but not type 2 T cell-dependent immune response in vivo. J. Immunol. 163:5116–5124, 1999.
93. Malmberg K-J, Arulampalam V, Ichihara F, Petersson M, Seki K, Andersson, T, Lenkei R, Masucci G, Pettersson S, and Kiessling R. Inhibition of activated/memory (CD45RO+) T cells by oxidative stress associated with block of NFκB activation. J. Immunol. 167:2592–2601, 2001.
94. Guerder S, Rincon M, and Schmitt-Verhults A-M. Regulation of activator protein-1 and NF-κB in CD8+ T cells exposed to peripheral self-antigens. J. Immunol. 166:4399–4407, 2001.
95. Finke JH, Rayman P, George R, Tannenbaum CS, Kolenko V, Uzzo R, Novick AC, and Bukowski RM. Tumor-induced sensitivity to apoptosis in T cells from patients with renal cell carcinoma: role of nuclear factor-kappaB suppression. Clin. Cancer Res. 7(3 Suppl):940s–946s, 2001.
96. Bloom BR, Salgame P, and Diamond B. Revisiting and revising suppressor T cells. Immunol. Today. 13:131–136, 1992.
97. Clerici M, and Shearer GM. The TH1/TH2 hypothesis of HIV infection: new insights. Immunol. Today. 15:575–581, 1994.
98. Yoneda Y, and Yoshida R. The role of T cells in allografted tumor rejection: IFN-gamma released from T cells is essential for induction of effector macrophages in the rejection site. J. Immunol. 160:6012–6017, 1998.
99. Kemp RA, and Ronchese F. Tumor-specific Tc1, but not Tc2, cells deliver protective antitumor immunity. J. Immunol. 167:6497–6502, 2001.
100. Hu MM, Urba WJ, and Fox BA. Gene-modified tumor vaccine with therapeutic potential shifts tumor-specific T cell response from a type 2 to a type 1 cytokine profile. J. Immunol. 15:3033–3341, 1998.
101. Goto S, Sato M, Kaneko R, Itoh M, Sato S, and Takeuchi S. Analysis of Th1 and Th2 cytokine production by peripheral blood mononuclear cells as a parameter of immunological dysfunction in advanced cancer patients. Cancer Immunol. Immunother. 48:435–442, 1999.
102. Bellone G, Turletti A, Artusio E, Mareschi K, Carbone A, Tibaudi D, Robecchi A, Emanuelli G, and Rodeck U. Tumor-associated transforming growth factor-beta and interleukin-10 contribute to a systemic Th2 immune phenotype in pancreatic carcinoma patients. Am. J. Pathol. 155:537–547, 1999.
103. Maeda H, and Shiraishi A. TGF-beta contributes to the shift toward TH2-type responses through direct and IL-10-mediated pathways in tumor-bearing mice. J. Immunol. 156:73–78, 1996.
104. Ortegel JW, Staren ED, Faber LP, Warren WH, and Braun DP. Modulation of tumor-infiltrating lymphocyte cytolytic activity against human non-small cell lung cancer. Lung. Cancer. 36:17–25, 2002.
105. Cottrez F, and Groux H. Regulation of TGF-beta response during T cell activation is modulated by IL-10. J. Immunol. 167:773–778, 2001.
106. Adris S, Klein S, Jasnis M, Chuluyan E, Ledda M, Bravo A, Carbone C, Chernajovsky Y, and Podhajcer O. IL-10 expression by CT26 colon carcinoma cells inhibits their malignant phenotype and induces a T cell-mediated tumor rejection in the context of a systemic Th2 response. Gene Ther. 6:1705–1712, 1999.
107. Huang S, Ullrich SE, and Bar-Eli M. Regulation of tumor growth and metastasis by interleukin-10: the melanoma experience. J. Interferon. Cytokine. Res. 19:697–703, 1999.
108. Groux H, Cottrez F, Rouleau M, Mauze S, Antonenko S, Hurst S, McNeil T, Bigler M, Roncarolo MG, and Coffman RL. A transgenic model to analyze the immunoregulatory role of IL-10 secreted by antigen-presenting cells. J. Immunol. 162:1723–1729, 1999.
109. Ribas A, Butterfield LH, Hu B, Dissette VB, Meng WS, Koh A, Andres KJ, Lee M, Amar SN, Glaspy JA, McBride WH, and Economou JS. Immune deviation and Fas-mediated deletion limit antitumor activity after multiple dendritic cell vaccinations in mice. Cancer Res. 60:2218–2224, 2000.
110. Muschen M, Moers C, Warskulat U, Even J, Niederacher D, and Beckmann MW. CD95 Ligand expression as a mechanism of immune escape in breast cancer. Immunology. 99:69–77, 2000.

111. Black PH. Shedding from the cell surface of normal and cancer cells. Adv. Cancer Res. 32:75–199, 1980.
112. Hakomori S. Tumor-associated carbohydrate antigens. Annu. Rev. Immunol. 2:103–126, 1984.
113. Hoon DS, Okun E, Neuwirth H, Morton DL, and Irie RF. Aberrant expression of gangliosides in human renal cell carcinomas. J. Urol. 150:2013–2018, 1993.
114. Ladisch S, Gillard B, and Wong C. Shedding and immunoregulatory activity of YAC-1 lymphoma cell gangliosides. Cancer Res. 43:3808, 1983.
115. Skipski VP, Katopodis N, Prendergast JS, and Stock CC. Gangliosides in blood serum of normal rats and Morris hepatoma 5123tc-bearing rats. Biochem. Biophys. Res. Commun. 67:1122–1127, 1975.
116. Kloppel TM, Keenan TW, Freeman MJ, and Morre DJ. Glycolipid-bound sialic acid in serum: increased levels in mice and humans bearing mammary carcinomas. Proc. Natl. Acad. Sci. USA 74:3011, 1977.
117. Li R, and Ladisch S. Shedding of human neuroblastoma gangliosides. Biochim. Biophys. Acta. 1083:57–64, 1991.
118. Heitger A, and Ladisch S. Gangliosides block antigen presentation by human monocytes. Biochim. Biophy. Acta. 1303:161–168, 1996.
119. Miller HC, and Esselman WJ. Modulation of the immune response by antigen reactive lymphocytes after cultivation with gangliosides. J. Immunol. 115:839–843, 1975.
120. Lu P, and Sharom FJ. Immunosuppression by YAC-1 lymphoma: role of shed gangliosides. Cell Immunol. 173:22–32, 1996.
121. Sharom FJ, Chiu AL, and Chu JW. Membrane gangliosides modulate interleukin-2-stimulated T-lymphocyte proliferation. Biochim. Biophys. Acta. 1094:35–42, 1991.
122. Garofalo T, Sorice M, Misasi R, Cinque B, Giammatteo M, Pontieri GM, Cifone MG, and Pavan A. A novel mechanism of CD4 down-modulation induced by monosialoganglioside GM3: involvement of serine phosphorylation and protein kinase Cd translocation. J. Biol. Chem. 273: 35153–35160, 1998.
123. Grayson G, and Ladisch S. Immunosuppression by human gangliosides. II. Carbohydrate structure and inhibition of human NK activity. Cell Immunol. 139:18–29, 1992.
124. Irani DN. Brain-derived gangliosides induce cell cycle arrest in a murine T cell line. J. Neuroimmunol. 87:11–16, 1998.
125. Kanda N. Gangliosides GD1a and GM3 induce interleukin-10 production by human T cells. Biochem. Biophys. Res. Commun. 256:41–44, 1999.
126. Estaquier J, and Ameisen JC. A role for T-helper type-1 and type-2 cytokines in the regulation of human monocyte apoptosis. Blood. 90:1618–1625, 1997.
127. Dhein J, Walczak H, Baumler C, Debatin KM, and Krammer PH. Autocrine T-cell suicide mediated by APO-1/(Fas/CD95). Nature. 373:438–441, 1995.
128. Radoja S, Saio M, and Frey AB. CD8+ tumor-infiltrating lymphocytes are primed for Fas-mediated activation-induced cell death but are not apoptotic in situ. J. Immunol. 166:6074–6083, 2001.
129. Uzzo RG, Rayman P, Kolenko V, Ckarj OE, Bloom T, Ward AM, Molto L, Tannenbaum C, Worford LJ, Bukowski R, Tubbs R, Hsi ED, Bander NH, Novick AC, and Finke JH. Mechanisms of Apoptosis in T cells from patients with renal cell carcinoma. Clin. Cancer Res. 5:1219–1229, 1999.
130. Nunez G, Benedict MA, Hu Y, and Inohara N. Caspases: the proteases of the apoptotic pathway. Oncogene. 17:3237–3245, 1998.
131. Boldin MP, Goncharov TM, Goltsev YV, and Wallach D. Involvement of MACH, a novel MORT1/FADD-interacting protease, in Fas/APO-1-and TNF receptor-induced cell death. Cell, 85:803–815, 1996.
132. Nagata S. Apoptosis by death factor. Cell. 88:355–365, 1997.
133. Ashkenazi A, and Dixit VM. Death receptors: Signaling and modulation. Science. 281:1305–1308, 1998.
134. Hirata H, Takahashi A, Kobayashi S, Yonebara S, Sawai H, Okazaki T, Yamamoto K, and Sasada M. Caspases are activated in a branched protease cascade and control distinct downstream processes in Fas-induced apoptosis. J. Exp. Med. 187:587–600, 1998.
135. Li P, Nijhawan D, Budihardjo I, Srinivasula SM, Ahmad M, Alnemri ES, and Wang X. Cytochrome c and dATP-dependent formation of Apaf-1/caspase-9 complex initiates an apoptotic protease cascade. Cell. 91:479–489, 1997.
136. Zou H, Henzel WJ, Liu X, Lutschg A, and Wang X. Apaf-1, a human protein homologous to C. elegans CED-4, participates in cytochrome c-dependent activation of caspase-3. Cell. 90:405–413, 1997.

137. Yang J, Liu XS, Bhalla K, Kim CN, Ibrado AM, Cai JY, Peng TI, Jones DP, and Wang XD. Prevention of apoptosis by Bcl2: release of cytochrome *c* from mitochondria blocked. Science. 275:1129–1132, 1997.
138. Kluck RM, Bossywetzel E, Green DR, and Newmeyer DD. The release of cytochrome *c* from mitochondria—a primary site for Bcl-2 regulation of apoptosis. Science. 275:1132–1136, 1997.
139. Jurgensmeier JM, Xie Z, Deveraux Q, Ellerby L, Bredesen D, and Reed JC. Bax directly induces release of cytochrome c from isolated mitochondria. Proc. Natl. Acad. Sci. USA. 95:4997–5002, 1998.
140. Srinivasula SM, Ahmad M, Fernandes-Alnemri T, and Alnemri ES. Autoactivation of procaspase-9 by Apaf-1-mediated oligomerization. Mol. Cell. 1:949–957, 1998.
141. Reed JC. Cytochrome c—can't live with it—can't live without it. Cell. 91:559–562, 1997.
142. Leithauser F, Dhein J, Mechtersheimer G, Koretz K, Bruderlein S, Henne C, Schmidt A, Debatin KM, Krammer PH, and Moller P. Constitutive and induced expression of APO-1, a new member of the nerve growth factor/tumor necrosis factor receptor superfamily, in normal and neoplastic cells. Lab. Invest. 69:415–429, 1993.
143. Rouvier E, Luciani MF, and Goldstein P. Fas involvement in Ca2+-independent T cell-mediated cytotoxicity. J. Exp. Med. 177:195–200, 1993.
144. Arase H, Arase N, and Saito T. Fas-mediated cytotoxicity by freshly isolated natural killer cells. J. Exp. Med. 181:1235–1238, 1995.
145. Russel JH. Activation-induced death o f mature T cell sin the regulation of immune responses. Curr. Opin. Immunol. 7:382–388, 1995.
146. Griffith TS, Brunner T, Fletcher SM, Green DR, and Gerguson TA. Fas ligand-induced apoptosis as a mechanism of immune privilege. Science. 270:1189–1191, 1995.
147. Schattner E, and Friedman SM. Fas expression and apoptosis in human B cells. Immunol. Res. 15:246–257, 1996.
148. van Parijs L, and Abbas A. Role of Fas-mediated cell death in the regulation of immune responses. Curr. Opin. Immunol. 8:355–361, 1996.
149. Whiteside TL, and Rabinowich H. The role of Fas/FasL in immunosuppression induced by human tumors. Cancer Immunol. Immunother. 46(4):175–184, 1998.
150. Cardi G, Heaney JHA, Schned AR, and Ernstoff MS. Expression of Fas (APO-1/CD95) in tumor-infiltrating and peripheral blood lymphocytes in patients with renal cell carcinoma. Cancer Res. 58:2078–2080, 1998.
151. Zaks TZ, Chappell DB, Rosenberg SA, and Restifo NP. Fas-mediated suicide of tumor-reactive T cells following activation by specific tumor: selective rescue by caspase inhibition. J. Immunol. 162:3272–3279, 1999.
152. Chappell DB, Zaks TZ, Rosenberg SA, and Restifo NP. Human melanoma cells do not express Fas (Apo-1/CD95) ligand. Cancer Res. 59:59–62, 1999.
153. Wischhusen J, Jung G, Radovanovic I, Beier C, Steinbach JP, Rimner A, Huang H, Schulz JB, Ohgaki H, Aguzzi A, Rammensee HG, and Weller M. Identification of CD70-mediated apoptosis of immune effector cells as a novel immune escape pathway of human glioblastoma. Cancer Res. 62:2592–2599, 2002.
154. Koyama S, Koike N, and Adachi S. Expression of TNF-related apoptosis-inducing ligand (TRAIL) and its receptors in gastric carcinoma and tumor-infiltrating lymphocytes: a possible mechanism of immune evasion of the tumor. J. Cancer Res. Clin. Oncol. 128:73–79, 2002.
155. De Maria R, Lenti L, Malisan F, d'Agostino F, Tomassini B, Zeuner A, Rippo MR, and Testi R. Requirement for GD3 ganglioside in CD95- and ceramide-induced apoptosis. Science. 277: 1652–1655, 1997.
156. Kristal BS, and Brown AM. Apoptogenic ganglioside GD3 directly induces the mitochondrial permeability transition. J. Biol. Chem. 274:3169–3175, 1999.
157. Mocellin S, Ohnmacht GA, Wang E, and Marincola FM. Kinetics of cytokine expression in melanoma metastases classifies immune responsiveness. Int. J. Cancer. 93:236–242, 2001.
158. Ronsin C, Chung-Scott V, Poullion I, Aknouche N, Gaudin C, and Triebel F. A non-AUG-defined alternate open reading frame of the intestinal carboxyl esterase mRNA generates an epitope recognized by renal cell carcinoma-reactive tumor-infiltrating lymphocytes in situ. J. Immunol. 163: 483–490, 1999.
159. Brossart P, Stuhler G, Flad T, Stevanovic S, Rammensee HG, Kanz L, and Brugger W. Her-2/neu-derived peptides are tumor associated antigens expressed by human renal cell and colon carcinoma lines and are recognized by in vitro induced specific cytotoxic T lymphocytes. Cancer Res. 58:732–736, 1998.

160. Zhang XH, Takenaka I, Sato C, and Sakamoto H. p53 and HER-2 alterations in renal cell carcinoma. Urology. 50:636–642, 1997.
161. Traversari C, van der Bruggen P, Luescher IF, Lurquin C, Chomez P, Van Pel A, De Plaen E, Amar-Costesec A, and Boon T. A nonapeptide encoded by human gene MAGE-1 is recognized on HLA-A1 by cytolytic T lymphocytes directed against tumor antigen MZ2-E. J. Exp. Med. 176:1453–1457, 1992.

3. NEW ALGORITHMS FOR THE STAGING OF KIDNEY CANCER

LEIBOVICI D., SELLA A.[1], SIEGEL I.Y., AND ZISMAN A.

From the Department of Urology and the Department of Oncology[1], Assaf-Harofeh Medical Center, affiliated to Sackler Faculty of Medicine, Tel Aviv University. Zerifin, 70300, Israel

INTRODUCTION

Malignant renal tumors account for 2.5% of the total cancer incidence and 2% of the total cancer mortality in the US.[1] Of them, renal cell carcinoma (RCC) is the most common. The estimated 5-year survival for patients with tumors confined to the kidney is 90–95%. Conversely, advanced RCC is associated with poor prognosis.[2–4] Radiotherapy and chemotherapy are not effective and immunotherapy is currently the adjuvant therapy available. Since the natural history of RCC is unpredictable, it is important to define staging systems that may guide the therapeutic approach towards the disease and predict outcomes. Staging systems, at general should efficiently communicate key tumor characteristics, aid clinicians in the appropriate selection of therapeutic options for an individual patient, stratify patients' risk of cancer progression or cancer death, and determine selection criteria for clinical trials. When a consensus regarding an accurate, universal staging system is possible, it allows outcome comparison between different demographic groups and therefore facilitates evaluation of treatment options and clinical research.

CONVENTIONAL SYSTEMS

The first documented staging system for RCC was composed by Flocks and Kadensky[5] based on physical characteristics of renal tumors and tumor spread. Flocks

Address for Correspondence: Amnon Zisman MD, The Urology Department, Assaf Harofeh Medical Center, Zerifin 70300, Israel. E-mail: zismana@asaf.health.gov.il

R.A. Figlin (ed.). KIDNEY CANCER. Copyright © 2003. Kluwer Academic Publishers. Boston. All rights reserved.

Table 1. Robson's staging system for RCC.[6]

Stage I	Tumor confined to kidney
Stage II	Tumor invades perinephric fat but confined to Gerota's fascia or adrenal
Stage IIIa	Tumor invades renal vein or inferior vena cava
Stage IIIb	Tumor involves regional lymph nodes
Stage IIIc	Tumor involves both local vessels and lymph nodes
Stage IVa	Tumor involves local organs (i.e. colon, pancreas)
Stage IVb	Distant metastases

Table 2. 1987 TNM staging system.[9]

Primary tumor (T)	
T0	No evidence of primary tumor
T1	Tumor = 2.5 cm and confined to the kidney
T2	Tumor >2.5 cm and confined to the kidney
T3	Tumor extends to perinephric fat, major vessels or adrenal but confined to Gerota's fascia
T3a	Tumor invading perinephric fat or adrenal gland
T3b	Tumor grossly invading inferior vena cava
T4	Tumor invades beyond Gerota's fascia
Lymph nodes (N)	
N0	No involvement of regional lymph nodes
N1	Metastasis into a single lymph node <2 cm
N2	Metastasis into a single lymph node 2–5 cm; or multiple nodes <5 cm
N3	Metastasis into lymph nodes >5 cm
Metastasis (M):	
M0	No distant metastases
M1	Distant metastases

and Kadenskys' system was modified by Robson et al who added a consideration for tumor vascular invasion (Table 1).[6] At first, the Robson staging system gained popularity but poor correlation with prognosis[7] led to a gradual shift towards the utilization of TNM system. For example, patients with Robson stage IIIa (extension into the renal vein) and with organ confined RCC had similar survival to those with disease confined to the renal capsule (stage I) or Gerota's fascia (stage II).

The Tumor Nodes and Metastasis system (TNM) composed by the International Union Against Cancer is notable for putting the accent on local growth, nodal spread, and distant metastasis and, therefore, meticulously classifies the extent of tumor involvement.[8] Initially it was considered to be too complex with too many staging categories. However, since it's introduction, the TNM system is continuously being refined and updated to be a useful tool, correlating with survival and disease free periods. The 1987 TNM system[9] (Table 2) was lastly updated in 1997.[10] Its main modifications were the inclusion of all tumors smaller than 7 cm in diameter into T1 category[10] as well as minor changes in the definitions of nodal spread and tumor thrombus involvement. This change in the cut-off point between 1987 and 1997 systems stemmed from the observation that there was no significant survival differ-

Table 3. UISS risk group assignment table. The UISS risk group (Left column) is determined using the correct combination of the 1997 TNM stage, Furman's grade and ECOG performance status in an individual patient. The corresponding 2 and 5-year survival estimates are shown in the right two columns. (Adapted with permission from Zisman, A, Pantuck, AJ, Dorey F et al. (2001). "Improved prognostication of RCC using an Integrated Staging System (UISS)." *JCO* 19(6): 1649–1657.[4])

UISS	1997 TNM stage	Furman's grade	ECOG performance status	2 year survival % (SE)	5 year survival % (SE)
I	I	1, 2	0	96 (2.5)	94 (2.5)
II	I	1, 2	1 or more	89 (3.8)	67 (6.4)
	I	3, 4	Any		
	II	Any	Any		
	III	Any	0		
	III	1	1 or more		
III	III	2–4	1 or more	66 (6.5)	39 (2.8)
	IV	1, 2	0		
IV	IV	3, 4	0	42 (3.5)	23 (3.1)
		1–3	1 or more		
V	IV	4	1 or more	9 (6.2)	0 (4.0)

UISS: UCLA integrated staging system, SE: standard error.

ence between TNM stage I and II when the 2.5 cm. cutoff point was applied[11,12] and that the prognosis of tumors confined to the renal parenchyma remain favorable up to size of 7 cm.

Since its introduction, the 1997 TNM system was subjected to validation efforts worldwide looking on its ability to predict patient outcome. At UCLA the 1997 TNM staging system was shown to be an independent predictor for survival as was shown for previous staging systems.[13–15] However, the discriminatory power of the 1997 TNM staging system was found to be lacking. In an analysis based on survival outcomes published in 2001, Zisman et al. reported that the 1997 TNM cut-off point (7.0 cm.) between T1 and T2 tumors is too high.[16] The various effects of 1997 TNM staging system were internally dissected. As a result lowering the tumor size cutoff between T1 and T2 disease to 4.5 cm. was suggested. Further analysis revealed that a sub-division of 1997 TNM T1 into T1a and T1b is not warranted in terms of survival and discriminatory power since the outcome of the proposed T1b (4–7 cm.) is not different from T2. This sub-division should perhaps be reserved in the future for other uses (i.e. to note incidental versus non-incidental T1 tumors in a similar fashion to stage T1c in carcinoma of prostate). In fact at the time of its composition based on data available in 1997,[17,18] workgroup number 3 on the TNM staging of renal cell carcinoma[10] forecasted such a trend and commented that, in future editions of the TNM classification, a sub- division of the1997 stage T1 into stage T1a and T1b using a 4 cm. cut-off value may be possible and advantageous for both prognostication and patient selection for nephron sparing surgery. This

Table 4. Significant explanatory variables in the multivariate analysis for metastatic (M1) and non-metastatic (M0) patients for entry into the Nadas equation, using the UCLA database (SE—standard error, ECOG PS—Eastern Cooperative Oncology Group Performance status). (Adapted with permission from Zisman, A, Pantuck, AJ, Dorey, F et al. (2002). "Mathematical model to predict individual survival for patients with renal cell carcinoma." *JCO* **20**(5): 1368–1374.[34])

	Variable	p	Hazard coefficient corrected by the bootstrap procedure	SE	95% confidence interval
N0M0 disease n = 241	ECOG PS (0 = 0; 1 or 2 or 3 = 1)	0.0001	1.088	0.286	0.567–1.689
	Fuhrman's grade (1, 2, 3, 4)	0.0001	0.568	0.161	0.251–0.883
N+/M1 disease n = 217	Number of symptoms (0, 1, 2, 3, 4 . . . n)	0.001	0.276	0.08	0.127–0.444
	Fuhrman's grade (1 − 3 = 0, 4 = 1)	0.039	0.494	0.227	0.065–0.956
	Immunotherapy given (0 = no, 1 = yes)	0.003	−0.591	0.189	−0.971−−0.233
	N + disease (0 = no, 1 = yes)	0.007	0.428	0.185	0.061–0.785
	T stage (1 − 2 = 0, 3 − 4 = 1)	0.015	0.479	0.206	0.097–0.904

recommendation is well supported by work done at the Cleveland clinic by Hafez et al[19] in which the survival after nephron sparing surgery was shown to be better in tumors that were 4 cm. and less in diameter. Others confirmed these findings by suggesting similar discriminatory cutoff value between 5–5.5 centimeters for the 1997 TNM T1/T2 category.[20,21]

FROM PROGNOSTIC FACTORS TO INTEGRATED STAGING SYSTEMS

Prognostic factors are classified according to the College of American Pathologists into three categories based on the scientific merit and clinical applicability.[22] *Category I:* Prognostic factors that are well established and are being used in patient management. This category includes clinical, anatomic and histological parameters such as grade and stage. *Category II (A):* Extensively studied biologically, *II (B):* Extensively studied clinically. Both Category II (A) and II (B) refer to a state in which the factor has yet to be rigorously validated clinically (i.e. symptomatic presentation, poor performance status, weight loss or hypercalcemia. *Category III* applies to those factors that show promise but do not meet the criteria for category I or II.

Although classification of patients according to histological subtype of RCC, nuclear grading and disease staging provides an estimate of prognosis, additional factors may affect the course of the disease. Analysis of large patient databases provides enough statistical power to allocate parameters that can further be analyzed

Table 5. One to six year basic survivorship representation
of metastatic (M1, with 1 symptom, no involvement of
the lymph nodes, 1997 T stage 1, grade 1 that received
immunotherapy) and non-metastatic RCC patients (M0, with
ECOG performance status = 0 and Fuhrman's grade = 1). (Adapted
with permission from Zisman, A, Pantuck, AJ, Dorey, F et al
(2002). "Mathematical model to predict individual survival for
patients with renal cell carcinoma." *JCO* **20**(5): 1368–1374.[34])

Time (years)	N0M0	N+/M1
0.5	0.983	0.939
1	0.968	0.873
2	0.951	0.770
3	0.921	0.684
4	0.910	0.631
5	0.894	0.586
6	0.889	0.523

by univariate and multivariate regression models to validate their individual and independent impact on patient outcome. Univariate analysis outlines the potential impact of one specific studied factor without regard to possible influence of other factors or a possible interplay of different factors. In contrast, multivariate analysis, allows for simultaneous assessment of several factors and their inter-relationship using the log-rank test for univariate analysis and the Cox proportional hazards model for multivariate analysis.[23] Thus, univariate analysis is used to reveal the value of a new potential prognostic factor, while multivariate analysis weighs the impact of each prognostic factor and determines its independence from other factors.

Identification of validated risk factors may allow for their integration into more accurate prognostic calculations for the individual patient. Many studies aimed to identify clinical features associated with patient outcome. Most studies found no association between demographic factors i.e. age, gender and race with survival. Performance status, a subjective estimate of overall well-being was clearly found to affect prognosis by most studies. Equivalently, weight loss is also a general indicator for health status, and was found to correlate with survival. Although both factors seem to measure the same parameter, multivariate analysis showed that they emerged as independent prognostic factors. In addition to performance status and weight loss, elevated ESR, serum c-reactive protein, fever, anemia, leukocytosis, serum LDH, serum calcium as well as serum alkaline phosphatase that has been assessed and were reported to have prognostic importance.[24–26]

The impact of prior therapy for RCC on patients' survival has been evaluated in many studies. While Radiotherapy has been consistently found not to induce a therapeutic effect on the disease course and patient outcome, Motzer et al, reported that prior radiotherapy had a negative effect on survival in univariate analysis.[26] Likewise, most studies agree that prior chemotherapy had no effect on outcome.[2,26] This reflects the resistance of RCC to both irradiation and chemotherapy. Several

Table 6. Elson algorithm for scoring prognostic factors for advanced RCC.

Variable	Score
Initial ECOG PS	Actual ECOG PS
Time from initial diagnosis	1 if <1 year
Number of metastatic sites	1 if >1 metastatic site
Weight loss	1 if weight loss present within the last 6 months
Prior chemotherapy	1 if received chemotherapy

Effective number of risk factors: The sum of all variable scores is summarized. The effective score equals the sum of all variables score minus 1 if number of metastatic sites score, prior chemotherapy and weight loss *all* equal 1. (Adapted with permission from Elson, PJ, Witte RS and Trump, DL (1988). "Prognostic factors for survival in patients with recurrent or metastatic renal cell carcinoma." *Cancer Res* **48**: 7310–7313.[2])

multivariate analysis studies found previous nephrectomy as an independent prognostic factor, while others confirmed it's value only in a univariate analysis,[26–28] but failed to prove an influence on outcome once other parameters were controlled in multivariate analyses.[2,29–33] Recently immunotherapy following cytoreductive surgery has been shown to have a protective value in a multivariate analysis.[34] Several disease related parameters including site and number of metastases, the interval between diagnosis and progression to metastatic state, were evaluated to determine their influence on outcome. While almost all studies confirmed the importance of metastasis in outcome prediction, the prognostic importance of the site of metastasis is not completely studied. A more consistent prognostic finding is the value of the total number of metastatic sites representing a crude estimate of tumor burden:[2,28,30,35] The relative risk of mortality increased 2–4 fold if more than a single metastatic site is present.[28,30] The disease free interval from initial diagnosis to metastasis is a significant determinant of prognosis. Patients with a short metastasis free interval have 50–90% increased risk of dying comparing with patients with longer intervals.

The histological type of RCC has not been generally found to have prognostic value, except for sarcomatoid tumors, which have been associated with a 3-fold mortality rate[31,36] as well as collecting duct RCC[37] and unclassified RCC.[38]

The abundance of prognostic factors renders the task of individual prognostication a cumbersome and complex one. To overcome this, integrated prognostic systems have been proposed. An integrated system is one that computes an array of independent prognostic factors to form a decision box, formula or nomogram that can be applied to predict outcome for the individual patient. Integrated staging systems are not unique to cancer. For an example such a system is used to predict patient's risk for postoperative pneumonia.[39] Up to 25% of early postoperative mortality may be attributed to postoperative pneumonia.[40] The process of refinement and validation of risk factors included accurate definition of the studied endpoint, inclusion of a multi-center database, definition of inclusion and exclusion criteria, development of a scoring system assigned to each factor (i.e. by multiplying the logistic regression model β-coefficients by 10 and rounding the result to the nearest integer) the overall risk is the sum of scores of all risk factors. In the postoperative pneumonia study, more than 106,000 patients undergoing surgery formed the study sample; of them 1.5% developed postoperative pneumonia. The analysis of preoperative and intraoperative characteristics defined risk factors. These risk factors were than validated by assessing the postoperative pneumonia risk index prospectively in a well-defined cohort of patients. The risk index can then be sub-divided into risk groups and any future patient can be classified to a specific risk group.

NEW ALGORITHMS FOR RCC

In the past 5 years few prognostic systems taking into account prognostic factors has been proposed for RCC.

Comprehensive Integrated Systems

At UCLA Zisman et al. developed an integrated staging system (UISS).[4] The medical records of 661 patients who underwent nephrectomy for RCC between 1989–1999 at University of California Los-Angeles were evaluated. 18 clinical variables were tested. Univariate and multivariate analyses were performed as well as bootstrapping and internal validation.[41] Lately the UISS was successfully validated using MD Anderson Cancer Center Kidney Cancer Database.[42] By combining for an individual patient the 1997 TNM stage, Fuhrman's nuclear grade and the ECOG performance status, one out of 5 risk groups is assigned to the patient by using the assignment table (Table 3). The expected survival is then predicted for each group accordingly (Figure 1). The UISS has an advantage in its simplicity and in its ability to predict prognosis for a given patient based on simple clinical data. Two thirds of the UISS components are already validated prognostic factors by themselves: The 1997 AJCC TNM stage and Fuhrman's grade are both College of American Pathologists type I prognostic factors whereas ECOG performance status is type I for metastatic disease and type IIA for patients with N0M0 disease. The UISS can pick-up survival differences imposed by different histological types of RCC and clearly discriminate between favorable disease (UISS I), Unfavorable (UISS V) and intermediate prognosis (UISS III) plus two intermediary categories (UISS II and IV). The basic UISS has been recently upgraded in two aspects. The allocation table was replace by two simpler decision boxes more convenient for office use and the outcomes detailed were expanded in order to make the system capable of predicting not only survival but also more relevant end points for both localized and metastatic patients. This algorithm integrates the complex interaction of multiple prognostic variables to generate patients stratification to risk groups and prognosticate outcome and survival and look at multiple points along the course of the disease such as at time of nephrectomy, time of local or systemic recurrence, and at completion of immunotherapy.[43,44] This was achieved by a prospective cohort study with outcome assessment based on chart review of 814 nephrectomized patients at UCLA. Based on UISS category and the presence of metastases, patients were

UCLA Integrated Staging System Risk group Assignment
for Patients with Renal Cell Carcinoma
LOCALIZED DISEASE (N0M0)

T Stage	1				2	3				4
Fuhrman's Grade	1-2		3-4			1		>1		⇓
ECOG PS	0	≥1	0	≥1		0	≥1	0	≥1	
RISK GROUP	Low		Intermediate						High	

To obtain a N0M0 patients risk group, begin at the top of the decision box and progress downward using patient 1977 AJCC T stage, Fuhrman's grade and ECOG performance status at diagnosis.

Reference Table

		Years after Nx	RISK GROUP		
			Low	Intermediate	High
Disease-Specific Survival (%)		1	100	97	89
		2	99	91	78
		3	95	88	64
		4	93	86	61
		5	91	80	55
Local Recurrence-Free Survival (%)		1	100	99	94
		2		99	89
		3		97	89
		4		97	85
		5		95	85
Systemic Failure-Free Survival (%)		1	97	89	76
		2	96	80	60
		3	95	77	49
		4	91	71	44
		5	91	71	40
*Early systemic Failure (≤6 mo)	Survival (%)	1		100	37
		2		67	28
		3		0	0
	Progression Free-Survival (%)	1		33	8
		2		0	0
		3		0	0
*Late systemic Failure >6 mo)	Survival (%)	1		79	76
		2		70	58
		3		70	36
		4		49	28
		5		36	15
	Progression Free Survival (%)	1		38	36
		2		19	15
		3		16	10
		4		0	0
		5		0	0

* From failure to death with immunotherapy treatment

Figure 1. Kaplan-Meier survival curve according to the UISS categories for 661 patients treated with nephrectomy or nephrectomy and immunotherapy at the University of California Los Angeles. Black triangles mark the 10 patients at risk point. (Adapted with permission from Zisman, A., Pantuck, AJ., Dorey F. et al. (2001). "Improved prognostication of RCC using an Integrated Staging System (UISS)." *JCO* 19(6): 1649–1657.[4])

divided into two sets of low (LR), intermediate (IR), and high-risk (HR) groups (localized LR, IR and HR and advanced LR, IR and HR). Two decision boxes integrating components of the 1997 TNM staging, tumor grade, and performance status were compiled for determining a risk group for an individual patient.

UCLA Integrated Staging System Risk group Assignment for Patients with Renal Cell Carcinoma
METASTATIC DISEASE

T Stage	N1M0	N2M0 or any M1						
Fuhrman's Grade		1		2		3		4
ECOG PS		0	≥1	0	≥1	0	≥1	0	≥1
RISK GROUP	Low	INTM	Low	Intermediate (INTM)				High

To obtain a metastatic patients risk group, begin at the top of the decision box and progress downward using patient 1977 AJCC N/M stage, Fuhrman's grade and ECOG performance status at diagnosis.

Reference Table

		RISK GROUP		
	Years	Low	Intermediate	High
Disease-Specific Survival following Nephrectomy (%)	1	87	63	21
	2	65	41	11
	3	56	31	0
	4	37	23	0
	5	32	20	0
Survival Following Immunotherapy (%)*	1	85	62	25
	2	55	42	17
	3	47	32	0
	4	33	25	0
	5	26	23	0
Progression-Free-Survival Following Immunotherapy (%)*	1	45	30	0
	2	33	21	0
	3	25	19	0
	4	25	16	0
	5	25	12	0

* Assuming no more then 6 weeks delay between nephrectomy and immunotherapy.

Figure 2. UISS decision box for determining risk group for patients with localized disease (N0M0) and corresponding outcome data

Following the determination of risk group a clinical outcome may be allocated for an individual patient (Figures 2 and 3). Dividing RCC patients into these 6 risk groups permits comprehensive outcome prediction. As the role of surgery alone to localized disease, IMT alone, or combination of surgery and IMT for metastatic patients have become more clearly defined, further progress is needed in identifying the appropriate candidates for each approach: According to the UCLA data, surgery alone is an adequate treatment for cure in NM-LR patients. The use of adjuvant IMT is questionable in NM patients with early recurrences (≤6 months after nephrectomy) and requires prospective studies. Immediate post nephrectomy adjuvant IMT may be indicated in NM-HR (and perhaps NM-IR patients) since the current results with deferred therapy are disappointing. Adjuvant IMT after cytoreductive nephrectomy in M-LR N+M0 patients may improve their survival. Furthermore, cytoreductive surgery and IMT yield a 25% and 12% 5-year freedom

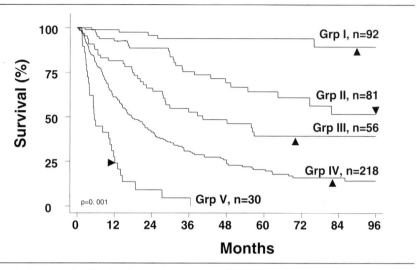

Figure 3. UISS decision box for determining risk group for patients with advanced disease (non-N0M0) and corresponding outcome data

from progression in M-LR and M-IR patients, respectively, but exert negligible impact on the progression of M-HR patients.

The UCLA Kidney Cancer Database was also used to create a mathematical model for the prediction of individual patient outcome by analyzing an array of clinical prognostic factors[34] and phrasing the impact of the significant ones into an exponential formula. Time to death of RCC was the primary tested endpoint. Applying univariate and multivariate analysis for 20 parameters separately for localized and advanced disease pointed out independent prognostic factors, that were further coded and incorporated into two functions based on the Nadas equation. Work performed by Arthur Nadas during the 1970's on the subject of proportional hazard functions led to the development of exponential formulas that were able to describe survival by integrating the influence of multiple hazards coefficients related to a given event on top of calculated basic survival. These formulas are capable of synthesizing the relative risk of multiple variables into a single probability.[45,46] Formulas were developed for non-metastatic and metastatic patients, using the independent risk factors that were found to be significant in the multivariate analysis (localized: ECOG performance status and grade, advanced: grade, T stage, number of presenting symptoms, nodal involvement and immunotherapy (protective)). In order to describe patients survival at a given time point during the follow-up (S_t), $S_t = S_b{}^c$ where: S_b = baseline survivorship estimates (given in the form of a fraction between 0–1), $c = e^{(\beta1+\beta2+\beta3+\ldots+\beta n)}$ where β = (Coded Cox explanatory variable value) × (Cox coefficient- "boot strap value"). Incorporation of the significant variables into the Nadas equation led to the phrasing of two formulas for localized (N0M0) and advanced (non-N0M0) disease at presentation.

Table 7. Elson's system risk groups prognosis.

Effective number of risk factors	Risk group	3 months survival %	1 year survival %	Median survival (months)
0, 1	1	92	52	12.8
2	2	87	31	7.7
3	3	76	18	5.3
4	4	54	9	3.4
5	5	35	1	2.1

(Adapted with permission from Elson, PJ, Witte RS and Trump, DL (1988). "Prognostic factors for survival in patients with recurrent or metastatic renal cell carcinoma." *Cancer Res* **48**: 7310–7313.[2])

For patient with localized disease Survival (%) = $100\,S_b\;e^{((1.09\times ECOG\;P.S.)+(0.57\times(grade-1))}$ whereas for advanced disease Survival (%) = $100\,S_b\;e^{((0.49\times grade)+(0.48\times T\;stage)+(0.28\times No.\;of\;symptoms)+(0.43\times node\;positive\;disease)-(0.59\times immunotherapy))}$. The basic survivalships (S_b) are detailed in Table 5. ECOG performance status is coded 0 (normal) or 1 (abnormal for ECOG PS 1 and up), node positive disease is coded 1 if positive and immunotherapy is coded 1 if given. The above mathematical tool was internally validated by comparison to standard Kaplan-Mayer survival charts and corrected for overestimation by using the bootstrap method. The various UCLA methods detailed are useful and powerful for surgical patients and apply postoperatively.

Systems Exclusive for Metastatic Patients

Most of the integrative prognostic systems used for metastatic patients relay on scoring systems. The first system of this kind was introduced in 1988 by Elson et al and was based on a group of 680 patients.[2] Using a multivariate analysis initial performance status, time from initial diagnosis, number of metastatic sites, weight loss and prior chemotherapy (Table 6) were found important risk factors for patients with advanced RCC. Five risk groups were aggregated based on a scoring algorithm using the aforementioned variables (Table 7). Since Elson's publication few more similar systems based on data from 1358 patients were proposed, most of which found performance status as a key variable.[25,29,30,33,47] Motzer et al. studied the risk factors of 670 patients with advanced RCC that participated in 24 clinical trials at the Memorial Sloan Kettering Cancer Center between 1975 and 1996.[26] The studied endpoint was survival time, and the clinical features assessed included number of metastatic sites, Karnofsky performance status, prior treatment (radiotherapy, chemotherapy or immunotherapy), prior nephrectomy, time interval between diagnosis and initiation of treatment, and baseline hemoglobin concentration, serum albumin, serum alkaline phosphatase, serum lactate dehydrogenase and serum calcium. Following a univariate and multivariate analysis supplemented with a bootstrap correction 5 variables found to remain and serve as significant risk factors for poor survival: elevated serum lactate dehydrogenase (cut off point 300 U/L), low hemoglobin concentration (cut off point 13 g/dL for males and 11.5 g/dL for females), high corrected serum calcium (cut off 10 mg/dL), low Kranofsky performance status (cut off point 80) and primary in place (Table 8). According to the calculated cutoff values of these parameters, and the absence of nephrectomy, a Cox model was fit and risk groups were defined: patients with no risk factors—favorable risk, those with 1–2 risk factors—intermediate risk and those with more than 3 risk factors—poor risk group. The corresponding 1 and 3-year survival for the 3 risk groups are detailed in Table 9. The study model was externally validated using data from 175 patients. One of the advantages of the Motzer system is that risk may be assessed preoperatively based on simple lab data.

Systems Dedicated for Localized Disease

Kattan et al, developed a nomogram to predict recurrence free survival following nephrectomy in non-metastatic RCC patients.[48] Their database included 836 tumors resected from 807 patients during 8.5 years at Memorial Sloan Kettering Cancer Center. Following exclusion, 612 patients who underwent unilateral partial or radical nephrectomy for localized RCC entered the analysis. The clinico-pathologic factors studied included: tumor size, presentation (incidental of symptomatic), histology and pathologic stage. The histological tumor type was assigned according to the Heidelberg system.[49] Any recurrence of RCC was considered as treatment failure. The Cox proportional hazards model was applied to create a nomogram (Figure 4) similar in its principles to the Kattan nomograms for prostate cancer.[50–54]

It was suggested that the nomogram may be used not only in patient counseling, but also to assist in defining patients at low risk for recurrence who might benefit from a less stringent follow up regime, or alternatively define patients at increased recurrence risk who might be eligible for clinical trials studying adjuvant therapy.

ON THE HORIZON—MOLECULAR MARKERS TO FORM MOLECULAR STAGING SYSTEMS

Molecular tumor markers for cancer at general and for RCC in particular are anticipated to have an immense impact on the way cancer is being diagnosed and treated. Molecular tumor markers provide not only prognostic information to aid in the identification of patients at risk for recurrence or metastasis but could open avenues to targeted therapy as well. The completion of the human genome sequencing and development of robust research technologies such as gene chip technologies promises rapid identification of new molecular markers. The evolving science of biostatistics assures that the enormous data collected using this technology may be translated into meaningful results pointing to specific genes of great significance. Currently, many markers relating to tumor proliferation, growth, angiogenesis and adhesion molecules as well as others, are being evaluated for their potential as prognostic factors and are discussed in other chapters in this book. Some are promising but clinical trials are needed to validate their usefulness in clinical practice.

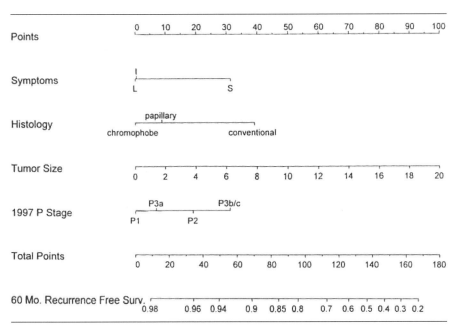

Figure 4. Kattan normogram for recurrence of renal cell carcinoma based on 601 patients treated with nephrectomy at Memorial Sloan-Kettering Cancer Center **Instructions for Physician**: locate the patient's symptoms (I = incidental, L = local, S = systemic); on the symptom axis. Draw a line straight upwards to the points axis to determine how many points towards recurrence the patient receives for his symptoms. Repeat this process for the other axes, each time drawing straight towards the Points axis. Sum the points achieved for each predictor and locate this sum on the Total Points axis. Draw a line straight down to the patient's probability of remaining recurrence free for 5 years assuming that he or she does not die from another cause first. **Instructions to Patient**: "Mr. X, if we had 100 men or women exactly like you, we could expect between ⟨predicted percentage from nomogram − 10%⟩ and ⟨predicted percentage + 10%⟩ to remain free of their disease for 5 years following surgery, though recurrence after 5 years is still possible. (Adapted with permission from Kattan, M.W., Reuter, V., Motzer, R.J." A postoperative prognostic nomogram for renal cell carcinoma" J Urol 166(1): 63–7.[48]).

Table 8. MSKCG prognostic system for patients with advanced RCC. After completing patient's values answer the assignment question in the "Yes" or "No" column by using X. In the hyphen box sum the number of X's. The number in the hyphen box equals the number of risk factors.

Variable	Patient value	Assignment question	Yes	No
LDH		Above 300 U/L		
Hemoglobin		Above 13 for male		
		Above 11.5 in female		
Corrected Calcium		Above 10 mg/dL		
Karnofsky PS		Below 80		
Prior nephrectomy				
	Number of risk factors			

(Adapted with permission from Motzer, R, Mazumbar, M, Bacik, J et al. (1999). "Survival and prognostic stratification of 670 patients with advanced renal cell carcinoma." *J Clin Oncol* **17**: 2530–2540.[26])

Table 9. MSKCC prognostic system for patients with advanced RCC. Survival data.

Number of risk factors	1 year survival %	2 year survival %	3 year survival %	Median survival (months)
0	71	45	31	20
1–2	42	17	7	10
3–4–5	12	3	0	4

(Adapted with permission from Motzer, R, Mazumbar, M, Bacik, J et al. (1999). "Survival and prognostic stratification of 670 patients with advanced renal cell carcinoma." *J Clin Oncol* **17**: 2530–2540.[26])

We anticipate that few of these markers will find their way into future classifications and staging systems and will aid in directing patients management and therapy.

IN CONCLUSION

The value of prognostication lies far beyond the capability to instruct an individual patient on his or her prospects of survival. It also allows for more accurate definition of disease status and permits a less biased data analysis for communication between caregivers and researchers. The more precisely can a patient's status be defined, the easier it becomes to assign the appropriate treatment modality and to weigh their impact on the course of disease.

The science of forecasting outcome has gone a long way from separate simple analyses of a few clinical and pathologic determinants to a complex computing comprehensive array of data that encompasses clinical, disease related parameters, therapy dependent parameters and new genetic and molecular indicators. To make practical use of the multitude of available independent prognostic factors, integrated prognostic systems have been developed that compute multiple parameters and define risk groups. Finally, mathematical modeling of independent risk factors may improve the ability to make more accurate predictions for an individual patient.

REFERENCES

1. Greenlee RT, Murray T, Bolden S et al, Cancer statistics, 2000. CA. Cancer. J. Clin. 50:7, 2000.
2. Elson PJ, Witte RS, and Trump DL, Prognostic factors for survival in patients with recurrent or metastatic renal cell carcinoma. Cancer. Res. 48:7310, 1988.
3. Figlin RA, Renal cell carcinoma: management of advanced disease. J. Urol. 161:381, 1999.
4. Zisman A, Pantuck A, Dorey F et al, Improved prognostication of RCC using an Integrated Staging System (UISS). J. Clin. Oncol. 19:1649, 2001.
5. Flocks R and Kadesky M, Malignant neoplasms of the kidney: analysis of 353 patients followed 5 years or more. Tr. Am. Ass. Gen. Surg., 49:105, 1958.
6. Robson C, Churchill B, and Anderson W, The results of radical nephrectomy for renal carcinoma. J. Urol. 101:297, 1969.
7. Pantuck A, Zisman A, and Belldegrun A, RCC 2000: Changing the natural history of renal cell carcinoma. J. Urol. 166:1611, 2001.
8. Bassil B, Dosoretz DE, and Prout GR, Jr., Validation of the tumor, nodes and metastasis classification of renal cell carcinoma. J. Urol. 134:450, 1985.
9. Hermanek P and Sobin L, eds. TNM classification of malignant tumors. 4 ed. UICC international union against cancer, UICC monograph series. Springer-Verlag: Berlin, New-York. 148, 1987.

10. Guinan P, Sobin L, Algaba F et al, TNM staging of renel cell carcinoma: Workgroup no.3—Union International Contre le Cancer (UICC) and the American Joint Committee on Cancer (AJCC). Cancer. 80:992, 1997.
11. Guinan P, Frank W, Saffrin R et al, Staging and survival of patients with renal cell carcinoma. Semin. Surg. Oncol. 10: 1994.
12. Hermanek P and Schrott K, Evaluation of the new tumor, nodes and metastases classification of renal cell carcinoma. J. Urol. 144:238, 1990.
13. Skinner D, Colvin R, Vermillion C et al, Diagnosis and management of renal cell carcinoma. A clinical and pathological study of 309 cases. Cancer. 28:1165, 1971.
14. Maldazys J and deKernion J, Prognostic factors in metastatic renal carcinoma. J. Urol. 136:376, 1986.
15. Thrasher J and Paulson D, Prognostic factors in renal cancer. Urol. Clin. North. Am. 20:247, 1993.
16. Zisman A, Pantuck A, Chao D et al, Reevaluation of the 1997 TNM classification for RCC: T1 and T2 cut-off point at 4.5 cm rather then 7 cm better correlates with clinical outcome. J. Urol. 166:54, 2001.
17. Licht M, Novick A, and Goormastic M, Nephron sparing surgery in incidntal vs. suspected renal cell carcinoma. J. Urol. 152:39, 1994.
18. Lerner S, Hawkins C, Blute M et al, Disease outcome in patients with low stage renal cell carcinoma treated with nephron sparing or radical surgery. J. Urol. 155:1868, 1996.
19. Hafez KS, Fergany AF, and Novick AC, Nephron sparing surgery for localized renal cell carcinoma: impact of tumor size on patient survival, tumor recurrence and TNM staging. J. Urol. 162, 1999.
20. Kinouchi T, Saiki S, Meguro N et al, Impact of tumor size on the clinical outcomes of patients with Robson State I renal cell carcinoma. Cancer. 85:689, 1999.
21. Igarashi T, Tobe T, Nakatsu HO et al, The impact of a 4 cm. cutoff point for stratification of T1N0M0 renal cell carcinoma after radical nephrectomy. J. Urol. 165:1103, 2001.
22. Srigley JR, Hutter RV, Gelb AB et al, Current prognostic factors–renal cell carcinoma: Workgroup No. 4. Union Internationale Contre le Cancer (UICC) and the American Joint Committee on Cancer (AJCC). Cancer. 80:994, 1997.
23. Cox DR and Oakes D, Analysis of survival data. New York: Chapman and Hall, 1990.
24. Ljungberg B, Landberg G, and Alamdari FI, Factors of importance for prediction of survival in patients with metastatic renal cell carcinoma, treated with or without nephrectomy. Scand. J. Urol. Nephrol. 34:246, 2000.
25. Lopez Hanninen E, Kirchner H, and Atzpodien J, Interleukin-2 based home therapy of metastatic renal cell carcinoma: risks and benefits in 215 consecutive single institution patients. J. Urol. 155:19, 1996.
26. Motzer R, Mazumbar M, Bacik J et al, Survival and prognostic stratification of 670 patients with advanced renal cell carcinoma. J. Clin. Oncol. 17:2530, 1999.
27. Minasian LM, Motzer RJ, Gluck L et al, Interferon alfa-2a in advanced renal cell carcinoma: treatment results and survival in 159 patients with long-term follow-up. J. Clin. Oncol. 11:1368, 1993.
28. Landonio G, Baiocchi C, Cattaneo D et al, Retrospective analysis of 156 cases of metastatic renal cell carcinoma: evaluation of prognostic factors and response to different treatments. Tumori. 80:468, 1994.
29. de Forges A, Rey A, Klink M et al, Prognostic factors of adult metastatic renal carcinoma: a multivariate analysis. Semin. Surg. Oncol. 4:149, 1988.
30. Palmer PA, Vinke J, Philip T et al, Prognostic factors for survival in patients with advanced renal cell carcinoma treated with recombinant interleukin-2. Ann. Oncol. 3:475, 1992.
31. Mani S, Todd MB, Katz K et al, Prognostic factors for survival in patients with metastatic renal cancer treated with biological response modifiers. J. Urol. 154:35, 1995.
32. Citterio G, Bertuzzi A, Tresoldi M et al, Prognostic factors for survival in metastatic renal cell carcinoma: retrospective analysis from 109 consecutive patients. Eur. Urol. 31:286, 1997.
33. Fossa SD, Kramar A, and Droz JP, Prognostic factors and survival in patients with metastatic renal cell carcinoma treated with chemotherapy or interferon-alpha. Eur. J. Cancer. 30A:1310, 1994.
34. Zisman A, Pantuck A, Dorey F et al, Mathematical model to predict individual survival for patients with renal cell carcinoma. J. Clin. Oncol. 20:1368, 2002.
35. Neves RJ, Zincke H, and Taylor WF, Metastatic renal cell cancer and radical nephrectomy: identification of prognostic factors and patient survival. J. Urol. 139:1173, 1988.
36. Kanamaru H, Li B, Miwa Y et al, Immunohistochemical expression of p53 and bcl-2 proteins is not associated with sarcomatoid change in renal cell carcinoma. Urol. Res. 27:169, 1999.
37. Chao D, Zisman A, Pantuck A et al, Collecting duct cell carcinoma: Clinical study of a rare tumor. J. Urol. 167:71, 2001.

38. Zisman A, Chao D, Pantuck A et al, Unclassified renal cell carcinoma: Clinical features and prognostic impact of a new histologic subtype. J. Urol. (In press). 2002.
39. Arozullah AM, Khuri SF, Henderson WG et al, Development and validation of a multifactorial risk index for predicting postoperative pneumonia after major noncardiac surgery. Ann. Intern. Med. 135:847, 2001.
40. Brooks-Brunn JA, Postoperative atelectasis and pneumonia: risk factors. Am. J. Crit. Care. 4:340, 1995.
41. Zisman A, Pantuck A, Figlin R et al, Validation of the UCLA integrated Staging System (UISS) for patients with renal cell carcinoma. J. Clin. Oncol. 19:3792, 2001.
42. Slaton J, Zisman A, Belldegrun A et al, Validation of UCLA Integrated Staging System (UISS) as a predictor for survival in patients undergoing nephrectomy for renal cell carcinoma. In AUA Annual Meeting. 2002. Orlando, FL.
43. Zisman A, Pantuck A, Wieder J et al, Risk group assessment and clinical outcome algorithm to predict the natural history of patients with surgically resected renal cell carcinoma. (submitted for publication). 2002.
44. Zisman A, Pantuck A, Chao H et al, UISS-based clinical algorithm to predict outcome of patients with localized and advanced renal cell carcinoma. In AUA Annual Meeting. 2002. Orlando FL.
45. Nadas A, On proportional hazard functions. Technometrics. 12:413, 1970.
46. Lee E, Statistical methods for survival data analysis. Belmont, CA: Lifetime learning publications. 289, 1980.
47. Jones M, Philip T, Palmer P et al, The impact of interleukin-2 on survival in renal cancer: a multivariate analysis. Cancer. Biother. 8:275, 1993.
48. Kattan MW, Reuter V, Motzer RJ et al, A postoperative prognostic nomogram for renal cell carcinoma. J. Urol. 166:63, 2001.
49. Kovacs G, Akhtar M, Beckwith BJ et al, The Heidelberg classification of renal cell tumours [editorial]. J. Pathol. 183:131, 1997.
50. Kattan MW, Potters L, Blasko JC et al, Pretreatment nomogram for predicting freedom from recurrence after permanent prostate brachytherapy in prostate cancer. Urology. 58:393, 2001.
51. Kattan MW, Zelefsky MJ, Kupelian PA et al, Pretreatment nomogram for predicting the outcome of three-dimensional conformal radiotherapy in prostate cancer. J. Clin. Oncol. 18:3352, 2000.
52. Kattan MW, Wheeler TM, and Scardino PT, Postoperative nomogram for disease recurrence after radical prostatectomy for prostate cancer. J. Clin. Oncol. 17:1499, 1999.
53. Kattan MW, Eastham JA, Stapleton AM et al, A preoperative nomogram for disease recurrence following radical prostatectomy for prostate cancer. J. Natl. Cancer. Inst. 90:766, 1998.
54. Kattan MW, Stapleton AM, Wheeler TM et al, Evaluation of a nomogram used to predict the pathologic stage of clinically localized prostate carcinoma. Cancer. 79:528, 1997.

4. BASIC BIOLOGY AND CLINICAL BEHAVIOR OF RENAL CELL CARCINOMA

KEN-RYU HAN, ALLAN J. PANTUCK, AND ARIE S. BELLDEGRUN

From the Department of Urology, University of California School of Medicine, Los Angeles, CA

INTRODUCTION

Renal cell carcinoma (RCC) accounted for over 31,000 new cases of cancer and led to approximately 12,000 deaths in the United States in 2001.[1] Nearly one-third of RCC cases present with metastatic disease and approximately 30% of those treated for localized disease eventually relapse.[2] Renal cell carcinoma occurs twice as often in men and most commonly occurs during the fifth through seventh decades of life, but has been reported in younger patients.[2]

Renal cell carcinomas are comprised of a family of distinct tumors which are thought to arise from different segments of renal tubular epithelium, the majority of which arise from the proximal tubules. The majority of these tumors are highly vascular and have the propensity to spread by multiple routes, including direct invasion into the perinephric tissues, hematogenously through the renal vein and inferior vena cava, and via the lymphatic tissues. It is unclear at this time what molecular mechanisms dictate an individual tumor's pattern of spread.

Once metastatic disease develops, the prognosis for long-term survival is poor. As a result, understanding the factors that impact the biologic behavior of RCC is essential for patient assessment, treatment planning, prediction of disease outcome, and assignment to clinical trials. These factors, which may be involved in tumor pro-

Address for Correspondence: Arie S Belldegrun, MD, University of California School of Medicine, Department of Urology, 10833 Le Conte Avenue, Room 66-118 CHS, Los Angeles, CA 90095-1738.
E-mail: abelldegrun@mednet.ucla.edu

R.A. Figlin (ed.). KIDNEY CANCER. Copyright © 2003. Kluwer Academic Publishers. Boston. All rights reserved.

liferation, invasion, and metastasis may dictate future therapeutic strategies. For RCC, tumor grade and stage remain the most useful predictors of clinical outcome and behavior. However, other important clinical, radiographic, and pathologic features contribute to our understanding and ability to predict the biologic behavior of kidney cancers. Finally, with progress in the understanding of the molecular biology and genetics of RCC, newer biomolecular markers are becoming available and are being investigated for their ability to enhance our outcome analysis capabilities. This chapter will examine the various factors that affect the development, progression, and clinical behavior of RCC.

HISTOLOGY

In the past, there was confusion regarding the terminology for the various histologic patterns recognized for RCC. Currently, there is a good consensus and the newer classifications reflect not only histology, but also advances in our understanding of the genetic alternations associated with each subtype of RCC. There are four main histological subtypes of RCC recognized as a result of a collaborative effort by an international workshop including the Union Internationale Contre le Cancer (UICC) and the American Joint Committee on Cancer (AJCC) in 1997 that took place in Rochester, Minnesota.[3,4] Each subtype has distinctive characteristics and biology.

Clear Cell Adenocarcinomas

Clear cell or conventional carcinomas account for 70–80% of RCC's and arise in the proximal tubules.[3,5,6] On gross inspection, clear cell RCC tumors have a yellowish-appearance secondary to their high lipid content.[7] On microscopic analysis, clear cells have a round or polygonal appearance and have abundant cytoplasm containing cholesterol, glycogen, and lipids. The clear content of the cells are a result of the lipids being dissolved by solvents prior to histologic sectioning in paraffin. The tumors also have a prominent meshwork of fine vascular structures between the tumor cells.[8]

Clear cell carcinomas come in both hereditary and sporadic forms. Herediatary clear cell RCC is seen in approximately 40 to 45% of individuals with von Hippel-Landau disease (VHL).[5] Patients with VHL disease have germline mutations in the VHL gene, which resides on the short arm of chromosome 3p25.[7] The VHL gene also plays a significant role in sporadic, non-familial clear cell RCC. Up to 60% of these patients have also been found to have VHL mutations.[9]

Papillary Renal Cell Carcinomas

Papillary RCC accounts for 10 to 15% of renal neoplasms and also arise from the proximal tubules.[5,6,10,11] The architecture of these tumors may be papillary, tubular, tubulo-papillary, or solid.[5] The cytoplasm of these tumors may have either basophilic or eosinophilic staining.[5] Recently Delahunt and Eble proposed to classify these tumors as type I (chromophil-basophilic) and type II (chromophil-eosinophilic).[12] Type I (basophilic) tumors have smaller cells and less cytoplasm.

Similar to clear cell adenocarcinomas, these tumors are felt to arise from the proximal renal tubular epithelium and occur in both hereditary and sporadic forms.[7] Mutations in the tyrosine kinase domain of the c-MET proto-oncogene (chrmosome 7q34) have been implicated in the development of hereditary papillary RCC.[13] These hereditary (type I), basophilic tumors often present with multi-focal, bilateral tumors.[5]

MD Anderson recently recently studied the biological significance of the c-MET proto-oncogene.[14] Immunohistochemical analysis of 55 papillary RCC specimens revealed that 80% of these tumors' cytoplasm expressed c-MET protein. Tumors expressing the c-MET protein presented with higher stage tumors (p = 0.004). Patients without c-MET expression demonstrated a trend towards better survival rates, but the association failed to achieve statistical significance (p = 0.07).[14]

The sporadic papillary renal cell carcinomas demonstrate polysomes in 80% of cases. Common karyotypic findings include trisomy of chromosomes 7, 16, and 17, as well as the long arm of the Y chromosome in men.[5]

Chromophobe Renal Cell Carcinomas

Chromophobe tumors arise from the intercalated cells of the collecting ducts and account for only 5% of cases.[6,15] Similar to papillary tumors, there are two histologic variants within the chromophobe type: typical(classic) and eosinophilic.[7] The typical or classic variant displays reticular features, while the eosinophilic variant demonstrates a granular appearance due to high mitochondrial content. Both types of cells are typically large with distinct cell borders.[16] Genetically, chromophobe tumors are characterized by monosomy of multiple chromosomes, including, 1, 2, 6, and 10.[7]

Chromophobe tumors have been recently been reported with increased frequency in patients with Birt Hogg Dube Syndrome (BHDS).[17] This syndrome is an inherited (autosomal dominant) familial syndrome that results in cutaneous lesions called fibrofolliculomas, which are benign tumors. However, patients with BHDS have an increased risk of multifocal-bilateral tumors, including both subtypes of chromophobe tumors.

Collecting Duct Carcinomas

Finally, collecting duct, medullary carcinoma of the kidney, or Bellini's duct carcinoma is a rare and aggressive variant arising in the medullary collecting ducts that accounts for less than 1% of renal tumors. Grossly, the tumor is often located centrally in or near the renal pelvis and appears gray-white.[18] Microscopically, they consist of irregular, ductlike structures or papillary architecutre surrouded by abundant, loose, demoplastic stroma.[18] since the papillary appearance of these tumors make distinction from papillary RCC difficult, immunohistochemical studies with antibodies to high molecular weight cytokeratins and lectins are often necessary. These antigens are widely expressed in distal tubule cells.[18] Furthermore, vimentin activity is usually very weak or negative.

Collecting duct carcinomas occur almost exclusively in African-American men with sickle cell trait or disease.[7,19] These tumors are very aggressive and tend to develop metastases very rapidly.[20] In addition, these tumors tend to occur in younger men and usually present with stage IV disease.[18] A recent review of 6 patients revealed that 5 patients presented with TNM stage IV disease and average survival was only 11.5 months (7 to 17).[18] In another study of 34 patients, average survival from the time of surgery was only 15 weeks (3–52 weeks).[6,21] Surgical extirpation alone rarely results in cure and a large proportion of patients cannot tolerate immunotherapy.[18]

Renal Cell Carcinoma, Unclassified

Renal cell carcinoma, unclassified is a category created to include renal epithelial tumors that cannot be readily classified in the previously described histologic types. As a result, this group represents a heterogenenous group of tumors that includes tumors with extensive necrosis and minimal viable unclassifiable tumor, mucin-producing tumors, and tumors with sarcomatoid change in which the epithelial elements cannot be classified.[15] Unclassified RCC is a highly aggressive tumor with a great propensity to spread to the lymph nodes and develop osseous metastases, leading to a grim prognosis.[22]

Prognostic Significance of Histologic Subtypes

Recent literature has investigated the clinical behavior of each of these subtypes and their effects on recurrence and survival. Most notably, Memorial Sloan-Kettering used Cox proportional hazards regression analysis to consruct a postoperative nomogram model based on the pathological data and disease followup of 601 patients who were treated for RCC with nephrectomy.[23] This nomogram can be used to predict the 5-year probability of recurrence and was discussed in detail in the previous chapter (Ch 3, Dr. A Zisman). In this nomogram, Kattan et al concluded that chromphobe tumors had a slightly decreased chance of recurrence when compared to papillary tumors. Both tumors had a significantly decreased risk of recurrence when compared to clear cell tumors.

These findings were corroborated recently by Amin et al in a review of 405 cases of renal tumors.[15] In this review, clear cell tumors (N = 255) tended to be symptomatic more often and presented at an advanced stage and a higher rate of metastatic disease at presentation.[15] The 5-year disease-specific survival (DSS) was 76% compared to 100% for chromphobe tumors (N = 24) and 86% for papillary (N = 75). The five-year recurrence rates were 94%, 88%, and 70% for chromophobe, papillary, and clear cell tumors, respectively.

These two studies support the notion that chromophobe tumors have the best prognosis, followed by papillary tumors, and then clear cell tumors. There is one variant of clear cell that may have a better prognosis than its conventional clear cell counterparts, however. Cystic RCC may have a lower potential for recurrence and metastatic disease.[6] According to Bielsa et al, the majority of the tumors in their review presented with a lower grade and stage.[24] Other studies have also confirmed low recurrence and metastatic potential.[25] More recently, the Mayo clinic presented a review of 24 cases of cystic RCC followed from 1969 to 1997. Twenty of 24 (83%) of the patients had T1 diseaese and 22 (92%) had no evidence of disease at a mean follow up 77.6 months.[26]

Sarcomatoid Component

Sarcomatoid tumors are no longer considered a distinct histologic sub-type of RCC, but rather represents a relatively rare, high grade form of RCC typified by a spindle cell growth pattern that is seen in less than 5% of RCC and bodes for a generally poor outcome.[27] Clinically, sarcomatoid RCC is characterized by its locally aggressive nature, metastatic potential, and poor prognosis.[28–30] Surgical resection alone often does not appear to significantly affect its clinical course since tumors with sarcomatoid features are commonly metastatic or locally advanced at the time of diagnosis. The reported median survival of sarcomatoid patients from the time of diagnosis is 3.8 to 6.8 months with no treatment.[28,31] When stratified by T stage, sarcomatoid variant patients were found to have a mean survival of 49.7 months for stage I and 6.8 months for stage II–IV.[32,33]

More recently, Amin et al reported a 5-year DSS of 24% for unclassified renal tumors, which includes tumors with sarcomatoid components.[15] In addition, any tumors with sarcomatoid change (N = 25) had a 35% 5-year DSS in this study. Finally, in a review of 25 patients with sarcomatoid tumors and metastatic disease from UCLA, Cangiano and colleagues reported that patients (N = 9) receiving hi-dose interleukin-2 (IL-2) had significantly improved survival when compared to patients who did not. At a mean follow-up of 21 months, nearly 80% of patients who received high-dose IL-2 remained alive. By comparison, patients who did not receive high-dose IL-2 had a median survival of only 6 months.[34]

Summary

There are five main classifications of RCC. Chromophobe tumors portend to a slightly better prognosis when compared to papillary tumors. Both of these tumors have a favorable clinical behavior when compared to the most common of the RCC subtypes, clear cell carcinoma. Collecting duct carcinomas and unclassified renal cell carcinomas have the worst prognosis, while patients with any evidence of sarcomatoid features also tend to do worse. Table 1 summarizes histologic subtypes and their likely cells of origin.

HYPOXIA AND NECROSIS

The roles of hypoxia and necrosis in the tumorigenesis of kidney cancer and other cancers are slowly evolving. Hypoxia has been implicated as an important component in tumor progression and spread. Furthermore, hypoxia is a vital factor in the emergence of necrosis.[35] The latter parameter has been recently demonstrated to be a prognostic factor for poor outcome in breast cancer and renal cancer.[15,36,37]

The development of solid tumors may be explained by a two-step model. In the first stage, as tumors begin to grow, they adapt mechanisms to overcome the hypoxia

Table 1. Summary of histologic classification.

Histologic type	Origin	Variants
Clear cell (70–80% of RCC)	Proximal tubules	A) *Sporadic*—up to 60% may have VHL mutation B) *Hereditary*—Up to 40% of patients with VHL disease will develop clear cell RCC
Papillary (10–15% of RCC)	Proximal tubules	A) *Type 1*—basophilic cytoplasm; can be seen in hereditary papillary RCC = c-MET proto-oncogene (chromosome 7) B) *Type 2*—eosinophilic cytoplasm; can be seen in hereditary leiomyomatosis in women
Chromophobe (3–5%)	Intercalated cells of collecting ducts	A) Typical/Classical B) Eosinophilic/ Granular Both types can be seen in Birth Hogg Dube Syndrome
Collecting duct Very rare	Medulla of collecting ducts	Usually seen in African-Americans with sickle cell disease or trait
Unclassified RCC		For any tumors not fitting any of the above histologic criteria

★ All of the above tumors may undergo sarcomatoid differentiation.

associated with outgrowing their blood supply. In the second stage, the hypoxia triggers changes in gene expression that allows for cells to adapt to the hypoxia.[38]

These changes lead to a microenvironment within and around the tumor characterized by low oxygen, high hydrostatic pressure, and an acidic extracellular pH.[38] Defects in VHL allows stabilization of HIF-1, especially in a hypoxic environment. Stabilization of HIF-1 subsequently leads to increased levels of several target genes, including vascular endothelial growth factor (VEGF), glucose transporters, and surface transmembrane carbonic anhydrases.[38]

Areas of necrosis have been correlated with carbonic anhydrase IX (CA9) expression. This gene is hypoxia-inducible and is upregulated by hypoxia-inducible factor-1.[35] Increased CA9 has been associated with perinecrotic regions of several tumor types.[38,39] Further details on the role of CA9 in RCC can be found in the molecular markers section. However, the role of necrosis as a prognostic factor has recently emerged as an important parameter in renal tumors.

In one study, a multivariate analysis that included TNM stage, Fuhrman grade, histologic subtype, size, and vascular invasion, demonstrated that the presence of necrosis in the tumor carried a hazard ratio of 3.1 ($p < 0.001$) and was a poor predictor of DSS.[15] In another study, necrotic tumors were twice as likely to metastasize when compared to tumors that did not exhibit necrosis.[36]

STAGE

Tumor stage reflects the anatomic spread and involvement of disease. The stage of the tumor is recognized by most as being the most important prognostic factor for patients with RCC and has the greatest impact upon its clinical behavior.[40] The first formal staging system for RCC was proposed by Flocks and Kadesky in 1958 and was based upon the physical characteristics of the tumor and the location of tumor spread.[41] Robson later modified these criteria in 1969 by proposing that staging should also take vascular involvement into account.[42] This staging system became widely used but was later demonstrated not to directly correlate with prognosis.[40,43]

Currently, the two most commonly used staging systems in use are Robson's modification of the system described by Flocks and Kadesky[42] and the Tumor-Node-Metastasis (TNM) system proposed by the International Union Against Cancer. With the advent of the TNM staging system, more accurate classification of the extent of tumor involvement was achieved.[44] The TNM system is notable for its systematic emphasis on local spread, nodal spread, and distant metastasis. Further subdividing Robson's criteria, this staging system was initially considered too complex, hampered by an excessive number of staging categories. However, the system was refined and simplified in 1992, organizing stage groupings according to tumor size, vascular spread, lymph node involvement, and metastasis. With these changes, this staging system was found to be a significant prognostic indicator, correlating with survival and disease free periods throughout all stage categories.[45,46]

In 1997, these criteria were altered to mirror the improved results attained with the management of RCC. This fifth edition of the TNM system was the result of a collaborative effort by an international workshop that included the UICC and the AJCC.[47] The T1 stage was expanded from less than 2.5 cm to include tumors measuring less than 7 cm since it was noted that the lower size cut-off did not generate statistically significant survival differences.[48,49] In addition, tumor thrombus located above the diaphragm, previously staged T4, was changed to stage T3c. Similarly, thrombus involvement of the IVC below the diaphragm, previously staged T3c, was changed to T3b along with renal vein involvement.[47]

Table 2 depicts the fifth edition of the TNM staging system in its current format. Using the 1997 TNM to predict survival, Tsui et al, reported 5-year DSS rates of 91%, 74%, 67%, and 32% for stages I through IV, respectively.[50] Other investigators have reported similar survival results for the respective TNM stages.[49,51–53] In addition, analysis of survival in terms of T stage demonstrated survival rates of 83%, 57%, 42%, and 28% for T1, T2, T3, and T4, respectively.[50] Multivariate analysis in this study cohort demonstrated that overall TNM stage, grade, and Eastern Cooperative Oncology Group (ECOG) score represent the most important prognostic factors for RCC.

TUMOR SIZE

Both the Robson and TNM staging systems include tumors confined to the renal capsule, although the Robson system does not take primary tumor size into account. Recognition of a size-dependent survival difference, perhaps due to microscopic metastasis, favors the use of the TNM system.[54] The TNM system currently categorizes any tumors less than or equal 7 cm as T1; however, recent studies have suggested that the breakpoint for T1 tumors should be decreased.[53,55–58]

Table 2. Tumor, nodes, and metastasis staging system for renal cell carcinoma according to the 1997 UICC/AJCC consensus classification.[47]

T1	Tumor less than or equal to 7.0 cm in greatest dimension, limited to the kidney
T2	Tumor greater than 7.0 cm in greatest dimension, limited to the kidney
T3a	Tumor invades adrenal gland or perinephric tissues, but confined by Gerota's fascia
T3b	Tumor extends into the renal vein or into the inferior vena cava below the level of the diaphram
T3c	Tumor extends into the vena cava above the level of the diaphgram
T4	Tumor extends beyond Gerota's fascia
N0	No regional lymph node metastasis
N1	Metastasis to a single regional lymph node
N2	Metastasis to a more than one regional lymph node
M0	No evidence of distant metastasis
M1	Distant metastasis

Using the T, N, M components to set the 1997 TNM stage.

Stage I	T1	N0	M0
Stage II	T2	N0	M0
Stage III	T1, T2	N1	M0
	T3	N0, N1	M0
Stage IV	T4	N0, N1	M0
	Any T	N2	M0
	Any T	Any N	M1

Based on classic autopsy studies, Bell first reported an association between tumor size and prognosis for patients with RCC based on 160 cases of renal tumors in 30,000 autopsies, noting an increased propensity for the development of metastasis for tumors greater than 3 centimeters.[59] Grignon et al have further demonstrated that tumor size by itself is an independent, significant predictor of patient outcome.[60] The optimal breakpoint in size criteria to stage localized RCC remains controversial.

In a review of 485 patients who underwent nephron sparing surgery, the Cleveland Clinic reported a greater than 90% 10-year DSS in 310 patients with tumors smaller than 4 cm.[57] By comparison, the 10-year DSS in patients with tumors measuring 4 to 7 cm (125 patients) was 71% and dropped to 62% in patients with tumors over 7 cm (50 patients). They concluded that cancer-free survival is significantly better in patients with tumors 4 cm or less and recommended subdividing T1 tumors into T1a (4 cm or less) and T1b (4 to 7 cm).

The Mayo clinic recently published its recommendations based on a review of 840 pathologic T1 tumors. In their analysis, a tumor size cutoff of 5 cm had the highest risk ratio for predicting DSS in patients with clear cell RCC.[56] This cutoff of 5 cm was determined based on univariate and multivariate Cox proportional hazards that determined that tumors greater than 5 cm carried a risk ratio of 4.93 ($p < 0.001$).[56] Grade 1 and 2 tumors smaller than 5 cm had a 97% 10-year DSS compared to 85% for tumors 5 cm to 7 cm. For patients with grade 3 and 4 tumors, the DSS at 10 years was 92% for tumors less than 5 cm compared to 59% for tumors 5 to 7 cm.[56]

Table 3. Fuhrman grading scheme of renal cell carcinoma.[63]

Grade	Characteristics Nuclei	Nucleoi	Size
1	Round and uniform contour	Absent or minute	10 μm nuclei
2	Irregular contour	Visible at 400×	15 μm nuclei
3	Very irregular contour	Visible at 100×	20 μm nuclei
4	Bizarre and irregular	Chromatin	At least 20 μm

Finally, Zisman et al at UCLA also evaluated the 1997 TNM classification and found that a cutoff point of 4.5 cm predicted clinical outcome better than a cutoff point of 7 cm. Using Cox model analysis, 11 potential cutoff points between 1 and 10 cm were evaluated. A cutoff point of 4.5 cm revealed a hazard ratio of 4.99 (p = 0.0001) and was found to be most predictive of clinical outcome.[58] Other investigators have suggested cutoff points of 5.5 cm,[53] 8 cm,[61] and 10 cm.[62] An international conference is set to occur in Paris in 2002 which will likely lead to a change in the definitions of T1 and T2 disease.

TUMOR GRADE

Second in importance only to tumor stage, nearly all histopathologic, tumor-grading systems have shown independent prognostic value in studies in which grade was included as a variable.[62–65] The first report on the correlation between grading and patient outcome was published in the United States in 1932.[66]

Although microscopic grading has provided no additional prognostic value when tumor stage is accounted for, nuclear grading has shown to be a valuable prognostic indicator of patient survival. In 1971, Skinner et al directed attention to the correlation between nuclear features and survival.[64] These observations were later expanded into a four-tier scheme based on nuclear size, conspicuousness of nucleoli, shape, and content as proposed by Fuhrman that remains the most commonly used system in North America.[63] Table 3 depicts the original Fuhrman grading scheme. Unfortunately, controversy still exists concerning the inter-observer reproducibility of grading as well as disagreement regarding relevant breakpoints between the different grades and survival.

The 1997 UICC/AJCC international consensus conference on renal cell carcinoma also took up the issue of grading.[67] The conference proposed the development of a new grading scheme that is easier to apply and is based on patient outcome, suggesting the combination of the first two grades in Fuhrman's system to convert it into a three grade system. Such a system has not yet been developed. Using the current system, fewer than 10% of cases are grade 1, grade 2 and 3 each represent approximately 35% of cases, and about 20% are grade 4.[62] At UCLA, the 5-year DSS rates based on tumor grade was recently reported to be 89% for grade 1, 65% for grade 2, and 46.1% for grades 3 and 4.[50]

Mayo clinic stratified their patients according to low-grade (grades 1 and 2) and high-grade (3 and 4) tumors. In patients who had tumors measuring over 5 cm in size, the 5-year DSS was 85% for low-grade tumors versus 59% for hi-grade tumors.[56] In another recent review of 405 cases, grade 1, 2, 3, and 4 tumors had 5-year DSS of 100%, 94%, 80%, and 35%, respectively.[15]

NODAL STATUS

Regional lymphadenopathy appears to have tremendous impact on patient response to immunotherapy (IMT) as well as prognosis. The clinical outcomes and responses to IMT of 180 patients at UCLA with metastatic disease who were either regional node-positive or node-negative were analyzed. In those patients with metastatic disease, there was a 31% response rate with IL-2 in patients without regional nodes compared to only a 3% response rate in patients with pathologic evidence of regional nodes.[68]

Survival was significantly improved by administration of IL-2 (p = 0.03) in patients without regional lymph node involvement. Patients with positive nodes had a median survival time of 10 months regardless of whether or not they received IMT. Those patients with negative nodes and receiving IMT had prolonged survival with a median time to death of 19 months compared to 12 months in those patients who did not receive IMT.[68]

In contrast, Vasselli et al found no significant difference in IL-2 response rates with or without lymphadenopathy in their retrospective study of 154 patients with metastatic RCC.[69] However, in their multivariate analysis, lymphadenopathy was a better predictor of survival than performance status.

Finally, at the 2001 Society of Urologic Oncology, the role of lymph node dissection was examined and presented. Pantuck et al showed that lymph node dissection does not provide survival benefit in patients without nodal disease.[68] However, in patients with evidence of nodal disease, lymph node dissection improved median survival from 9 months to 14 months (p = 0.0002).

In summary, with regards to lymph node dissection, there is limited staging value in patients with clinically negative nodes. Furthermore, there is no therapeutic value. However, patients with clinical evidence of nodal involvement should undergo lymph node dissection for several reasons. Pathologic confirmation of nodal involvement provides prognostic value since patients with nodal involvement fare significantly worse. At UCLA, lymph node dissection in patients with pathologic evidence of nodal involvement has been demonstrated to provide survival benefit.[68] Lymph node dissection can be achieved with little added morbidity and should be performed when technically feasible as part of an integrated treatment plan including surgery and immunotherapy in properly selected patients.

PATIENT PERFORMANCE STATUS

The Karnofsky and Eastern Cooperative Oncology Group (ECOG) patient performance status (PS) scales are convenient common denominators for the overall impact of multiple objective and subjective symptoms and signs on patients. These scales are often used as eligibility criteria for high dose interleukin-2 (IL-2) immunotherapy regimens as well as for entry into clinical trials. The ECOG scores are based on the activity levels of patients, ranging from a score of 0 (fully active) to 4 (bedridden).[70] Several studies have demonstrated that ECOG is a good prognostic factor for patients with metastatic RCC at presentation and can help guide decision making in regards to treatment.[71–73]

Recently, it has been suggested that the utility of ECOG as a prognostic factor can be extended to all stages of RCC.[74] RCC patients with ECOG values ≥1 were found to have a significantly lower five-year survival of 51% as compared to the 81% five-year survival for patients with an ECOG of 0. This difference was found to be an independent prognostic factor of survival. It is not surprising that ECOG PS is an important prognostic variable since it makes intuitive sense as patients with RCC that are more symptomatic and debilitated by the cancer most likely have more advanced, metastatic disease.[27]

OTHER PATIENT-RELATED FACTORS

A number of other clinical characteristics have been identified as having an impact on the clinical behavior and subsequent survival in patients with advanced RCC. These include, in addition to initial performance status, time from diagnosis to metastasis, location and number of metastatic sites as well as weight loss and whether the patient has undergone a nephrectomy or still has the primary tumor in place.[70,75–78]

In 1988, Elson et al developed a scoring system to determine prognosis for patients with advanced RCC, stratifying patients into 5 groups based on ECOG performance status, time from diagnosis to metastasis, weight loss, prior chemotherapy, and number of metastatic sites.[70] Expected median survival ranged from 2.1 to 12.8 months depending on the number of risk points and prognostic group. Citterio et al, using a similar approach, identified prognostic subgroups based on ECOG performance status and blood hemoglobin level.[71]

Most recently, Motzer et al have developed a model based on the study of 670 patients with advanced RCC treated at Memorial Sloan-Kettering Cancer Center defining the relationship between pre-treatment clinical features and survival.[79] Median overall survival was 10 months, and 5 pretreatment features were identified to be associated with a shorter survival as determined by multivariate analysis. These included low Karnofsky performance status, high serum lactate dehydrogenase (LDH) levels (>1.5 times normal), low hemoglobin (< lower limit or normal), hypercalcemia (>10 mg/dl), and absence of prior nephrectomy. Poor risk patients with three or more risk factors had a median survival time of only 4 months, whereas median survival improved to 20 months in patients with zero risk factors. Further details on this study are found in Chapter 8 (Dr. Motzer).

Incidental versus Symptomatic Presentation. RCC progression can be indolent, growing to various sizes before becoming clinically apparent. The location of the kidneys in the retroperitoneum tends to delay detection of symptoms until the tumor involves adjacent structures or involves the collecting system. Fortunately, more and more cases of RCC are being detected incidentally with the increased use of ultrasound and abdominal computed tomography (CT) for other reasons in otherwise asymptomatic patients.[6,80]

Several studies looking at the clinical significance of early detection of RCC prior to the onset symptoms demonstrated that incidental RCCs tended to be smaller, lower stage lesions that yielded better survival outcomes than RCC tumors detected in symptomatic patients.[81,82]

The records of 633 consecutive patients undergoing either radical or partial nephrectomy for RCC at the UCLA Medical Center between 1987 and 1998 were reviewed.[50] Ninety-five of 633 (15%) of patients had incidentally discovered tumors, while the other 538 patients (85%) presented with signs and symptoms. Patient age and sex distributions were similar in the two groups. In this retrospective analysis, incidental tumors were significantly lower in both stage and grade than tumors that produced symptoms. Furthermore, these clinically and histologically less aggressive lesions led to better survival rates and decreased recurrence rates. The 5-year DSS rate was found to be significantly higher for incidental tumors (85.3%) than for symptomatic lesions (62.5%). It is noteworthy that when stage was adjusted for, the differences in survival between incidental versus symptomatic presentation disappeared. The improved survival in incidentally detected tumors was attributed to earlier diagnoses of lower stage, lower grade, and smaller tumors.

THE UCLA INTEGRATED STAGING SYSTEM (UISS)

The UCLA Integrated Staging System (UISS) combines pathological staging information with some of these additional prognostic variables in order to better stratify patients into prognostic categories using statistical tools that can accurately define an individual patient's probability of survival.[74] A staging system with 5 categories based on the most significant explanatory variables, namely TNM stage, grade, and ECOG performance status.

The projected 2 and 5 year survival for patients in UISS group I are: 96% and 94%, II: 89% and 67%, III: 66% and 39%, IV: 42% and 23%, and 9% and 0% for group V, respectively. This novel system for staging and predicting survival for patients with RCC is simple to use, superior to stage alone in differentiating patients' survival, any may prove to be an important prognostic tool for counseling patients with various stages of kidney cancer. Details of this staging system can be found in Chapter 3 (Dr. Zisman's chapter).

The UISS was recently simplified further in an effort to better predict patient outcome. Based on metastatic status, patients were categorized into low, intermediate, and high-risk groups for both non-metastatic (NM) or localized disease and metastatic (M) disease. Patients in the NM low-risk, intermediate-risk, and high-risk groups had overall 5-year survivals of 84%, 72%, and 44%, respectively.[83] In patients with M low-risk, intermediate-risk, and high-risk, the overall 5-year survival rates were 30%, 19%, and 0%, respectively.[83]

Table 4. College of American Pathologists classification scheme of prognostic factors.[85]

Category	Definition
I	Well supported by the literature and used in patient management. Examples include grade, stage, histology.
IIA	Factors studied biologically. Has not been rigorously validated to be of clinical value.
IIB	Studied clinically. Has not been rigorously validated to be of clinical value.
III	Factors that show promise, but do not meet criteria in I or II

• adapted from.[85]

Finally, Zisman et al recently used the Nadas equation to construct a mathematical model to predict individual survival for patients with renal cell carcinoma.[84] Using the Nadas equation allows any multivariate analysis to be carried one step further and delineate the interplay of a number of significant variables associated with survival. By using this mathematical model, Zisman et al reported that Fuhrman grade and Eastern Cooperative Oncology Group performance status were significant variables in patients with localized or non-metastatic disease. For patients with metastatic disease, Fuhrman's grade, 1997 T stage, number of symptoms, nodal involvement, and immunotherapy were all independent predictors of survival.[84]

MOLECULAR MARKERS AS PROGNOSTIC FACTORS

Molecular tumor markers for renal cell carcinoma are expected to have an enormous impact on the diagnosis and treatment of RCC. Tumor markers provide not only prognostic information to aid in the identification of patients at risk for recurrence or metastasis but could hold the key to targeted therapeutic interventions as well. Currently, many markers relating to tumor proliferation, growth, angiogenesis and loss of cell adhesion are being evaluated for their potential as prognostic factors. Some are promising but clinical trials are needed to validate their usefulness in clinical practice. Table 4 summarizes the classification scheme used by the College of American Pathologists to define the scientific merit and clinical relevance of prognostic factors.[85] Table 5 lists the molecular markers that are discussed next.

DNA ploidy has been extensively studied clinically for it prognostic value Aneuploid DNA content pertains to a cell population in which the DNA index differs from diploid. Deviation from the normal diploid pattern is evidence of genomic instability that may generate clones with enhanced survival and metastatic capacity.[86] Determinations may be made by flow cytometry or image analysis. The histological variants of RCC which have demonstrated aneuploidy include collecting duct, chromophobe and papillary carcinoma. Changes in ploidy in papillary carcinoma correlates with grade, stage and prognosis.[87] Most, but not all, studies of RCC have shown good correlation between DNA ploidy and other prognostic parameters such as grade and stage. Therefore, its usefulness in RCC prognosis, at this time, is still inconclusive.

Table 5. Potential candidates for prognostication of RCC.

Prognostic factor	Unfavorable feature	CAP category
DNA ploidy	Deviation from normal diploid pattern	IIB (clinical)
Proliferation markers		
AgNOR	Increase in AgNOR proteins may be seen in aneuploid tumors	IIB
Ki-67	Increased levels may be associated with unfavorable grade and decreased survival	IIB
PCNA	Increased levels may be associated with increased recurrence rates and decreased survival	III
Apoptosis markers		
p53	Mutation leads to inhibition of apoptosis	III
bcl-2	Overexpression of bcl-2 inhibits apoptosis	III
p21	Also controls cell cycling	III
Clusterin	Increased levels may portend to worse prognosis by inhibiting apoptosis	III
Surface markers		
CA-125	Elevated levels may predict for poor prognosis	III
E-cadherin	No value thus far	III
Carbonic anhydrase 9	Increased levels may confer survival benefit, especially in those with metastatic disease	III
Angiogenesis		
VEGF	No value thus far	III

Abbreviations
CAP   = College of American Pathologists.
AgNOR = Silver-stained nucleolar organizer regions.
PCNA   = Proliferating cell nuclear antigen.
VEGF   = Vascular endothelial growth factor.

Proliferation Markers

Tumor markers of cellular proliferation such as AgNOR score, Ki-67 and proliferating cell nuclear antigen (PCNA) are also being investigated as prognostic markers. AgNORs are chromosomal DNA loops encoding ribosomal RNA detectable by silver staining. An increase in AgNOR proteins may be due to an increased demand for ribosomal biogenesis which occurs in aneuploid tumors.[88] In a multivariate analysis, the AgNOR score correlated with grade and survival and therefore added significant prognostic value.[89–92]

Ki-67 is a nuclear antigen that is present in all cycling human cells and is a marker for active cell proliferation. Immunohistochemical staining of Ki-67 provides an index that estimates the growth fraction of a population of cells. Labeling indices of Ki-67 correlates with grade and survival in RCC, providing additional prognostic indication of biological aggressiveness.[93–95]

Proliferating cell nuclear antigen (PCNA), like Ki-67, is also a marker for predicting biological aggressiveness of renal cell tumors. PCNA expression has been correlated with recurrence[93] and survival.[96]

Apoptosis Markers

Potential markers associated with apoptosis include p53, bcl-2, p21, and clusterin. p53 overexpression has been found in a wide variety of cancers. Normal, wild type p53 binds DNA and causes cell cycle arrest, allowing for DNA repair or apoptosis in cells damaged beyond repair. However, mutations in p53 may lead to tumor progression in certain cancers. However, unlike bladder cancer, the role of p53 remains undefined. Several series have not confirmed p53 to be a significant prognostic factor.[97–99]

Bcl-2 is involved with inhibition of apoptosis and its overexpression has been proposed to block programmed cell death, leading to a proliferation of malignant cells. However, the role of bcl-2 in RCC remains unclear and several studies evaluating its prognostic value have not found bcl-2 to be a useful marker.[97,100,101]

Similar to p53, p21 controls cell cycling in quiescent cells. However, just like p53 and bcl-2, its role in RCC has been limited.[6] In a recent study of 118 cases, multivariate analysis demonstrated that p21 had no prognostic value and was expressed in 6.8% of cases.[102]

Finally, clusterin is the latest of the apoptosis-related molecules to be investigated in RCC. Miyake et al recently studied the RNA of 93 nonpapillary RCC's via Northern blot analysis.[103] They compared 48 cases with strong clusterin mRNA expression to 45 cases with either weak or nonexistent expression. Strong clusterin expression was associated with increased T stage and increased recurrence risk. Furthermore, multivariate analyses revealed that strong expression of clusterin was an independent predictor of increased recurrence and decreased overall survival.[103]

Carbonic Anhydrase

The MN/CA9/G250 protein, a member of the carbonic anhydrase family, is a tumor-associated antigen that has selective high expression in RCC.[104,105] In one study, MN/CA9/G250 expression was seen in 42 of 49 (86%) RCC samples, but in only 2 of 22 (9%) normal kidney and none of five oncocytoma samples.[106] Similarly, immunohistochemical analysis in another study demonstrated strong expression in 128/147 (87.1%) of RCCs, in contrast to the lack of expression observed in normal tissues.[107]

Furthermore, MN/CA9/G250 expression appears to be selective for clear cell subtypes with 92% positive staining by immunohistochemistry. There are limited studies of MN/CA9/G250 as prognostic factor. Tumours of low clinical stage showed a striking increase in MN/CA9/G250 expression, and high MN/CA9/G250 expression was associated with a good patient outcome.[106]

Recent work from UCLA has demonstrated that increased expression of CA9 may confer survival benefit in patients with metastatic clear cell RCC.[108] Survival tree analysis determined that a cut-off of 85% CA9 staining provided the most accurate prediction of survival. Low CA9 staining (<85%) was an independent poor prognostic factor for patients with metastatic RCC (HR 3.10, $p < 0.001$).[108] Variables analyzed in the multivariate analysis included ECOG PS, tumor stage, grade, and nodal involvement.

Even more impressively, patients with high-risk localized disease (i.e. T3/T4 disease), but high CA9 levels had similar survival rates to patients with low-risk, low-CA9 expression patients. Patients in the former group had a median survival of 16.7 months, while the low-risk, but low CA9 patients had a median survival of 12.2 months.[108] Based on their preliminary findings, Bui et al predicted that CA9 may eventually a role in both the prognostication and treatment of patients with RCC.

Microsatellite Analysis

Aberrations in repetitive genomic elements known as microsatellite sequences have been increasingly used as diagnostic markers for detection of cancers such as breast, bladder, and lung cancer.[109] Microsatellite alterations are tumor-specific changes that have been used to detect cancer cells in bodily fluids such as serum, urine, and sputum. A recent publication investigated a panel of 28 microsatellite markers to assess loss of heterozygosity (LOH) and microsatellite instability in the urine, serum, and tumors of DNA of 30 patients with clinically organ-confined RCC. In this study, the frequency of microsatellite alterations (loss of heterozygosity) found in the preoperative serum of patients with renal masses was an independent predictor of disease recurrence.[109]

In another microsatellite analysis, Presti et al correlated allelic loss of chromosomes 8p, 9p, and 14q with clinical outcome in locally advanced clear cell carcinoma.[110] The authors analyzed 72 P3N0 radical nephrectomy specimens and detected the following: LOH on chromosome 3p in 60 of 64 (94%), on 8p in 19 of 59 (32%), on 9p in 21 of 67 (33%) and on 14q in 18 of 70 (26%). Twenty-four of 72 (33%) had recurrence. On univariate analysis, patients with LOH on chromosomes 8p and 9q were at highest risk for recurrence. Even more impressively, multivariate analysis revealed that LOH was a more powerful predictor of recurrence than grade.[110]

Vascular Endothelial Growth Factor

Cell markers associated with metastatic potential such as vascular endothelial growth factor (VEGF) have been recognized as an important factor in the angiogenesis, vascularization, and growth of tumors. However, several analyses have not shown VEGF to be an independent prognostic factor despite the detection of elevated levels in patients having tumors with venous invasion.[111,112]

Recently, investigators have demonstrated that tumors that spread via lymphatics may do so with the aid of VEGF-D.[113] In this study, Stacker et al used SCID mice to demonstrate that VEGF-D can induce both tumor angiogenesis and lymphangiogenesis whereas VEGF induces only angiogenesis. It remains to be seen whether tumors expressing increased levels of VEGF-D and therefore a potentially increased propensity to develop nodal metastases may behave more aggressively.

CONCLUSION

For tumor-related prognostic factors, tumor grade and stage remain the most useful available predictors of clinical outcome. The TNM staging system more accurately classifies the extent of tumor involvement and relates directly to prognosis. Furthermore, tumor grading is second in importance only to stage and provides independent prognostic value based on nuclear size, shape and content. Important patient-related prognostic factors include symptomatic presentation, weight loss, performance status, laboratory findings and response to treatment.

Molecular markers are the next frontier in prognostic factors. Although statistical significance and independence from other factors has been shown for several biomolecular markers such as AgNOR, Ki-67 and PCNA, there have been delays due to reproducibility and lack of clinical validation to allow them to be used directly for patient management. On the other hand, molecular marker profiles will, hopefully, soon be ready for widespread use. The markers available are highly promising as prognostic tools but still need critical clinical validation.

REFERENCES

1. Jemal A, Thomas A, Murray T, Thun M. Cancer statistics, 2002. CA Cancer J Clin 2002; 52:23–47.
2. Figlin RA. Renal cell carcinoma: management of advanced disease. J Urol 1999; 161:381–6; discussion 386–7.
3. Storkel S, Eble JN, Adlakha K, et al. Classification of renal cell carcinoma: Workgroup No. 1. Union Internationale Contre le Cancer (UICC) and the American Joint Committee on Cancer (AJCC). Cancer 1997; 80:987–9.
4. Union Internationale Contre le Cancer (UICC) and the American Joint Committee on Cancer (AJCC). Workshop on Diagnosis and Prognosis of Renal Cell Carcinoma. Rochester, Minnesota, March 21–22, 1997. Cancer 1997; 80:973–1000.
5. Zambrano NR, Lubensky IA, Merino MJ, Linehan WM, Walther MM. Histopathology and molecular genetics of renal tumors toward unification of a classification system. J Urol 1999; 162: 1246–58.
6. Bui MH, Zisman A, Pantuck AJ, Han K, Wieder J, Belldegrun A. Prognostic factors and molecular markers for renal cell carcinoma. Expert Reviews in Anticancer Therapy 2001; 1:565–75.
7. Pantuck AJ, Zisman A, Belldegrun A. Biology of renal cell carcinoma: changing concepts in classification and staging. Semin Urol Oncol 2001; 19:72–9.
8. Said JW, Thomas G, Zisman A. Kidney Pathology: Current classification of renal cell carcinoma. Current Urology Reports 2002; 3:25–30.
9. Linehan W, Zbar B, Bates S, Zelefsky M, Yang J. Cancer of the kidney and ureter. In: DeVita S, Hellman S, SA R, eds. Cancer Principles and Practice of Oncology. Philadelphia: Lippincott-Raven, 2001:1362–96.
10. Thoenes W, Storkel S, Rumpelt HJ. Histopathology and classification of renal cell tumors (adenomas, oncocytomas and carcinomas). The basic cytological and histopathological elements and their use for diagnostics. Pathol Res Pract 1986; 181:125–43.
11. Kovacs G. Papillary renal cell carcinoma. A morphologic and cytogenetic study of 11 cases. Am J Pathol 1989; 134:27–34.
12. Delahunt B, Eble JN. Papillary renal cell carcinoma: a clinicopathologic and immunohistochemical study of 105 tumors. Mod Pathol 1997; 10:537–44.
13. Schmidt L, Duh FM, Chen F, et al. Germline and somatic mutations in the tyrosine kinase domain of the MET proto-oncogene in papillary renal carcinomas. Nat Genet 1997; 16:68–73.
14. Sweeney P, El-Naggar AK, Lin SH, Pisters LL. Biological Significance of C-met Over Expression in Papillary Renal Cell Carcinoma. J Urol 2002; 168:51–5.
15. Amin MB, Tamboli P, Javidan J, et al. Prognostic Impact of Histologic Subtyping of Adult Renal Epithelial Neoplasms: An Experience of 405 Cases. Am J Surg Pathol 2002; 26:281–91.
16. Nagashima Y. Chromophobe renal cell carcinoma: clinical, pathological and molecular biological aspects. Pathol Int 2000; 50:872–8.
17. Schmidt LS, Warren MB, Nickerson ML, et al. Birt-Hogg-Dube syndrome, a genodermatosis associated with spontaneous pneumothorax and kidney neoplasia, maps to chromosome 17p11.2. Am J Hum Genet 2001; 69:876–82.

18. Chao D, Zisman A, Pantuck AJ, et al. Collecting duct renal cell carcinoma: clinical study of a rare tumor. J Urol 2002; 167:71–4.
19. Davis CJ, Jr., Mostofi FK, Sesterhenn IA. Renal medullary carcinoma. The seventh sickle cell nephropathy. Am J Surg Pathol 1995; 19:1–11.
20. Kennedy SM, Merino MJ, Linehan WM, Roberts JR, Robertson CN, Neumann RD. Collecting duct carcinoma of the kidney. Hum Pathol 1990; 21:449–56.
21. Avery RA, Harris JE, Davis CJ, Jr., Borgaonkar DS, Byrd JC, Weiss RB. Renal medullary carcinoma: clinical and therapeutic aspects of a newly described tumor. Cancer 1996; 78:128–32.
22. Zisman A, Chao DH, Pantuck AJ, et al. Unclassified renal cell carcinoma: clinical features and prognostic impact of a new histologic subtype. Journal of Urology In press.
23. Kattan MW, Reuter V, Motzer RJ, Katz J, Russo P. A postoperative prognostic nomogram for renal cell carcinoma. J Urol 2001; 166:63–7.
24. Bielsa O, Lloreta J, Gelabert-Mas A. Cystic renal cell carcinoma: pathological features, survival and implications for treatment. Br J Urol 1998; 82:16–20.
25. Sherman ME, Silverman ML, Balogh K, Tan SS. Multilocular renal cyst. A hamartoma with potential for neoplastic transformation? Arch Pathol Lab Med 1987; 111:732–6.
26. Corica FA, Iczkowski KA, Cheng L, et al. Cystic renal cell carcinoma is cured by resection: a study of 24 cases with long-term followup. J Urol 1999; 161:408–11.
27. Pantuck AJ, Zisman A, Belldegrun AS. The changing natural history of renal cell carcinoma. J Urol 2001; 166:1611–23.
28. Sella A, Logothetis CJ, Ro JY, Swanson DA, Samuels ML. Sarcomatoid renal cell carcinoma. A treatable entity. Cancer 1987; 60:1313–18.
29. Tomera KM, Farrow GM, Lieber MM. Sarcomatoid renal carcinoma. J Urol 1983; 130:657–9.
30. Oda H, Machinami R. Sarcomatoid renal cell carcinoma. A study of its proliferative activity. Cancer 1993; 71:2292–8.
31. Farrow GM, Harrison EG, Jr., Utz DC, ReMine WH. Sarcomas and sarcomatoid and mixed malignant tumors of the kidney in adults. I. Cancer 1968; 22:545–50.
32. Selli C, Hinshaw WM, Woodard BH, Paulson DF. Stratification of risk factors in renal cell carcinoma. Cancer 1983; 52:899–903.
33. Ro JY, Ayala AG, Sella A, Samuels ML, Swanson DA. Sarcomatoid renal cell carcinoma: clinicopathologic. A study of 42 cases. Cancer 1987; 59:516–26.
34. Cangiano T, Liao J, Naitoh J, Dorey F, Figlin R, Belldegrun A. Sarcomatoid renal cell carcinoma: biologic behavior, prognosis, and response to combined surgical resection and immunotherapy. J Clin Oncol 1999; 17:523–8.
35. Chia SK, Wykoff CC, Watson PH, et al. Prognostic significance of a novel hypoxia-regulated marker, carbonic anhydrase IX, in invasive breast carcinoma. J Clin Oncol 2001; 19:3660–8.
36. Lau W, Blute M, Cheville J. Pathologic stage T1 renal cell carcinoma: prognostic value of tumor subtype, size, and Fuhrman grade after radical nephrectomy. Urology 2002; in press.
37. Fisher ER, Anderson S, Redmond C, Fisher B. Pathologic findings from the National Surgical Adjuvant Breast Project protocol B-06. 10-year pathologic and clinical prognostic discriminants. Cancer 1993; 71:2507–14.
38. Ivanov S, Liao SY, Ivanova A, et al. Expression of hypoxia-inducible cell-surface transmembrane carbonic anhydrases in human cancer. Am J Pathol 2001; 158:905–19.
39. Olive PL, Aquino-Parsons C, MacPhail SH, et al. Carbonic anhydrase 9 as an endogenous marker for hypoxic cells in cervical cancer. Cancer Res 2001; 61:8924–9.
40. Pantuck AJ, Zisman A, Belldegrun A. Biology of renal cell carcinoma: changing concepts in classification and staging. Seminars in Urologic Oncology 2001; 19:72–9.
41. Flocks R, Kadesky M. Malignant neoplasms of the kidney: analysis of 353 patients followed 5 years or more. Trans Am Assoc Genitouri Surg 1958; 49:105.
42. Robson CJ, Churchill BM, Anderson W. The results of radical nephrectomy for renal cell carcinoma. Journal of Urology 1969; 101.
43. Belldegrun AS, deKernion JB. Renal Tumors. In: Walsh PC, Retik AB, Vaughan JED, Wein AJ, eds. Campbell's Urology. Vol. 3. Philadelphia: W.B. Saunders Co., 1998:2283–326.
44. Bassil B, Dosoretz DE, Prout GR, Jr. Validation of the tumor, nodes and metastasis classification of renal cell carcinoma. J Urol 1985; 134:450–4.
45. Hofmockel G, Tsatalpas P, Muller H, et al. Significance of conventional and new prognostic factors for locally confined renal cell carcinoma. Cancer 1995; 76:296–306.
46. Ruiz JL, Hernandez M, Martinez J, Vera C, Jimenez-Cruz JF. Value of morphometry as an independent prognostic factor in renal cell carcinoma. Eur Urol 1995; 27:54–7.

47. Guinan P, Sobin LH, Algaba F, et al. TNM staging of renal cell carcinoma: Workgroup No. 3. Union International Contre le Cancer (UICC) and the American Joint Committee on Cancer (AJCC). Cancer 1997; 80:992–3.
48. Hermanek P, Schrott KM. Evaluation of the new tumor, nodes and metastases classification of renal cell carcinoma. J Urol 1990; 144:238–41; discussion 241–2.
49. Guinan P, Frank W, Saffrin R, Rubenstein M. Staging and survival of patients with renal cell carcinoma. Semin Surg Oncol 1994; 10:47–50.
50. Tsui KH, Shvarts O, Smith RB, Figlin RA, deKernion JB, Belldegrun A. Prognostic indicators for renal cell carcinoma: a multivariate analysis of 643 patients using the revised 1997 TNM staging criteria. J Urol 2000; 163:1090–5; quiz 1295.
51. Javidan J, Stricker HJ, Tamboli P, et al. Prognostic significance of the 1997 TNM classification of renal cell carcinoma. J Urol 1999; 162:1277–81.
52. Stein JP, Kaji DM, Eastham J, Freeman JA, Esrig D, Hardy BE. Blunt renal trauma in the pediatric population: indications for radiographic evaluation. Urology 1994; 44:406–10.
53. Kinouchi T, Saiki S, Meguro N, et al. Impact of tumor size on the clinical outcomes of patients with Robson State I renal cell carcinoma. Cancer 1999; 85:689–95.
54. Gelb AB, Shibuya RB, Weiss LM, Medeiros LJ. Stage I renal cell carcinoma. A clinicopathologic study of 82 cases. Am J Surg Pathol 1993; 17:275–86.
55. Igarashi T, Tobe T, Nakatsu HO, et al. The impact of a 4 cm. cutoff point for stratification of T1N0M0 renal cell carcinoma after radical nephrectomy. J Urol 2001; 165:1103–6.
56. Lau WK, Cheville JC, Blute ML, Weaver AL, Zincke H. Prognostic features of pathologic stage T1 renal cell carcinoma after radical nephrectomy. Urology 2002; 59:532–7.
57. Hafez KS, Fergany AF, Novick AC. Nephron sparing surgery for localized renal cell carcinoma: impact of tumor size on patient survival, tumor recurrence and TNM staging. J Urol 1999; 162: 1930–3.
58. Zisman A, Pantuck AJ, Chao D, et al. Reevaluation of the 1997 TNM classification for renal cell carcinoma: T1 and T2 cutoff point at 4.5 rather than 7 cm. better correlates with clinical outcome. J Urol 2001; 166:54–8.
59. Bell E. A classification of renal tumors with observations on the frequency of the various types. Journal of Urology 1938; 39:238.
60. Grignon DJ, Ayala AG, el-Naggar A, et al. Renal cell carcinoma. A clinicopathologic and DNA flow cytometric analysis of 103 cases. Cancer 1989; 64:2133–40.
61. Green LK, Ayala AG, Ro JY, et al. Role of nuclear grading in stage I renal cell carcinoma. Urology 1989; 34:310–5.
62. Medeiros LJ, Gelb AB, Weiss LM. Renal cell carcinoma. Prognostic significance of morphologic parameters in 121 cases. Cancer 1988; 61:1639–51.
63. Fuhrman SA, Lasky LC, Limas C. Prognostic significance of morphologic parameters in renal cell carcinoma. Am J Surg Pathol 1982; 6:655–63.
64. Skinner DG, Colvin RB, Vermillion CD, Pfister RC, Leadbetter WF. Diagnosis and management of renal cell carcinoma. A clinical and pathologic study of 309 cases. Cancer 1971; 28:1165–77.
65. Thrasher JB, Paulson DF. Prognostic factors in renal cancer. Urol Clin North Am 1993; 20:247–62.
66. Hand J, Broders A. Carcinoma of the kidney: the degree of malignancy in relation to factors bearing on prognosis. Journal of Urology 1932; 28:199.
67. Medeiros LJ, Jones EC, Aizawa S, et al. Grading of renal cell carcinoma: Workgroup No. 2. Union Internationale Contre le Cancer and the American Joint Committee on Cancer (AJCC). Cancer 1997; 80:990–1.
68. Pantuck AJ, Zisman A, Chao D, et al. Regional lymphadenopathy during cytoreductive nephrectomy predcits IL-2 failure in patients with metastatic renal cell carcinoma. Proceedings of ASCO 2001; 20:172A.
69. Vasselli JR, Yang JC, Linehan WM, White DE, Rosenberg SA, Walther MM. Lack of retroperitoneal lymphadenopathy predicts survival of patients with metastatic renal cell carcinoma. J Urol 2001; 166:68–72.
70. Elson P, Witte R, Trump D. Prognostic factors for survival in patients with recurrent or metastatic renal cell carcinoma. Cancer Research 1988; 48:7310–13.
71. Citterio G, Bertuzzi A, Tresoldi M, et al. Prognostic factors for survival in metastatic renal cell carcinoma: retrospective analysis from 109 consecutive patients. Eur Urol 1997; 31:286–91.
72. Fallick ML, McDermott DF, LaRock D, Long JP, Atkins MB. Nephrectomy before interleukin-2 therapy for patients with metastatic renal cell carcinoma. J Urol 1997; 158:1691–5.

73. Mani S, Todd MB, Katz K, Poo WJ. Prognostic factors for survival in patients with metastatic renal cancer treated with biological response modifiers. J Urol 1995; 154:35–40.
74. Zisman A, AJ P, FD, et al. Improved prognostication using a novel integrated staging system (UISS) for renal cell carcinoma. Journal of Urology 2001; 165:660A.
75. Belldegrun A, Shvarts O, Figlin RA. Expanding the indications for surgery and adjuvant inter-leukin-2-based immunotherapy in patients with advanced renal cell carcinoma. Cancer J Sci Am 2000; 6 Suppl 1:S88–92.
76. Klugo RC, Detmers M, Stiles RE, Talley RW, Cerny JC. Aggressive versus conservative management of stage IV renal cell carcinoma. J Urol 1977; 118:244–6.
77. Dekernion JB, Ramming KP, Smith RB. The natural history of metastatic renal cell carcinoma: a computer analysis. J Urol 1978; 120:148–52.
78. Maldazys JD, deKernion JB. Prognostic factors in metastatic renal carcinoma. J Urol 1986; 136: 376–9.
79. Motzer RJ, Mazumdar M, Bacik J, Berg W, Amsterdam A, Ferrara J. Survival and prognostic stratification of 670 patients with advanced renal cell carcinoma. J Clin Oncol 1999; 17: 2530–40.
80. Homma Y, Kawabe K, Kitamura T, et al. Increased incidental detection and reduced mortality in renal cancer—recent retrospective analysis at eight institutions. Int J Urol 1995; 2:77–80.
81. Konnak JW, Grossman HB. Renal cell carcinoma as an incidental finding. J Urol 1985; 134:1094–6.
82. Thompson IM, Peek M. Improvement in survival of patients with renal carcinoma—the role of the serendipitously detected tumor. J Urol 1988; 140:487–90.
83. Zisman A, Pantuck AJ, Wieder JA, et al. Risk group assessment and clinical outcome algorithm to predict the natural history of surgically resected renal cell carcinoma. Submitted for publication 2002.
84. Zisman A, Pantuck AJ, Dorey F, et al. Mathematical model to predict individual survival for patients with renal cell carcinoma. J Clin Oncol 2002; 20:1368–74.
85. Srigley JR, Hutter RV, Gelb AB, et al. Current prognostic factors—renal cell carcinoma: Workgroup No. 4. Union Internationale Contre le Cancer (UICC) and the American Joint Committee on Cancer (AJCC). Cancer 1997; 80:994–6.
86. Bonsib SM. Risk and prognosis in renal neoplasms. A pathologist's prospective. Urol Clin North Am 1999; 26:643–60, viii.
87. Shishikura Y, Suzuki M. Clinicopathologic study of 97 cases of small renal cell carcinomas using DNA flow cytometric analyses. Pathol Int 1996; 46:947–52.
88. Gelb AB. Renal cell carcinoma: current prognostic factors. Union Internationale Contre le Cancer (UICC) and the American Joint Committee on Cancer (AJCC). Cancer 1997; 80:981–6.
89. Yasunaga Y, Shin M, Miki T, Okuyama A, Aozasa K. Prognostic factors of renal cell carcinoma: a multivariate analysis. J Surg Oncol 1998; 68:11–18.
90. Tannapfel A, Hahn HA, Katalinic A, Fietkau RJ, Kuhn R, Wittekind CW. Prognostic value of ploidy and proliferation markers in renal cell carcinoma. Cancer 1996; 77:164–71.
91. Delahunt B, Ribas JL, Nacey JN, Bethwaite PB. Nucleolar organizer regions and prognosis in renal cell carcinoma. J Pathol 1991; 163:31–7.
92. Delahunt B. Histopathologic prognostic indicators for renal cell carcinoma. Semin Diagn Pathol 1998; 15:68–76.
93. Onda H, Yasuda M, Serizawa A, Osamura RY, Kawamura N. Clinical outcome in localized renal cell carcinomas related to immunoexpression of proliferating cell nuclear antigen, Ki-67 antigen, and tumor size. Oncol Rep 1999; 6:1039–43.
94. Rioux-Leclercq N, Turlin B, Bansard J, et al. Value of immunohistochemical Ki-67 and p53 determinations as predictive factors of outcome in renal cell carcinoma. Urology 2000; 55:501–5.
95. Jochum W, Schroder S, al-Taha R, et al. Prognostic significance of nuclear DNA content and proliferative activity in renal cell carcinomas. A clinicopathologic study of 58 patients using mitotic count, MIB-1 staining, and DNA cytophotometry. Cancer 1996; 77:514–21.
96. Morell-Quadreny L, Clar-Blanch F, Fenollosa-Enterna B, Perez-Bacete M, Martinez-Lorente A, Llombart-Bosch A. Proliferating cell nuclear antigen (PCNA) as a prognostic factor in renal cell carcinoma. Anticancer Res 1998; 18:677–82.
97. Sejima T, Miyagawa I. Expression of bcl-2, p53 oncoprotein, and proliferating cell nuclear antigen in renal cell carcinoma. Eur Urol 1999; 35:242–8.
98. Gelb AB, Sudilovsky D, Wu CD, Weiss LM, Medeiros LJ. Appraisal of intratumoral microvessel density, MIB-1 score, DNA content, and p53 protein expression as prognostic indicators in patients with locally confined renal cell carcinoma. Cancer 1997; 80:1768–75.

99. Bot FJ, Godschalk JC, Krishnadath KK, van der Kwast TH, Bosman FT. Prognostic factors in renal-cell carcinoma: immunohistochemical detection of p53 protein versus clinico-pathological parameters. Int J Cancer 1994; 57:634–7.
100. Vasavada SP, Novick AC, Williams BR. P53, bcl-2, and Bax expression in renal cell carcinoma. Urology 1998; 51:1057–61.
101. Hofmockel G, Wittmann A, Dammrich J, Bassukas ID. Expression of p53 and bcl-2 in primary locally confined renal cell carcinomas: no evidence for prognostic significance. Anticancer Res 1996; 16:3807–11.
102. Aaltomaa S, Lipponen P, Ala-Opas M, Eskelinen M, Syrjanen K, Kosma VM. Expression of cyclins A and D and p21(waf1/cip1) proteins in renal cell cancer and their relation to clinicopathological variables and patient survival. Br J Cancer 1999; 80:2001–7.
103. Miyake H, Hara S, Arakawa S, Kamidono S, Hara I. Over expression of clusterin is an independent prognostic factor for nonpapillary renal cell carcinoma. J Urol 2002; 167:703–6.
104. Liao SY, Aurelio ON, Jan K, Zavada J, Stanbridge EJ. Identification of the MN/CA9 protein as a reliable diagnostic biomarker of clear cell carcinoma of the kidney. Cancer Res 1997; 57:2827–31.
105. Opavsky R, Pastorekova S, Zelnik V, et al. Human MN/CA9 gene, a novel member of the carbonic anhydrase family: structure and exon to protein domain relationships. Genomics 1996; 33:480–7.
106. Murakami Y, Kanda K, Tsuji M, Kanayama H, Kagawa S. MN/CA9 gene expression as a potential biomarker in renal cell carcinoma. BJU Int 1999; 83:743–7.
107. Uemura H, Cho M, Nakagawa Y, et al. [MN/CA IX antigen as a potential target for renal cell carcinoma]. Hinyokika Kiyo 2000; 46:745–8.
108. Bui MH, Seligson D, Han K-R, et al. Carbonic anhydrase IX is an independent predictor of survival in advanced renal clear cell carcinoma; implications for prognosis and therapy. Submitted for publication 2002.
109. Gonzalgo ML, Eisenberger CF, Lee SM, et al. Prognostic significance of preoperative molecular serum analysis in renal cancer. Clin Cancer Res 2002; 8:1878–81.
110. Presti JC, Jr., Wilhelm M, Reuter V, Russo P, Motzer R, Waldman F. Allelic loss on chromosomes 8 and 9 correlates with clinical outcome in locally advanced clear cell carcinoma of the kidney. J Urol 2002; 167:1464–8.
111. MacLennan GT, Bostwick DG. Microvessel density in renal cell carcinoma: lack of prognostic significance. Urology 1995; 46:27–30.
112. Jacobsen J, Rasmuson T, Grankvist K, Ljungberg B. Vascular endothelial growth factor as prognostic factor in renal cell carcinoma. J Urol 2000; 163:343–7.
113. Stacker SA, Caesar C, Baldwin ME, et al. VEGF-D promotes the metastatic spread of tumor cells via the lymphatics. Nat Med 2001; 7:186–91.

II. KIDNEY CANCER: SURGICAL APPROACHES

5. NEPHRON–SPARING SURGERY FOR RENAL CELL CARCINOMA

ITHAAR H. DERWEESH, M.D.

Postgraduate Fellow, Glickman Urological Institute, The Cleveland Clinic Foundation

ANDREW C. NOVICK, M.D.

Chairman, Glickman Urological Institute, The Cleveland Clinic Foundation, and Professor of Surgery, Cleveland Clinic Lerner College of Medicine of Case Western University

INDICATION FOR NEPHRON–SPARING SURGERY

Accepted indications for nephron-sparing surgery include situations in which radical nephrectomy would render the patient anephric, with subsequent immediate need for dialysis. This encompasses patients with bilateral RCC or RCC involving a solitary functioning kidney. The latter circumstance may result from unilateral renal agenesis, prior removal of the contralateral kidney, or irreversible impairment of contralateral renal function. Nephron-sparing surgery is also indicated in patients with unilateral RCC and a functioning opposite kidney, when the opposite kidney is affected by a condition that might threaten its future function, such as calculus disease, chronic pyelonephritis, renal artery stenosis, ureteral reflux, or systemic diseases such as diabetes and nephrosclerosis.[1]

Recent studies have clarified the role of nephron-sparing surgery in patients with localized unilateral RCC and a normal contralateral kidney. The data indicate that radical nephrectomy and nephron-sparing surgery provide equally effective curative treatment for such patients who present with a single, small (≤4 cm), and clearly localized RCC. More recent data further suggest that NSS provides a long-term renal functional advantage over radical nephrectomy in such patients with a normal opposite kidney. The results of nephron-sparing surgery are less satisfactory in patients with larger (>4 cm) or multiple localized RCCs, and radical nephrectomy remains the treatment of choice in such cases when the opposite kidney is normal.

R.A. Figlin (ed.). KIDNEY CANCER. Copyright © 2003. Kluwer Academic Publishers. Boston. All rights reserved.

Table 1. Results of Nephron-Sparing Surgery for Renal Cell Carcinoma.

Series	# Patients	Local Tumor Recurrence	5-Year Cancer-Specific Survival
Steinbech, 1992[2]	121	4.1%	90%
Lerner, 1996[3]	185	5.9%	89%
Belldegrun, 1999[4]	146	2.7%	93%
Cleveland Clinic, 1999[5]	485	3.2%	92%

CLINICAL RESULTS FOLLOWING NEPHRON-SPARING SURGERY

The technical success rate with NSS is excellent, and long-term patient survival free of cancer is comparable to that obtained after radical nephrectomy, particularly for low-stage RCC (Table 1).[2-5] The major disadvantage of NSS for RCC is the risk of postoperative local tumor recurrence in the operated kidney which has occurred in 3–6% of patients. These local recurrences are most likely a manifestation of undetected microscopic multifocal RCC in the remnant kidney. The risk of local tumor recurrence after radical nephrectomy has not been studied, but it is presumably very low.

We recently reviewed the results of NSS for treatment of localized sporadic RCC in 485 patients managed at the Cleveland Clinic prior to December 1996.[5] A technically successful operation with preservation of function in the treated kidney was achieved in 476 patients (98%). The overall and cancer-specific five-year patient survival rate in the series was 81% and 93%, respectively. Recurrent RCC developed postoperatively in 44 of 485 patients (90%). Sixteen of the patients (3.2%) developed local recurrence in the remnant kidney, while 28 patients (5.8%) developed metastatic disease.

More recently, we received the long-term (10 year) results of NSS in 107 patients with localized sporadic RCC treated prior to 1988.[6] All patients were followed for a minimum of 10 years or until death. Cancer-specific survival was 88.2% at 5 years, and 73% at 10 years. Long-term preservation of renal function was achieved in 100 patients (93%). These results attest that NSS is an effective therapy for localized RCC which can provide both long-term tumor control and preservation of renal function.

NEPHRON-SPARING SURGERY WITH A NORMAL CONTRALATERAL KIDNEY

Although radical nephrectomy remains the standard treatment for localized RCC in patients with an anatomically and functionally normal opposite kidney, a growing number of authors are reporting excellent results with nephron-sparing surgery in this setting. A recent article detailed the outcome of NSS in 315 reported patients with unilateral localized RCC and a normal opposite kidney.[7] The mean cancer-specific survival rate was 95% at approximately three years of follow-up, and there were only two cases of postoperative tumor recurrence. Significantly, the mean tumor size in most of these reports was <3.5 cm. Clearly, patient selection on the basis of small tumor size was a significant factor accounting for favorable outcome after NSS in these studies.

In a study from the Cleveland Clinic, we reviewed the outcome of NSS in 216 patients with sporadic RCC.[8] Our findings confirmed that extended cancer-free survival was significantly improved in patients with small (<4 cm) tumors compared to larger ones. Other factors associated with significantly improved survival were unilateral renal involvement, low pathological tumor stage, and the presence of a single tumor. There were no postoperative tumor recurrences and the cancer-specific five-year survival rate was 100% in patients with small (<4 cm), unilateral stage $T_1N_0M_0$ RCC.

The aforementioned data suggested that NSS may be an acceptable therapeutic approach in patients who have a single, small (<4 cm) RCC and a normal contralateral kidney. To test this hypothesis, we conducted a subsequent study wherein the outcome following radical nephrectomy versus NSS was evaluated in 88 patients with a single, small (<4 cm), localized, unilateral, sporadic RCC.[9] The radical (n = 42) and nephron-sparing (n = 46) surgical groups were well-matched for patient age, sex, renal function, diabetes, hypertension, tumor-size, tumor location, and tumor stage. All patients in both groups had low pathological stage RCC. A single patient in each group developed recurrent RCC postoperatively. The cancer-specific five-year survival rate for patients in the radical and nephron-sparing surgical groups was 97% and 100%, respectively. More recently, Lerner and associates from the Mayo Clinic reported the results of a similar study comprising patients with solitary, small (<4 cm), low-stage RCC; the five-year cancer-specific survival rate following radical nephrectomy versus NSS was 96% versus 92%, respectively.[3] A subsequent study from the Cleveland Clinic showed that there are no significant biological differences between centrally versus peripherally located small, solitary, unilateral RCCs and that treatment with NSS or radical nephrectomy is equally effective regardless of tumor location in these patients.[10]

The data from these studies affirm that radical nephrectomy and nephron-sparing surgery provide equally effective curative treatment for patients with a single, small, unilateral, localized RCC. Other studies have further shown that the cost of nephron-sparing surgery is equivalent to that of radical nephrectomy,[11] and that quality of life is improved following nephron-sparing surgery in these patients.[12] Finally, recent data comparing the long-term (>10 years) development of renal dysfunction following elective NSS versus radical nephrectomy now suggest that progressive renal insufficiency is significantly less after NSS in patients with a normal contralateral kidney.[13] Therefore, patients with a single, small, unilateral, localized RCC may now be considered suitable candidates for nephron-sparing surgery even when the opposite kidney is completely normal.

FOLLOW-UP AFTER NEPHRON-SPARING SURGERY

Patients who undergo nephron-sparing surgery for RCC are advised to return for initial follow-up 4–6 weeks postoperatively. At that time, a serum creatinine mea-

Table 2. Recommended Postoperative Surveillance After
Nephron-Sparing Surgery for Sporadic Localized Renal Cell Carcinoma.

Pathologic Tumor Stage	History, Exam, Chest Blood Tests*	X-Ray	Abdominal CT Scan
T_1	Yearly	—	—
T_2	Yearly	Yearly	Every 2 yrs
T_3	Yearly	Yearly	Every 6 mos for 2 yrs, then every 2 yrs

* Medical history, physical examination, and measurement of serum calcium, alkaline phosphatase, liver function, and renal function.

surement and intravenous pyelogram are obtained to document renal function and anatomy; in patients with impaired overall renal function, a renal ultrasound or MRI study is obtained instead of an intravenous pyelogram.

We recently completed a detailed analysis of tumor recurrence patterns after nephron-sparing surgery for sporadic localized RCC in 327 patients at the Cleveland Clinic.[14] The purpose of this study was to develop appropriate guidelines for long-term surveillance after nephron-sparing surgery for RCC. Recurrent RCC occurred postoperatively in 38 patients (11.7%), including 13 patients (4.0%) who developed local tumor recurrence and 25 patients (7.6%) who developed metastatic disease. The incidence of postoperative local tumor recurrence and metastatic disease according to initial pathologic tumor state was as follows: 0% and 4.4% for T_1RCC, 2.0% and 5.3% for T_2RCC, 8.2% and 11.5% for T_{3a}RCC, and 10.6% and 14.9% for T_{3b}RCC. The peak postoperative intervals for developing local tumor recurrence were 6–24 months (in T_3RCC patients) and more than 48 months (in T_2RCC patients).

The above data indicate that surveillance for recurrent malignancy after nephron-sparing surgery for RCC can be tailored according to the initial pathological tumor stage. The recommended surveillance scheme is depicted in Table 2. All patients should be evaluated with a medical history, physical examination, and selected blood studies on a yearly basis. The latter should include serum calcium, alkaline phosphatase, liver function tests, blood urea nitrogen, serum creatinine, and electrolytes. A 24-hour urinary protein measurement should be obtained in patients with a solitary remnant kidney to screen for hyperfiltration nephropathy.[15] Patients who have proteinuria may be treated with a low-protein diet and a converting enzyme inhibitor agent, which appear to be beneficial in preventing glomerulopathy caused by reduced renal mass.[16]

The need for postoperative radiographic surveillance studies varies according to the initial pathological tumor (pT) stage. Patients who undergo nephron-sparing surgery for pT_1 RCC do not require radiographic imaging postoperatively in view of the very low risk of recurrent malignancy. A yearly chest radiograph is recommended after nephron-sparing surgery for pT_2 or pT_3 RCC because the lung is the most common site of postoperative metastasis in both groups. Abdominal or retroperitoneal tumor recurrence is uncommon in pT_2 patients, particularly early after nephron-sparing surgery, and these patients require only occasional follow-up abdominal CT scanning; we recommend that this be done every two years in this category. Patients with pT_3 RCC have a higher risk of developing local tumor recurrence, particularly during the first two years after nephron-sparing surgery, and they may benefit from more frequent follow-up abdominal CT scanning initially; we recommend that this be done every six months for two years and every two years thereafter.

REFERENCES

1. Licht MR and Novick AC. 1993. Nephron-sparing surgery for renal cell carcinoma. Urology 149: 1–7.
2. Steinbach F, Stockle M, Muller SC, Thuroff JW, Melchior SW, et al. 1992. Conservative surgery of renal cell tumors in 140 patients: 21 years of experience. J Urol 148:24–9, discussion 29–30.
3. Lerner SE, Hawkins CA, Blute ML, Grabner A, Wollan PC, et al. 1996. Disease outcome in patients with low stage renal cell carcinoma treated with nephron sparing or radical surgery. J Urol 155:1868–73.
4. Belldegrun A, Tsui KH, deKernion JB and Smith RB. 1999. Efficacy of nephron-sparing surgery for renal cell carcinoma: analysis based on the new 1997 Tumor-Node-Metastasis Staging System. J Clin Oncol 17:2868–75.
5. Hafez KS, Fergany AF and Novick AC. 1999. Nephron-sparing surgery for localized renal cell carcinoma: impact of tumor size on patient survival, tumor recurrence and TNM staging. J Urol 162: 1930–3.
6. Fergany AF, Hafez KS and Novick AC. 2000. Long-term results of nephron-sparing surgery for localized renal cell carcinoma: 10-year follow-up. J Urol 163:442–5.
7. Novick AC. 1995. Partial nephrectomy for renal cell carcinoma. Urology 36:149–52.
8. Licht MR, Novick AC, Goormastic M. 1994. Nephron-sparing surgery in incidental versus suspected renal cell carcinoma. J Urol 152:39–42.
9. Butler BP, Novick AC, Miller DP, Campbell SA and Licht MR. Management of small unilateral renal cell carcinomas: radical versus nephron-sparing surgery. Urology 45:34–40, discussion 40–41.
10. Hafez KS, Novick AC and Butler BP. 1998. Management of small solitary unilateral renal cell carcinomas: impact of central versus peripheral tumor location. J Urol 159:1156–60.
11. Uzzo RG, Wei JT, Hafez K, Kay R, Novick AC. 1999. Comparison of direct hospital costs and length of stay for radical nephrectomy versus nephron-sparing surgery in the management of localized renal cell carcinoma. Urology 54:994–98.
12. Clark PE, Schover LR, Uzzo RG, Hafez KS, Rybicki LA and Novick AC. 2000. Quality of life and psychological adaptation following surgery for localized renal cell carcinoma: impact of the amount of remaining renal tissue. J Urol 163:157.
13. Lau W, Blute ML, Zincke H. 2000. Matched comparison of radical nephrectomy versus elective nephron-sparing surgery for renal cell carcinoma: evidence for increased renal failure rate on long-term follow-up (>10 years). J Urol 163:153.
14. Hafez KS, Novick AC and Campbell SC. 1997. Patterns of tumor recurrence and guidelines for follow-up after nephron-sparing surgery for sporadic renal cell carcinoma. J Urol 157:2067–70.
15. Novick AC, Gephardt G, Guz B, Steinmuller D and Tubbs RR. 1991. Long-term follow-up after partial removal of a solitary kidney. NEJM 325:1058–62.
16. Novick AC and Schreiber JM, Jr. 1995. Effect of angiotensin-converting enzyme inhibition on nephropathy in patients with a remnant kidney. Urology 46:785–89.

6. LAPAROSCOPIC RADICAL NEPHRECTOMY AND MINIMALLY INVASIVE SURGERY FOR KIDNEY CANCER

NICOLETTE K. JANZEN, M.D., KENT T. PERRY, M.D., AND PETER G. SCHULAM, M.D., PH.D.

University of California Los Angeles, Los Angeles, CA 90095

INTRODUCTION

Radical nephrectomy has long been the gold standard for the management of renal tumors since Robson and colleagues reported increased survival in that group as compared to those who underwent simple nephrectomy.[1] Over the last decade, however, the surgical management of renal tumors has changed with emergence of laparoscopy as an alternative to open surgery. The short-term benefits of laparoscopic radical nephrectomy (LRN) in the form of reduced morbidity were clearly established soon after its inception. However, the long-term benefits and particularly the oncological efficacy of LRN were not established until very recently. Mature data from several groups provide evidence that LRN appears to have equivalent oncological efficacy to open radical nephrectomy, establishing it as a new standard of care in select cases.

At the same time that the benefits of laparoscopic surgery were becoming evident, a growing trend toward the implementation of nephron-sparing surgery was being established. The widespread use of abdominal CT, ultrasound and MRI has led to an increase in the number of incidentally detected renal masses. Prior to the use of these imaging modalities, renal cell carcinomas less than 3 cm in diameter accounted for approximately 5% of cases.[2] At present, 10–40% of renal tumors are discovered when less than 3 cm in size. Reluctance to perform radical nephrectomy for small bilateral tumors or small unilateral renal tumors in patients with a solitary kidney and/or compromised renal function led to the development of the open partial nephrectomy.[3,4] Large series studies have confirmed similar 5-year cancer-specific survival rates between partial and radical nephrectomy. Consequently, the indications for partial nephrectomy were expanded to include those patients with a normally functioning contralateral kidney.[5]

Given the broad acceptance of laparoscopy and the principle of nephron-sparing surgery, the logical next step was to consider laparoscopic partial nephrectomy for select cases. Due to the technical limitations of obtaining hemostasis and preventing urinary extravasation, laparoscopic partial nephrectomy remains technically demanding. However, it is an accepted treatment option for most open partial nephrectomy candidates and its application is primarily limited by the experience and technical skills of the laparoscopic surgeon.

Other minimally invasive nephron-sparing modalities for the management of select renal tumors are being investigated. These include cryoablation, radiofrequency ablation (RFA), and high-intensity focused ultrasound (HIFU). Renal ablative surgery is unique in that it attempts to destroy the renal tumor tissue in situ rather than curing by extirpation. It can be applied either percutaneously or laparoscopically. These modalities are still considered experimental, however, promising data suggests that they are likely to evolve into accepted forms of treatment.

LAPAROSCOPIC RADICAL NEPHRECTOMY

Historical Perspective

Prior to its widespread use for nephrectomy, laparoscopy was implemented in urology mainly as a diagnostic tool in the evaluation of the non-palpable testis.[6,7] It was also used to perform pelvic lymph node dissection for staging purposes in patients with prostate cancer.[8] In the field of gynecology, laparoscopy was used for visual diagnosis of certain conditions, biopsies, and minor operations such as tubal ligation and lysis of adhesions. It was not until the introduction and rapid acceptance of laparoscopic cholecystecomy for gallbladder disease that interest in performing major operations laparoscopically occurred.[9] Laparoscopic nephrectomy, unlike previous applications, presented a great challenge to surgeons because of the need to ligate large vascular structures and to remove a structure much larger than the port sites. After performing feasibility studies in animal models, Clayman and colleagues performed the first laparoscopic radical nephrectomy at Washington University in St. Louis in June, 1990 on an 85-year-old female with a 3-cm solid right renal mass.[10] Since then, numerous variations in technique have evolved.

Techniques

With the laparoscopic removal of the kidney for a renal mass, a radical or total nephrectomy may be performed which is essentially the same procedure that is employed in the open approach. Radical nephrectomy as defined by Robson and colleagues can be performed laparoscopically and includes en bloc removal of the kidney and adrenal, Gerota's fascia, pararenal fat and hilar lymph nodes. Total nephrectomy is performed in the same manner except the adrenal gland is left intact.

With the patient in the flank position, LRN can be performed either via the transperitoneal (TP) or the retroperitoneal (RP) approach. Pneumoperitoneum is achieved via a Veress needle or Hasson cannula. An initial 12-mm trocar is placed after which additional trocars are placed under direct vision.

Using the transperitoneal approach, access to the retroperitoneum begins by incising the white line of Toldt from the pelvic brim to the liver (for a right nephrectomy) or spleen (for a left nephrectomy). Reflection medially of the colon provides access to the renal hilum. The adrenal is spared or resected en bloc with the specimen depending on its preoperative appearance on imaging studies and the location and size of the renal mass. The renal artery, then renal vein are ligated. Next, the ureter is identified and ligated and any remaining retroperitoneal attachments are divided in order to obtain a free specimen.[11]

Hand-assistance is possible with the laparoscopic transperitoneal approach by employing an airtight device that fits around the surgeon's arm. An incision slightly larger than the size of the surgeon's glove is made in the midline and a self-sealing gasket is placed in the incision and secured to the abdominal wall. The surgeon is then able to insert and remove a gloved hand via this gasket. Hand-assisted laparoscopy (HAL) evolved to lessen the degree of difficulty of the laparoscopic procedure by enabling tactile feedback, manual dissection and spatial orientation.[12] Benefits include a comparable morbidity and valuable assistance to surgeons in-training who have little laparoscopic experience.[13] Shorter operative times have also been demonstrated when surgeons employ the hand-assisted approach,[14,15] though this probably is a reflection of laparoscopic experience.

The retroperitoneal approach (RP) is an alternative method of kidney retrieval made possible by the introduction of the atraumatic balloon dilation technique described by Gaur.[16] With the retroperitoneal approach, the patient is in the lateral decubitus position. A 2-cm incision is made posterior to the tip of the 12th rib and carried through the lumbodorsal fascia and into the pararenal space. A trocar-mounted balloon is inflated to displace the kidney anteromedially to create room in the retroperitoneum for additional trocars and instruments. Alternatively, blunt dissection is used to create space in the area.[17] The renal pedicle is located using the medial border of the psoas as a guide. The renal vein, then artery are dissected free and ligated. On the left side, the gonadal, ascending and adrenal vein must be ligated and cut in order to finish the renal vein dissection. The adrenal gland is routinely removed en bloc with the specimen on the left side, though on the right, it may be preserved. The remainder of the attachments of Gerota's fascia to the retroperitoneum are dissected and the ureter is clipped and divided until the specimen is completely freed.[11]

The ideal method of specimen retrieval is controversial. Intact retrieval is favored by groups who cite superior pathological specimen delivery and a theoretical decreased risk of tumor recurrence/tumor seeding. Alternatively, specimen morcellation or fragmented retrieval is advocated by others who cite improved cosmesis, a reduction in incisional hernia, decreased analgesic requirements and a minimal risk of peritoneal contamination with appropriate technique.[11,18,19] Specimen morcella-

Table 1. Long-term outcomes of laparoscopic versus open radical nephrectomy.

	Ono et al[30] 2001		Chan et al[29] 2001		Portis et al[28] 2002	
Technique	Open	Lap	Open	Lap	Open	Lap
No. patients	46	103	54	67	69	64
Follow-up (months)	39	29	44	35.6	69	54
Mean operating time (min)	198	286	193	256	128	287
Mean mass size (cm)	3.3	3.1	5.4	5.1	6.2	4.3
No. conversions	NA	4	NA	1	NA	NA
Mean hospital stay (days)	NA	NA	7.2	3.8	7.4	4.8
No. complications (%)	4 (8)	13 (13)	8 (15)	10 (15)	NA	NA
No. local recurrences (%)	0 (0)	1 (1)	0 (0)	0 (0)	1 (1)	1 (2)
No. metastasis (%)	3 (7)	3 (3)	3 (6)	4 (6)	9 (13)	3 (5)
5-year survival	95.6%	95%	75%	86%	89%	81%
5-year disease-free survival	89.7%	95.1%	86%	95%	92%	98%

tion, however, has resulted in cases where no tumor could be found on pathological evaluation.[20,21] And, of two reported cases of port-site recurrence, both occurred in cases where specimen morecellation was performed.[22,23] The overall effect of a small incision is most likely insignificant in terms of morbidity compared to the risk of violation of the bag and tumor seeding.[24] Therefore, the method that we prefer is removal of the specimen in an endocatch bag via a short infraumbilical Pfannenstiel incision.

Oncological Efficacy

Just over a decade has passed since the introduction of LRN for the management of renal masses. Early studies have confirmed the immediate benefits of laparoscopic nephrectomy both for benign and malignant disease when compared to open nephrectomy. Numerous advantages exist including decreased operative blood loss, postoperative analgesic use, and hospital stay as well as earlier return to full activity.[21,25–27] Of greater importance, however, is the oncological effectiveness of LRN as compared to open radical nephrectomy.

To date, no prospective randomized study comparing the laparoscopic approach with the open approach has been conducted. Three recently published retrospective studies with long-term follow-up have provided important results demonstrating equivalent outcomes between LRN and open radical nephrectomy. See Table 1. This should not be surprising given the fact that they are virtually the same operation merely employing different approaches.

Portis and colleagues report on a group of patients with the longest follow-up published to date.[28] In their multi-center study, 64 patients with pathologically confirmed renal cell carcinoma (RCC) treated by laparoscopic nephrectomy (median follow-up 54 months) were compared to 69 patients with clinical T1 or T2 lesions treated by open radical nephrectomy (median follow-up 69 months). Lesions treated by open nephrectomy were slightly larger on average than those treated laparoscopically on preoperative imaging (6.2 cm versus 4.3 cm); however, pathological specimen weight and Fuhrman grade were similar. No statistically significant difference in 5-year recurrence free survival was noted between the two groups which was 92% and 91% for laparoscopic and open radical nephrectomy respectively. 5-year cancer specific survival was 98% and 92% respectively.

Chan and colleagues studied 67 patients with clinical T1/T2, Nx, Mx pathologically confirmed RCC who underwent laparoscopic radical nephrectomy and compared this group to 54 patients who underwent open radical nephrectomy with pathologically confirmed T1/T2, Nx, Mx disease.[29] In all but one case, the transperitoneal approach was used. Specimen morcellation prior to removal was performed in 40 of the laparoscopic cases. All patients were followed for at least 12 months and mean follow-up in the laparoscopic group was 35.6 months and 44 months in the open group. No port site recurrence was reported in any case. In 59/67 patients, there was no evidence of local recurrence or metastatic disease. Two patients died of metastatic disease, one of unknown disease. Two patients with known metastatic disease died of other causes (MI and automobile accident), and two patients died of severe CHF at 1 and 64 months. For the laparoscopic and open radical nephrectomy, the 5-year calculated disease-free survival rates were 95% and 86%, and the calculated actuarial survival rate was 86% and 75% respectively.

Ono and colleagues compared LRN with open radical nephrectomy in 149 patients with small localized tumors <5 cm in diameter.[30] 103 patients were treated with laparoscopy with a median follow-up of 29 months and 46 underwent open nephrectomy with a median follow-up of 39 months. No port site seeding occurred in any patient. In the laparoscopic group, three patients were diagnosed with metastatic disease in months 3, 19, and 61. Two patients died without evidence of metastatic disease or local recurrence at months 34 and 45. One patient had a local recurrence at month 43. 5-year disease-free and patient survival rates were 95.1 and 95% compared to 89.7% and 95.6% for the group of patients treated with open radical nephrectomy.

Follow-up with 10-year data is forthcoming and is necessary to definitively conclude equivocal cancer control outcomes between the laparoscopic and open approaches. However, five-year data demonstrates equivalent efficacy and we optimistically await 10-year data that we expect will be similar to the 5-year data.

Patient Selection

The indications for laparoscopic radical/total nephrectomy include all patients who are candidates for open nephrectomy with the exception of patients with severe chronic obstructive pulmonary disease. T1, T2 and T3 tumors have all been successfully removed with the laparoscopic approach. Successful laparoscopic removal of tumors involving the renal vein and inferior vena cava have been reported.[31,32]

Reduced estimated blood loss, decreased narcotic utilization postoperatively, decreased length of hospitalization, and earlier return to full activity make the laparo-

Table 2. Complications of cryoablation in larger clinical studies.

	Bishoff et al, 1998[78]	Rodriguez et al, 2000[79]	Gill et al, 2000[54]	Rukstalis et al, 2001[68]
No. patients	9	7	32	29
Technique	Lap	Open/lap	Lap	Open
Urinary extravasation	0	0	0	0
Postop hemorrhage	0	0	0	0
Renal capsule fracture with intraop control	0	0	0	4
Renal failure requiring dialysis	0	0	0	3
Liver laceration	0	0	1	0
Postop congestive heart failure	0	0	0	1
Pelvic vein thrombosis	0	1	0	0
Recurrence	0	0	0	1

Perc-percutaneous; Lap-laparoscopy; Postop-postoperative; Intraop-intraoperative.

scopic approach advantageous over open surgery for all patients, especially high-risk operative candidates including those with obesity and those older than 80 years.[33,34]

Recent data advocating pre-immunotherapy cytoreductive surgery for patients with metastatic disease has brought this group into focus as candidates for the laparoscopic approach.[35,36] This is particularly appealing when one considers the possibility of a decrease in delay until immunotherapy can be given due to a decrease in convalescent time with laparoscopic surgery.

Potential Complications

The incidence and severity of complications between open and laparoscopic nephrectomy are comparable.[37,38] Nevertheless, complications are not rare events and laparoscopy should appropriately be regarded as major surgery. Total complication rates for LRN have been reported between 8% and 37% as compared to 24%–55% for open radical nephrectomy.[17,21,39,40] Reported intraoperative complications include vascular injury to the renal pedicle or inferior vena cava, splenic laceration, bowel injury, and pneumothorax. Bowel injury, vascular injury and adhesions account for the majority of conversions to open nephrectomy which have been reported in 0%–10% of cases.[17,21,28,29] Conversion rates have been noted to decline with increased operator experience.[41] A single intraoperative death has been reported.[39] This occurred in a 54-year old male who developed acute hypoxia and suffered cardiac arrest possibly attributable to a CO_2 embolus. Blood transfusion rates range from 2%–12%.[17,21,29] Postoperative complications are similar to those seen in open cases such as ileus, hematoma, incisional or port site hernia, bowel injury, and pulmonary embolus.

Limitations

The widespread application of any new technology depends in part on an acceptable risk profile, reasonable cost and ease of implementation. As previously described,

LRN has demonstrated equal if not decreased complication rates and is superior to open surgery with regards to decreased post-operative pain, earlier return to full activity and decreased length of hospitalization.

At present, laparoscopic radical nephrectomy is more expensive than its open counterpart. Estimated cost differentials of 15% to 29% favoring the open approach were reported at two institutions.[11,42] Accounting for the greatest increase in cost differential is increased operative time. Although LRN is associated with a decreased length of hospital stay and decreased narcotic use, the cost-savings associated with these advantages does not offset the cost of increased operative time. Average operative times in several series of LRN range from 207 to 345 minutes compared to 121 to 186 minutes for open radical nephrectomy. Some authors advocate HAL as a way to achieve more efficient operative times, however, we believe that as more experience is gained with LRN, times will become equivalent.

Meraney and colleagues were recently able to demonstrate a cost-savings associated with laparoscopic nephrectomy and nephroureterectomy over the open counterparts.[43] Cost savings in the laparoscopic group resulted from a substantial improvement in operative time as well as a decreased length of hospital stay.

Finally, the cost of surgical training in the operating room are high due to increased operative times. Training with both bench and video trainers may improve the cost-effectiveness of laparoscopic versus open training. As such, the need for improving operator experience during residency training is paramount.

THERMAL THERAPY IN THE TREATMENT OF RENAL MASSES

Historical Perspective

Cryosurgery is a form of thermal therapy that focuses on the destructive response to cold and that is based on the use of freezing temperatures to elicit necrosis in tissues exposed to a severe cryogenic injury. The roots of cryosurgery can be traced to the 19th century when James Arnott[44] hypothesized that freezing temperatures attained using iced salt solutions could be used to destroy tissue in 1845. Cryotherapy underwent an evolution in terms of materials used to convey the therapy, i.e. solidified carbon dioxide and liquid nitrogen. The application remained limited to the treatment of lesions accessible lesions such as on the skin and cervix until a century later when Cooper[45] in 1961 made improvements to the cryotherapy delivery apparatus. In the urologic arena, cryotherapy was directed at the treatment of prostate cancer and BPH throughout the 1960's but was abandoned due to unacceptable rates of local complications. However, Onik and colleagues[46] sparked renewed interest in cryosurgery as a treatment modality for malignancies in the 1980's and are credited with confirming the ability of ultrasound to monitor tissue destruction through the freezing process.

Cryosurgery represents an improvement in the age-old application of cold for destruction of tissue. RFA and HIFU are newer modalities developed in the 1990's that rely on thermotherapy for tissue destruction. Thermotherapy refers to tissue damage taking place by heating tissue to temperatures of 45°C and above. Investigation into the application of RFA to RCC followed its successful use in the treatment of other conditions including hepatocellular carcinoma,[47] osteoid osteoma,[48] undesirable endometrium,[49] as well as aberrant myocardial conductive pathways.[50]

While fundamentally different in their mechanisms of tissue destruction, advances in each of the minimally invasive ablative techniques for renal masses were made possible by advances in imaging capabilities. The success of CT, ultrasound and MRI imaging in monitoring the delivery of therapy and the post-treatment radiographic appearance of the treated lesions has been instrumental in the clinical utility of minimally invasive ablative procedures.

Cryosurgery

Equipment

The cryoprobe is the device used to deliver into target tissues the freezing temperatures necessary for tissue destruction. These are vacuum-insulated instruments which become cool when circulated with a cryogen such as liquid nitrogen ($-195°C$). In a recently developed application, pressurized argon gas is circulated through a probe and permitted to depressurize through a narrow nozzle located at the probe tip. This results in the cooling of surrounding tissue to $-187°C$. Probes are available in a variety of models and diameters (1.5–8 mm) suitable for open, laparoscopic and percutaneous use.

Cryobiology

Cryosurgery causes tissue destruction by immediate and delayed mechanisms.[51] The freezing of tissue causes ice crystals to form in the extracellular space and inside the microvascular bed leading to an increase in the extracellular osmotic concentration. Water is drawn into the extracellular space leading to a cytotoxic hyperosmotic intracellular environment. Rapid freezing also leads to intracellular ice crystal formation which is cytotoxic. During the thaw phase, circulation is restored, but damage to endothelial cells leads to porous blood vessels with subsequent edema formation, vascular occlusion and thrombosis. Failure of the microcirculation results in further tissue necrosis. Achieving cytotoxic freezing temperatures is essential for successful cancer eradication. Uchida and colleagues[52] froze renal cancer cell lines for 60 minutes at $-5°C$ to $-30°C$ and found that 96% of RCC cells survived when cooled to above $-10°C$ whereas only 15% survived when cooled to below $-20°C$. Experimental and clinical reports in the treatment of non-urological malignancies show that tissue temperatures as low as $-40°$ to $-50°C$ are required to induce complete cell death.[51] Therefore, obtaining adequate margins is achieved by a proper location of the $-40°C$ isotherm at the tumor's margin. Campbell and colleagues[53] studied mongrel dogs using 3.4 mm cryoprobes in order to correlate between intrarenal temperatures and the sonographic appearance of the cryolesion. They found that the iceball needed to extend at least 3.1 mm beyond the sonographic edge of the tumor to ensure adequate cooling of the tissue to at least −20°C. Gill and colleagues[54] routinely extend the iceball 1 cm beyond the tumor edge to be assured complete tissue destruction within "free cryogenic margins".

Some investigators have speculated on the possibility of achieving even lower tissue temperatures by occluding the renal artery during cryoablation. Campbell and associates,[53] however, could not demonstrate a practical advantage of renal artery occlusion in a canine model.

Most investigators advocate repeating the freeze/thaw cycle in order to ensure adequate cell death in renal tissue. The rationale for repeating the freeze/thaw cycle stems from evidence for increased cytotoxicity in prostate and hepatocellular carcinoma. No direct comparison of the two approaches (single vs. repeat freeze/thaw cycle) in the treatment of RCC has been published to date.

The gross and microscopic appearance of cryoablated renal tissue has been studied in canine models.[55] Four hours following treatment, the tissue is grossly hemorrhagic with a sharp demarcation between treated and untreated tissue. This corresponds to vascular congestion, intratubular and interstitial hemorrhage, early nuclear pyknosis; at 8 days, a central region of coagulative necrosis and a 2 mm thick area of sublethal injury are evident; at 3 months, the region of necrosis is absorbed, and a 1 to 1.5 mm thick fibrosis layer corresponds to the area of sub-lethal injury. Untreated tissue remained normal both in the ipsilateral and contralateral kidneys. These findings were confirmed in a porcine model where a sharp line of demarcation between injured and normal tissue as well as swelling of tubular cells, mitochondria and luminal microvilli as well as variable margination of nuclear chromatin consistent with irreversible tissue damage were demonstrated by electron microscopy.[56]

Laparoscopic Cryosurgical Technique

The kidney may be approached either transperitoneally or retroperitoneally. The potential advantage of the retroperitoneal approach is a decreased risk of bowel injury and formation of adhesions. The retroperitoneal approach facilitates exposure of posterior lesions while the transperitoneal approach facilitates access to anterior lesions (See Figure 1). The most important factor in determining the approach chosen will be surgeon experience and preference. Intraoperative frozen needle biopsy of the lesion is obtained. Real time B-mode ultrasonography using a 7.5 MHz linear array probe is used with color flow Doppler to assess tumor size, depth of the parenchymal lesion and the relationship of the mass to the collecting system and major vessels. Multiple cryoprobes are places at 1 cm intervals along the periphery and base of the tumor in addition to the center of the tumor in order to create a wedge shaped lesion. Tip positioning is guided by ultrasound. Cryoablation is initiated by producing tip temperatures reaching −180°C. Freezing continues until the iceball is advanced 10 mm beyond the tumor edge. Ultrasound confirms normal blood flow to the surrounding kidney and obliteration of flow to the ablated lesion. Following a second freeze-thaw cycle, the probe tracts are inspected to ensure hemostasis.

Percutaneous Cryosurgical Technique

The percutaneous approach utilizes the Seldinger technique to position sheaths in the kidney under ultrasound, CT, or MRI guidance in the vicinity of renal lesions. Cryoprobes are then placed through these sheaths and cryoablation is initiated. Uchida and colleagues[52] were the first to report the clinical application of cryoablation to renal cell carcinoma utilizing a percutaneous technique with ultrasound guidance. Technical difficulties in monitoring the size of the ice ball have been reported.[57]

Monitoring

Intracorporeal ultrasonography is used for both laparoscopic and open approaches whereas open MRI is used for percutaneous cryoablation. Ultrasound is able to detect renal tumors, reliably guide a cryoprobe to the target lesion and monitor the characteristic change in appearance of cryotreated tissue. The cryolesion appears as a hypoechoic area with a hyperechoic rim that expands as the freezing process advances. During thawing, the echotexture of the lesion returns to normal. The lesion has frequently been described as an "iceball". Animal studies have shown excellent correlation between the lesion's ultrasonographic image and the lesion measured by calipers.[46,55]

Radiofrequency Ablation

Mechanism of Action

Radiofrequency energy can be used to rapidly create highly localized lesions via a *temperature-based* or an *impedance-based* system. Both systems rely on the creation of a closed electrical circuit. The cytotoxic mechanism is similar in both: desiccation due to high intracellular temperatures. High frequency current flows from a needle electrode to the surrounding tissue resulting in ionic agitation that leads to accelerated molecular friction that produces heat. Heat induces immediate cellular damage which leads to coagulative necrosis. Energy returns to the RF generator via a return pad that completes the circuit. A comparison of the two systems showed no difference in renal lesion formation.[58]

Following RF treatment, the macroscopic findings correlate with the microscopic findings.[59–61] Macroscopically, following saline RF treatment, kidneys demonstrate a gray-white area of necrosis surrounding a central cavity containing both areas of hemorrhage and necrotic debris. Clear demarcation between the induced lesion and the surrounding normal parenchyma is present. Shortly after RF ablation, intense stromal and epithelial edema with marked hypereosinophilia and pyknosis are present accompanied by microvascular thrombosis and coagulative necrosis. Chronic lesions demonstrate dense fibrosis.

Technique

Temperature-based systems were the first to be introduced for renal tissue RF ablation. Power ranging from 26W to 50W at a frequency ranging from 460kHz to 500kHz is delivered. RFA may be performed percutaneously or laparoscopically via

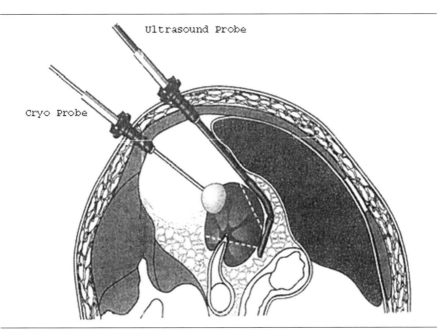

Figure 1. Schematic of laparoscopic cryoablation of right exophytic posterior renal mass using ultrasound guidance

a transperitoneal or retroperitoneal approach. Bipolar electrodes result in pillow-shaped or ovoid lesions. Monopolar needles are coupled with secondary hooks to create spherical lesions. An insulating shaft protects normal tissue. Tissue temperature measurements are made via thermocouples located at the tip of the needles. Electrode temperatures at approximately 100°C are generally required in order to assure a temperature of at least 60°C at the periphery of the ablated lesion.[60] Temperature-based systems are limited to a lesion diameter of 16 mm. Early tissue desiccation causing a rise in tissue impedance is responsible for this limitation. Multiprobe, hooked and bipolar arrays, intraparenchymal saline injection and internally cooled electrodes have all been developed to enhance the size of lesion created. In addition to the monopolar and bipolar devices described above, a probe with 4 needle tips or arrays with adjustable lengths can be used. Polascik and colleagues[60] introduced the modified technique of saline perfusion of tissue during radiofrequency ablation. This was found to prevent tissue desiccation resulting in increased volumes of ablated tissue. In addition, radiofrequency with saline perfusion allowed tissue ablation to occur in a predictable manner.

Crowley and colleagues[61] introduced an impedance-based system to overcome the limitations of conventional radiofrequency and studied its effects in a porcine model. RF was delivered both laparoscopically and percutaneously with CT guidance. The resistance of the tissue surrounding the electrode is monitored as RF energy flows to the return pad. RF energy is applied until the tissue becomes desiccated which then acts as an insulator and blocks further flow of energy to the return pad allowing the temperature at that particular location to rise and cause denaturation of intracellular proteins and hence cell death.

Monitoring

The ability of real time ultrasound to monitor the development of the RFA lesion is debatable. Polascik and colleagues reported that during saline infused RFA, a bubbling effect in the area of the treatment may be ultrasonographically imaged as an area of increased echogenicity.[62] Post-treatment lesions have been described as a distinct hyperechoic zone, an area of bright echogenic foci or a heterogeneous area of mild hyperechogenicity. Zlotta and colleagues[59] described similar findings. This point, however, is not settled as others have found that US was not useful for intraoperative monitoring.[61]

High Intensity Focused Ultrasound

Mechanism of Action

Extracorporeally applied high-intensity focused ultrasound is able to induce tissue lesions in vivo by focusing energy on to a small volume of tissue causing tissue temperatures to rise to approximately 90°C. Lesions are created by two types of physical insults: thermal and cavitational. The thermal effect is caused by heat which is produced as sound waves passing through the tissue are absorbed. The thermal effect is obtained by using low ultrasonic intensities over long periods of exposure. Cavitation results from high peak intensities over brief exposure periods. Cavitation occurs as a result of a process in which bubbles develop and acutely increase in size to the point that resonance is achieved. When the bubble suddenly collapses, high pressures ranging from 20,000–30,000 bars develop and cause damage to nearby cells.[63] Theoretically, the focusing ability of HIFU prevents surrounding tissues from experiencing thermal destruction.

Studies on the effects of HIFU on rat and canine kidneys and demonstrated lesions consistent with coagulative necrosis or cavitation depending on ultrasound duration and intensity.[63] The size of lesions also varied depending on the acoustic intensity and the number of firings. Histologically, affected cells demonstrate pale eosinophilic cytoplasm and separation from one another.[64] At the periphery of the lesions, areas of hemorrhage were noted in close proximity to normal appearing tissue. Susani and colleagues[65] attempted to study the gross and histologic effects of HIFU in two patients with RCC prior to nephrectomy; however, the area of treatment was undistinguishable from the large area of tumor necrosis.

Technique

Ultrasound energy is delivered via a highly focused transducer. The transducer is composed of a piezoelectric element that both images and delivers therapy. Its main theoretical advantage is that it may be performed extracorporeally without an intimate contact between the effector probe and the lesion.

Monitoring

A limitation of this technology is the difficulty in imaging lesions for the precise targeting of tissue destruction. Adams and colleagues induced experimental VX-2 kidney tumors in a rabbit model.[64] At the time of lesioning, it was impossible to accurately localize lesions for destruction. The group suggested integration of the HIFU technology with other imaging modalities such as duplex Doppler, CT or MRI as a possible means of precisely localizing renal tumors. Other groups have similarly described the limitation of ultrasound in demonstrating detectable tissue changes during or following the creation of lesions.[66,67]

Oncological Efficacy of Ablative Techniques

After cryosurgical treatment of renal masses, immediate post-operative and long-term efficacy is assessed by the radiographic appearance of lesions at various intervals. Radiographic response criteria has been defined as: *initial evidence of infarction and hemorrhage, subsequent obliteration or reduction in size of the renal mass and absence of growth on radiologic follow-up exams.*[68] Atypical enhancement on CT or MRI should not be considered a failure unless associated with persistence or growth of the mass. Gill, Novick and associates performed routine post-cryoablation biopsies in order to confirm adequate treatment.[54] In all 23 patients, no evidence of tumor was noted. Because of these consistent findings with their technique, the group essentially abandoned the practice of postoperative biopsy. Another investigator reported on one patient with an enhancing mass unchanged in size at 3 months post-op.[68] Biopsy showed a microscopic focus of grade 1 renal cell carcinoma and a repeated cryosurgery was eventually performed with good local control. In another series of 22 patients undergoing biopsy 6 months after laparoscopic renal cryoablation, RCC was detected in only one patient.[69] Shingleton and Sewell reported on percutaneous renal cryoablation of 5 tumors in 4 patients with von Hippel-Lindau disease. At follow-up of 2 to 23 months, no radiographic evidence of recurrence could be detected, however, two tumors required repeat cryoablation due to residual tumor.[70]

RFA results are limited to feasibility studies and lack long-term follow-up. Gervais and colleagues[71] utilized percutaneous RFA to treat nine renal masses in eight patients with CT-guidance or US-guidance. All patients had life expectancies less than 10 years and significant comorbidities. Those with metastatic disease were excluded. Seven of eight patients survived at least 6 months post-op. Four lesions required multiple RFA treatments based on follow-up imaging that demonstrated evidence of residual tumor. At a mean follow-up of 10.3 months, seven of the nine tumors were completely eradicated. Pavlovich and colleagues reported two month follow-up on 21 patients with Von-Hippel Lindau treated with percutaneous RFA for renal tumors <3 cm.[72] Five tumors demonstrated focal areas of persistent enhancement on CT suggestive of incomplete eradication.

For HIFU, technical problems of visualizing target organs and lesions and controlling lesion size formation have precluded clinical trials, consequently, the issue of oncological efficacy cannot be addressed. Additionally, the theoretical risk of promoting metastasis using HIFU has been raised as a concern. Early studies in animal models demonstrating an increased risk of metastasis with HIFU ablation of tumors, however, have not been validated in subsequent studies.[72]

Potential Complications

Cryosurgery and RFA have been relatively safe. No detrimental effects on renal function following these procedures have been reported.[73] Hemorrhage, thrombosis and urinary fistula formation are all potential risks of cryosurgery and RFA; however, few if any of these complications have been noted (See Table 2). Complications of RFA that have been reported in clinical studies include: incomplete ablation of a renal lesion requiring multiple treatments to treat lesion completely and postoperative hemorrhage.[60,71] Complications of cryosurgery and RFA noted in animal models, but not in humans included: freezing of the collecting system in a dog without evidence of urinary leakage or hemorrhage;[55] secondary UPJ stricture;[53] and urinoma.[61]

Cracking and bleeding of renal parenchyma during the thaw phase has been noted by some groups during open as well as laparoscopic cryoablation.[74] Electrocautery, surgical mesh, avitene plugs, thrombin-soaked gel foam, surgicell, and argon beam laser application have all been used to establish hemostasis in laparoscopic procedures when bleeding was encountered. The authors prefer to infuse fibrin glue into the probe tract while still frozen in order to prevent bleeding following thawing.

HIFU appears to have a number of associated adverse side effects demonstrated in animal models that has limited its clinical use in human kidneys. Chapelon and colleagues[63] showed that in 13/16 dogs, abdominal organ lesions occurred following HIFU. This was felt to be due to misfocusing of the target organ. Some improvement was achieved using ultrasound bi-dimensional scanner, however, in only 10/16 animals, a kidney lesion was obtained and 6 dogs suffered cutaneous burns. Adams and colleagues[64] also noted difficulty in tumor localization due to the movement of kidney during ventilation. Watkin et al[66] also reported poor targetability of renal lesions while using HIFU: only 67% of total shots fired were detected in the target area. Moreover, no change in the ultrasound appearance of the treated area following HIFU was noted making it difficult to evaluate complete destruction of renal lesions. Recently, Kohrmann and colleagues performed HIFU on three renal masses in a patient who refused open surgery.[72] Each tumor was treated individually in three sessions. Two renal carcinomas were completely ablated with no lesion outside the target area, however, the upper pole tumor was not affected due to absorption of ultrasound energy by the interposed ribs.

Limitations

Ablative techniques do not generate pathologic specimens that allow accurate histologic evaluation and therefore preclude accurate tissue diagnosis, staging and grading which are important for prognosis determination. Therefore, biopsy of perirenal fat as well as biopsy of the renal mass is advocated by some investigators. Reliability of such biopsies, however, has been called into question.[75] Moreover performing pretreatment biopsy during percutaneous procedures brings back to discussion the question of tract seeding.

Therefore, reliable freezing and complete eradication of tissue with achievement of adequate margins during the procedure needs to be ensured. Debate exists between two techniques of intraoperative monitoring: use of thermocouples as advocated by Kavoussi and Rodriguez versus following radiographic lesion appearance as advocated by Gill and Novick.[76]

Concern for achieving negative margins has led some investigators to modify their techniques in order to obtain pathological specimens. Gettman and colleagues[77] describe the use of RFA-assisted laparoscopic partial nephrectomy in 10 patients. All ablated lesions were excised and sent for pathological evaluation with negative margins reported in all cases. Other innovative modifications of ablative techniques are likely to follow. Currently, we are not convinced that ablative measures followed by tissue removal have a role.

CONCLUSION

The surgical management of renal masses over the last decade has changed significantly with the introduction and validation of the laparoscopic approach and nephron-sparing surgery for select renal masses. Just over a decade after its introduction, LRN has been validated at 5-year follow-up as an oncologically effective operation with significant advantages over the open approach. Indeed, laparoscopic radical nephrectomy is viewed by many at this time as the new standard of care for the treatment of renal masses in select cases. We are currently awaiting ten-year follow-up data which might be available by publication of this text. We are cautiously optimistic that the data will show equivalent efficacy. The different laparoscopic approaches should have no effect on oncological efficacy and the driving force behind which procedure is performed should be left to the judgment and experience of the surgeon.

Minimally invasive modalities for the treatment of RCC are being introduced as new nephron sparing approaches in an attempt to minimize operative time, morbidity and time to full recovery. The majority of candidates are those with unifocal, small, peripheral exophytic lesions located away from the collecting system. The most appealing approach is laparoscopic since it provides the best anatomic control. As for cryotherapy, the kidney is in a favorable location for treatment with less risk to adjacent structures. Another favorable aspect is that small renal cell carcinomas are usually unifocal.

Few large series with long-term results confirming the curative efficacy of ablative techniques have been conducted. Cryosurgery is the most studied modality. RFA studies have been limited to small series of patients with short-term follow-up or to case reports. The alarming complication rate demonstrated with HIFU in animal models warrants further investigation and refinement prior to widespread clinical use. Optimization of treatment modalities and refinement of techniques is ongoing. Long-term studies are needed to confirm a durable response as compared to partial and radical nephrectomy. Nevertheless, inclusion criteria in terms of size, location, and type of treatable lesions and patient selection are evolving.

Cryosurgery and RFA are generally reserved for lesions <4 cm which are exophytic. It is currently reserved for older patients with significant comorbidities. The role of percutaneous techniques is still under investigation. Radiographic follow-up is essential. The best modality (i.e. MRI, US, or CT) for tumor targeting, monitoring of therapy and follow-up is still unclear. Debate continues to exist as to the best method of ensuring adequate intraoperative tumor cryoablation: thermocouples vs. radiographic appearance of the lesion. Finally, the role of follow-up biopsy to ensure complete eradication of tumor needs has yet to be defined. In order for minimally invasive ablative measures to gain a place in nephron sparing approaches, these modalities should show equivalent efficacy and reduced morbidity relative to open partial nephrectomy. At this time these techniques should be reserved for selected patients. Laparoscopic partial nephrectomy is an alternative to the above nephron-sparing approaches that eliminates any questions about tumor kill while maintaining the low morbidity aspect of minimally invasive surgery.

REFERENCES

1. Robson CJ, Churchill BM, Anderson W: The results of radical nephrectomy for renal cell carcinoma. J Urol 1969; 101:297–301.
2. Smith SJ, Bosniak MA, Megibow AJ, et al.: Renal cell carcinoma: earlier discovery and increased detection. Radiology 1989; 170:699–703.
3. Palmer JM: Role of partial nephrectomy in solitary or bilateral renal tumors. Jama 1983; 249: 2357–2361.
4. Novick AC: Partial nephrectomy for renal cell carcinoma. Urol Clin North Am 1987; 14:419–433.
5. Novick AC, Streem S, Montie JE, et al.: Conservative surgery for renal cell carcinoma: a single-center experience with 100 patients. J Urol 1989; 141:835–839.
6. Cortesi N, Ferrari P, Zambarda E, Manenti A, Baldini A: Diagnosis of bilateral abdominal cryptorchidism by laparoscopy. Endoscopy 1976; 8:33.
7. Manson AL, Terhune D, Jordan G, et al.: Preoperative laparoscopic localization of the nonpalpable testis. J Urol 1985; 134:919.
8. Schuessler WW, Vancaillie TG, Reich H, Griffith DP: Transperitoneal endosurgical lymphadenectomy in patients with localized prostate cancer. J Urol 1991; 145:988–991.
9. McMahon AJ, Russell IT, Baxter JN, et al.: Laparoscopic versus mini-laparotomy cholecystectomy: a randomized trial. Lancet 1994; 343:135.
10. Clayman RV, Kavoussi LR, Soper NJ, et al.: Laparoscopic nephrectomy: initial case report. J Urol 1991; 146:278–282.
11. Portis AJ, Elnady M, Clayman RV: Laparoscopic radical/total nephrectomy: a decade of progress. J Endourol 2001; 15:345–354; discussion 375–346.
12. Litwin DE, Darzi A, Jakimowicz J, et al.: Hand-assisted laparoscopic surgery (HALS) with the Hand-Port system: initial experience with 68 patients. Ann Surg 2000; 231:715–723.
13. Batler RA, Campbell SC, Funk JT, Gonzalez CM, Nadler RB: Hand-assisted vs. retroperitoneal laparoscopic nephrectomy. J Endourol 2001; 15:899–902.
14. Wolf JS, Moon TD, Nakada SY: Hand assisted laparoscopic nephrectomy: comparison to standard laparoscopic nephrectomy. J Urol 1998; 160:22–27.
15. Shichman SJ, Wong JE, Sosa RE, Berlin BB: Hand assisted laparoscopic radical nephrectomy and nephroureterectomy: A new standard for the 21st century (abstract). J Urol 1999; 161 (suppl):23.
16. Gaur DD: Laparoscopic operative retroperitoneoscopy: use of a new device. J Urol 1992; 148:1137–1139.
17. Abbou CC, Cicco A, Gasman D, et al.: Retroperitoneal laparoscopic versus open radical nephrectomy. J Urol 1999; 161:1776–1780.

18. Elashry OM, Giusti G, Nadler RB, McDougall EM, Clayman RV: Incisional hernia after laparoscopic nephrectomy with intact specimen removal: caveat emptor. J Urol 1997; 158:363–369.
19. Walther MM, Lyne JC, Libutti SK, Linehan WM: Laparoscopic cytoreductive nephrectomy as preparation for administration of systemic interleukin-2 in the treatment of metastatic renal cell carcinoma: a pilot study. Urology 1999; 53:496–501.
20. Barrett PH, Fentie DD, Taranger LA: Laparoscopic radical nephrectomy with morcellation for renal cell carcinoma: the Saskatoon experience. Urology 1998; 52:23–28.
21. Dunn MD, Portis AJ, Shalhav AL, et al.: Laparoscopic versus open radical nephrectomy: a 9-year experience. J Urol 2000; 164:1153–1159.
22. Fentie DD, Barrett PH, Taranger LA: Metastatic renal cell cancer after laparoscopic radical nephrectomy: long-term follow-up. J Endourol 2000; 14:407–411.
23. Castilho LN, Fugita OE, Mitre AI, Arap S: Port site tumor recurrences of renal cell carcinoma after videolaparoscopic radical nephrectomy. J Urol 2001; 165:519.
24. Gettman MT, Napper C, Corwin TS, Cadeddu JA: Laparoscopic radical nephrectomy: prospective assessment of impact of intact versus fragmented specimen removal on postoperative quality of life. J Endourol 2002; 16:23–26.
25. McDougall E, Clayman RV, Elashry OM: Laparoscopic radical nephrectomy for renal tumor: the Washington University experience. J Urol 1996; 155:1180–1185.
26. Kavoussi LR, Kerbl K, Capelouto CC, McDougall EM, Clayman RV: Laparoscopic nephrectomy for renal neoplasms. Urology 1993; 42:603–609.
27. Ono Y, Katoh N, Kinukawa T, Matsuura O, Ohshima S: Laparoscopic radical nephrectomy: the Nagoya experience. J Urol 1997; 158:719–723.
28. Portis AJ, Yan Y, Landman J, et al.: Long-term followup after laparoscopic radical nephrectomy. J Urol 2002; 167:1257–1262.
29. Chan DY, Cadeddu JA, Jarrett TW, Marshall FF, Kavoussi LR: Laparoscopic radical nephrectomy: cancer control for renal cell carcinoma. J Urol 2001; 166:2095–2099; discussion 2099–2100.
30. Ono Y, Kinukawa T, Hattori R, et al.: The long-term outcome of laparoscopic radical nephrectomy for small renal cell carcinoma. J Urol 2001; 165:1867–1870.
31. Sundaram CP, Rehman J, Landman J, Oh J: Hand assisted laparoscopic radical nephrectomy for renal cell carcinoma with inferior vena caval thrombus. J Urol 2002; 168:176–179.
32. Savage SJ, Gill IS: Laparoscopic radical nephrectomy for renal cell carcinoma in a patient with level I renal vein tumor thrombus. J Urol 2000; 163:1243–1244.
33. Fazeli-Matin S, Gill IS, Hsu TH, Sung GT, Novick AC: Laparoscopic renal and adrenal surgery in obese patients: comparison to open surgery. J Urol 1999; 162:665–669.
34. Hsu TH, Gill IS, Fazeli-Matin S, et al.: Radical nephrectomy and nephroureterectomy in the octogenarian and nonagenarian: comparison of laparoscopic and open approaches. Urology 1999; 53:1121–1125.
35. Flanigan RC, Salmon SE, Blumenstein BA, et al.: Nephrectomy followed by interferon alfa-2b compared with interferon alfa-2b alone for metastatic renal-cell cancer. N Engl J Med 2001; 345:1655–1659.
36. Belldegrun A, Shvarts O, Figlin RA: Expanding the indications for surgery and adjuvant interleukin-2-based immunotherapy in patients with advanced renal cell carcinoma. Cancer J Sci Am 2000; 6 Suppl 1:S88–92.
37. Gill IS, Meraney AM, Schweizer DK, et al.: Laparoscopic radical nephrectomy in 100 patients: a single center experience from the United States. Cancer 2001; 92:1843–1855.
38. McDougall E: Minimally invasive therapy. J Urol 1995; 153:712–713.
39. Cadeddu JA, Ono Y, Clayman RV, et al.: Laparoscopic nephrectomy for renal cell cancer: evaluation of efficacy and safety: a multicenter experience. Urology 1998; 52:773–777.
40. Gill IS, Schweizer DK, Hobart MG, et al.: Retroperitoneal laparoscopic radical nephrectomy: The Cleveland clinic experience. J Urol 2000; 163:1665–1670.
41. Higashihara E, Baba S, Nakagawa K, et al.: Learning curve and conversion to open surgery in cases of laparoscopic adrenalectomy and nephrectomy. J Urol 1998; 159:650–653.
42. Hobart MG, Gill IS, Schweizer D, Bravo EL: Financial analysis of needlescopic versus open adrenalectomy. J Urol 1999; 162:1264–1267.
43. Meraney AM, Gill IS: Financial analysis of open versus laparoscopic radical nephrectomy and nephroureterectomy. J Urol 2002; 167:1757–1762.
44. Arnott J: Practical illustrations of the remedial efficacy of a very low or anaesthetic temperature in cancer. Lancet 1850; 2:257–259.

45. Cooper IS, Lee A: Cryostatic congelation: a system for producing a limited controlled region of cooling or freezing of biologic tissues. J Nerv Ment Dis 1961; 133:259–263.
46. Onik GM, Reyes G, Cohen JK, Porterfield B: Ultrasound characteristics of renal cryosurgery. Urology 1993; 42:212–215.
47. Rossi S, Di Stasi M, Buscarini E, et al.: Percutaneous Radiofrequency Interstitial Thermal Ablation in the Treatment of Small Hepatocellular Carcinoma. Cancer J Sci Am 1995; 1:73.
48. De Berg JC, Pattynama PMT, Obermaun WRI: Percutaneous computed-tomography-guided thermocoagulation for osteoid osteomas. Lancet 1995; 346:346–350.
49. Phipps JH, Lewis BV, Prior MV, Roberts T: Experimental and clinical studies with radiofrequency-induced thermal endometrial ablation for functional menorrhagia. Obstet Gynecol 1990; 76:876–881.
50. Calkins H, Langberg J, Sousa J, et al.: Radiofrequency catheter ablation of accessory atrioventricular connections in 250 patients. Abbreviated therapeutic approach to Wolff-Parkinson-White syndrome. Circulation 1992; 85:1337–1346.
51. Baust J, Gage AA, Ma H, Zhang CM: Minimally invasive cryosurgery–technological advances. Cryobiology 1997; 34:373–384.
52. Uchida M, Imaide Y, Sugimoto K, Uehara H, Watanabe H: Percutaneous cryosurgery for renal tumours. Br J Urol 1995; 75:132–136; discussion 136–137.
53. Campbell SC, Krishnamurthi V, Chow G, et al.: Renal cryosurgery: experimental evaluation of treatment parameters. Urology 1998; 52:29–33; discussion 33–24.
54. Gill IS, Novick AC, Meraney AM, et al.: Laparoscopic renal cryoablation in 32 patients. Urology 2000; 56:748–753.
55. Stephenson RA, King DK, Rohr LR: Renal cryoablation in a canine model. Urology 1996; 47: 772–776.
56. Nakada SY, Lee FT, Jr., Warner T, Chosy SG, Moon TD: Laparoscopic cryosurgery of the kidney in the porcine model: an acute histological study. Urology 1998; 51:161–166.
57. Long JP, Faller GT: Percutaneous cryoablation of the kidney in a porcine model. Cryobiology 1999; 38:89–93.
58. Gettman MT, Lotan Y, Corwin TS, et al.: Radiofrequency coagulation of renal parenchyma: comparison of effects of energy generators on treatment efficacy. J Endourol 2002; 16:83–88.
59. Zlotta AR, Wildschutz T, Raviv G, et al.: Radiofrequency interstitial tumor ablation (RITA) is a possible new modality for treatment of renal cancer: ex vivo and in vivo experience. J Endourol 1997; 11:251–258.
60. Walther MC, Shawker TH, Libutti SK, et al.: A phase 2 study of radio frequency interstitial tissue ablation of localized renal tumors. J Urol 2000; 163:1424–1427.
61. Crowley JD, Shelton J, Iverson AJ, et al.: Laparoscopic and computed tomography-guided percutaneous radiofrequency ablation of renal tissue: acute and chronic effects in an animal model. Urology 2001; 57:976–980.
62. Polascik TJ, Hamper U, Lee BR, et al.: Ablation of renal tumors in a rabbit model with interstitial saline-augmented radiofrequency energy: preliminary report of a new technology. Urology 1999; 53:465–472; discussion 470–462.
63. Chapelon JY, Margonari J, Theillere Y, et al.: Effects of high-energy focused ultrasound on kidney tissue in the rat and the dog. Eur Urol 1992; 22:147–152.
64. Adams JB, Moore RG, Anderson JH, et al.: High-intensity focused ultrasound ablation of rabbit kidney tumors. J Endourol 1996; 10:71–75.
65. Susani M, Madersbacher S, Kratzik C, Vingers L, Marberger M: Morphology of tissue destruction induced by focused ultrasound. Eur Urol 1993; 23 Suppl 1:34–38.
66. Watkin NA, Morris SB, Rivens IH, ter Haar GR: High-intensity focused ultrasound ablation of the kidney in a large animal model. J Endourol 1997; 11:191–196.
67. Hill CR, ter Haar GR: Review article: high intensity focused ultrasound–potential for cancer treatment. Br J Radiol 1995; 68:1296–1303.
68. Rukstalis DB, Khorsandi M, Garcia FU, Hoenig DM, Cohen JK: Clinical experience with open renal cryoablation. Urology 2001; 57:34–39.
69. Levin HS, Meraney AM, Novick AC: Needle biopsy histology of renal tumors 3–6 months after laparoscopic renal cryoablation. J Urol 2000; 163 (S):153a.
70. Shingleton WB, Sewell PE, Jr.: Percutaneous renal cryoablation of renal tumors in patients with von Hippel-Lindau disease. J Urol 2002; 167:1268–1270.
71. Gervais DA, McGovern FJ, Wood BJ, et al.: Radio-frequency ablation of renal cell carcinoma: early clinical experience. Radiology 2000; 217:665–672.

72. Kohrmann KU, Michel MS, Gaa J, Marlinghaus E, Alken P: High intensity focused ultrasound as noninvasive therapy for multilocal renal cell carcinoma: case study and review of the literature. J Urol 2002; 167:2397–2403.
73. Carvalhal EF, Gill IS, Meraney AM, et al.: Laparoscopic renal cryoablation: impact on renal function and blood pressure. Urology 2001; 58:357–361.
74. Cozzi PJ, Lynch WJ, Collins S, Vonthethoff L, Morris DL: Renal cryotherapy in a sheep model; a feasibility study. J Urol 1997; 157:710–712.
75. Zincke H, Dechet CB, Blute ML: Needle biopsy of solid renal masses. J Urol 1998; 159:169.
76. Gill IS, Novick AC: Letter to Editor. Urology 2001; 58:132–134.
77. Gettman MT, Bishoff JT, Su LM, et al.: Hemostatic laparoscopic partial nephrectomy: initial experience with the radiofrequency coagulation-assisted technique. Urology 2001; 58:8–11.
78. Bishoff JT, Chan DY, Chen RB: Laparoscopic renal cryoablation: acute and long-term clinical and pathological effects in animal and human studies [abstract]. J Endourol 1998; 12:S88.
79. Rodriguez R, Chan DY, Bishoff JT, et al.: Renal ablative cryosurgery in selected patients with peripheral renal masses. Urology 2000; 55:25–30.

7. ROLE OF NEPHRECTOMY IN METASTATIC KIDNEY CANCER

PAUL M. YONOVER, M.D., SAMEER K. SHARMA, M.D., AND ROBERT C. FLANIGAN, M.D.

Loyola University Stritch School of Medicine, Department of Urology, 2160 S. 1st Avenue, Room 245, Building 54, Maywood, IL 60153-5500.

INTRODUCTION

Overall, 30–50% of patients with renal cell carcinoma (RCC) will eventually develop metastatic cancer at some point during their illness. Approximately 20–30% of patients present with metastatic disease, while 20 to 40% undergoing nephrectomy for clinically localized RCC will develop clinically detectable metastases during postoperative surveillance.[1,2] Common sites of metastases are the lung, liver, bone, brain, and adrenal gland, with case reports detailing this cancer's capacity to manifest itself almost anywhere in the body. Metastatic RCC predicts a dismal prognosis, with a median survival of only 6 to 10 months and a 2-year survival of 10 to 20%[3] (Table 1).

Recent advances in biologic response modifier therapy (BMR) have brought new hope for a small percentage of patients and have also rekindled interest in cytoreductive nephrectomy.

EPIDEMIOLOGY

Annually in the United States RCC accounts for approximately 31,000 new cancer diagnoses and almost 11,900 cancer related deaths.[4] RCC is the seventh most common cancer. Less than 10% of patients with RCC present with the classic triad of flank pain, hematuria, and a palpable mass. Potential symptoms are derived from

Address for Correspondence: Robert, C. Flanigan, MD, Albert J. Spah, Jr. and Claire R. Spah Professor and Chair Department of Urology, Loyola University Stritch School of Medicine, 2160 S. 1st Avenue, Building 54, Maywood, IL 60153-5500

R.A. Figlin (ed.). KIDNEY CANCER. Copyright © 2003. Kluwer Academic Publishers. Boston. All rights reserved.

Table 1. Survival of patients with metastatic RCC.

| Author | No. of Patients | Survival (%) | |
		1 year	5 years
Riches et al, 1951[62]	409	33	0.5
Middleton, 1967[63]	141	10	0
Skinner et al, 1971[64]	77	—	0
Johnson et al, 1975[23]	93	26	—
Thompson et al, 1975[65]	65	22	0
Klugo et al, 1977[66]	64	12	3
Montie et al, 1977[27]	78	18	—
deKernion et al, 1978[67]	86	43	10
McNichols et al, 1981[68]	56	—	14
Bassil et al, 1985[8]	53	—	18
Golimbu et al, 1986[69]	88	—	2
Giuiliani et al, 1990[70]	50	—	7

Adopted from Kavolius et al: Resection of Metastatic Renal Cell Carcinoma. J Clin Onc 16(6):2261–2266, 1998.

paraneoplastic phenomena or directly due the growth of metastatic lesions that can produce to bone pain, cough, or neurologic symptoms. This protean array of symptoms can be nonspecific and the diagnosis of advanced RCC can be challenging. More recently, most RCC are being diagnosed incidentally due to an increase in the radiographic evaluation of patients with various abdominal complaints. Patients with advanced RCC remain likely to present symptomatically, especially with constitutional symptoms such as weight loss, anorexia, or malaise indicative of a poor prognosis.

PROGNOSTIC FACTORS

The prognosis for metastatic RCC is very poor with only a minority of patients achieving long-term survival, with median survival of a few to several months being typical for many subgroups of patients. Prognostic factors that clearly correlate with length of survival include performance status, sites of metastases, total burden of disease, metastasis-free interval, pathologic stage, tumor grade, and cell type. Other factors, including tumor size, age, race, sex, and associated paraneoplastic syndromes may be important prognostically.

PATHOLOGIC STAGE

The prognosis for patients with RCC is clearly stage related, with pathologic stage being the most powerful single prognostic factor for patients with localized RCC Using the older Robson classification schema, several large studies reported a five-year overall survival in patients with Stage IV disease to be between 2 and 20%.[5] Patients with any form of extrarenal extension display a significantly compromised prognosis.[5]

Lymph node involvement, like distant metastases, has an adverse impact on survival. In comparing patients with nodal involvement to those with distant metastatic disease, Libertino found no difference in overall five-year survival between the two groups.[6] Similarly, Bassil and colleagues reported a 0 to 5% ten-year survival for node positive patients.[7] The value of regional lymphadenectomy in conferring a survival benefit to some patients with limited nodal involvement remains controversial. Well-conducted prospective studies are much needed in this area.

NUCLEAR GRADE AND CELL TYPE

Grading systems for RCC, including the Fuhrman system, have correlated with prognosis for RCC. Recently published algorithms have improved prognostic power by incorporating tumor grade along with stage and other parameters.[8,9,10] Tumor histology is also very important. It is now clear that RCC is a heterogeneous disease consisting of several distinct subtypes that can be defined by cytogenetic, molecular, histologic, and ultrastructural features.[11,12] These subtypes include conventional RCC (clear cell and granular), papillary, chromophobic, and collecting duct carcinomas.[11] Sarcomatoid features can occur in any of these subtypes and is no longer classified as a distinct subtype of RCC, although the prognostic significance of sarcomatoid features has not changed with a median survival of less than 1 year.[11,12] In general, conventional RCC appears to have a graver prognosis than papillary or chromophobic subtypes, although high-grade and aggressive variants of the latter have been well described. Some authors have argued that stage for stage and grade for grade, there may not be a profound difference in prognosis.[13,14,15,16] In addition, there is emerging data that suggests that patients with papillary RCC may be more refractory to IL-2 based immunotherapy than are patients with clear cell tumors.

PATIENTS WITH ADVANCED RCC

Prognostic factors for patients with metastatic RCC are increasingly well defined and include performance status, metastasis-free interval, and sites (or burden) of disease. As with most other cancers, performance status correlates with outcome for advanced RCC by reflecting the state of debilitation and ability to tolerate aggressive therapeutic modalities. Median survival for patients with excellent performance status may range from 10–15 months, while those with poor performance status can only expect a median survival of 2–5 months.[2,17,18,19,20,21] The interval between nephrectomy and the development of metastatic disease also predicts a more indolent course.[22] Patients with pulmonary only metastases appear to have a more favorable prognosis. In contrast, patients with hepatic and CNS metastases have a worse prognosis, while those with bone metastases have an intermediate length prognosis.[22] Some have suggested that total burden of disease may be more important than disease location.[22] Other potentially useful prognostic factors for patients with metastatic RCC include hypercalcemia, weight loss, anemia, elevated ESR, and thrombocytosis.[2,22,23,24,25,85]

Table 2. Traditional indications for nephrectomy in metastatic RCC.

1) Palliative nephrectomy (rarely indicated)
2) Nephrectomy to induce spontaneous regression (no longer valid indication)
3) Nephrectomy plus embolization (no longer valid indication)
4) Nephrectomy plus metastasectomy with curative intent
5) Cytoreductive nephrectomy in preparation for immunotherapy
6) Nephrectomy after response to immunotherapy
7) Nephrectomy as a component of adoptive immunotherapy protocols

INDICATIONS FOR SURGERY IN PATIENTS WITH METASTATIC RCC

When considering the role for surgery in patients with metastatic RCC, a careful assessment of prognostic indicators must be made for each patient individually. Traditional indications for nephrectomy have included palliative nephrectomy, nephrectomy to induce spontaneous regression, nephrectomy combined with preoperative embolization, nephrectomy combined with metastasectomy for curative intent, cytoreductive nephrectomy, nephrectomy and/or metastasectomy to consolidate partial responses to systemic therapy, and nephrectomy as a component of adoptive immunotherapy protocols (Table 2).

PALLIATIVE NEPHRECTOMY

Patients with metastatic RCC rarely present with severe symptomotology directly related to their primary tumor. However, intractable hemorrhage and unrelenting flank pain are occasionally encountered. Large arteriovenous fistulas can also develop, and can lead to hypertension, cardiomegaly, and high output congestive heart failure. Finally, RCC's predilection for paraneoplastic manifestations is well recognized, and occasionally requires intervention. Nephrectomy has been advocated to palliate all of these symptoms, and in some cases it may be appropriate.[26] However, the outlook with nephrectomy alone in this setting is dismal, with approximately 50% of these patients dying of cancer progression within 4–12 months. Thus, it is difficult to justify the morbidity associated with open surgery alone for palliation when less invasive techniques, such as angioinfarction, may suffice.[1]

Recently, Montie and colleagues cautioned that the systemic effects attributed to RCC may be the result of metastases rather than the primary tumor, and hence, that palliative nephrectomy may thus not bring relief for the problem it is meant to alleviate.[27] Similarly, in an study examining the effects of nephrectomy on hypercalcemia associated with advanced RCC, Walther reported that surgical extirpation of the primary tumor helped reduce calcium levels in only 7 of 12 patients, while 4 patients actually suffered an increase in their serum calcium and 1 patient had no change.[28] Those patients who experienced a decrease in calcium levels after nephrectomy had no better survival than those who failed to respond, with both groups having a median survival of only 6 months.

Table 3. Spontaneous regression after nephrectomy.

Author	No. of Patients	No. of Patients with Regression (%)
Rafla et al, 1970[71]	14	0
Wagle & Seal, 1970[72]	80	2
Bottinger et al, 1970[73]	100	0
Mims et al, 1987[44]	57	1
Middleton, 1967[63]	33	0
Johnson et al, 1975[23]	43	0
Skinner et al, 1971[64]	77	1
Lokich & Harrision, 1975[75]	45	0
Montie et al, 1977[27]	25	0
TOTAL	**474**	**4 (0.8)**

Adopted from Couillard et al: Surgery of Renal Cell Carcinoma. Urol Clin of North Amer 20(2):263–275, 1993.

Historically, another argument against the liberal use of nephrectomy alone to treat symptomatic patients is the high operative mortality that has been observed. DeKernion noted a six percent mortality rate even after excluding debilitated patients, while other studies have reported mortality rates as high as 17% in this patient population.[29] *In summary, palliative nephrectomy not followed by other adjunctive therapy, is not warranted except in patients with significant symptomotology from the primary tumor, and will only be required in exceptional cases.*

SPONTANEOUS REGRESSION

One of the most difficult aspects of RCC is its unpredictable nature. Primary renal malignancies may on occasion remain stable for years without growing or metastasizing while even some metastatic lesions have been known to exhibit long periods of growth arrest or prolonged tumor doubling time. Spontaneous regression of distant metastases is rare, occurring in approximately 0.4 to 0.8% of patients, most commonly in patients with metastases to the lung.[26,30] (Table 3) In reality, some have suggested that many suspicious pulmonary lesions that regress may actually be benign conditions such as old granulomas, fungal lesions, or pulmonary infarcts. Most cases of reported spontaneous regression have not been biopsy-proven.[31] *True spontaneous regression of RCC appears to be a real phenomenon, but it is rare and should* **not** *be considered an indication for nephrectomy in patients with metastatic RCC.*

ANGIOINFARCTION PLUS NEPHRECTOMY

Historically, nephrectomy has also been combined with preoperative angioinfarction and postoperative hormonal therapy (medroxyprogesterone 400 mg intramuscularly twice weekly) for the treatment of patients with metastatic RCC.[32] Tumor antigens released from the infarcted tumor were postulated to provide a powerful stimulus to the host immune system. In one early study of 100 patients followed for at least

Table 4. Five-year survival of metastatic RCC after metastectomy.

Author	No. of Patients	5 year Survival (%)
Middleton, 1967[63]	59	34
Skinner et al, 1971[64]	41	29
Tolia & Whitmore, 1975[36]	17	35
Klugo et al, 1977[66]	10	50
Odea et al, 1978[76]	44	16
deKernion et al, 1978[67]	20	25
McNichols et al, 1981[68]	13	69
Jett et al, 1983[77]	44	27
Dernevik et al, 1985[78]	33	21
Kierney et al, 1994[35]	36	31
Kavolius et al, 1998[37]	141	44
Dinney et al, 1999[79]	173	29

Adopted from Kavolius et al: Resection of Metastatic Renal Cell Carcinoma. J Clin Onc 16(6):2261–2266, 1998.

12 months, an overall response rate of 28% (with complete response in 7 patients), and a median survival for responders in this series of 19 months was reported. Patients most likely to benefit from this protocol were those with pulmonary metastases only, displaying a 64% one-year survival rate.[32] In contrast, Kurth and colleagues reported on 25 patients treated with embolization and delayed nephrectomy, and observed only one complete response (lasting greater than 36 months) and 6 patients with stable disease (duration of 14 to 31 months). Seventy-two percent of the patients in this series died after a median of only 5.7 months.[33]

These provocative reports prompted a multi-institutional study by the Southwest Oncology Group (SWOG) that failed to document any significant efficacy for renal angioinfarction followed by nephrectomy.[34] Thirty patients with metastatic with a minimal follow-up was one year demonstrated no complete responses (only one partial remission that lasted 21 months before progression of disease). Furthermore, only 3 of 11 patients with metastases limited to the lung lived one year. A 21% one-year survival and a 7-month median survival was reported. Significant side effects of angioinfarction have been documented to include abdominal pain, nausea, vomiting, diarrhea, fever, ileus, and inadvertent embolization of peripheral vessels. *Renal, angioinfarction prior to nephrectomy should be reserved for controlling severe symptoms and used only in a limited manner, perhaps for patients with very large tumors or those with potentially difficult hilar dissections.*

NEPHRECTOMY WITH RESECTION OF METASTASES

The potential benefit for complete surgical resection of all tumor burden, including removal of both the primary renal mass as well as metastatic deposits in carefully selected patients with minimal volume metastatic RCC has been demonstrated by several series. (Table 4) Kierney described 41 patients in whom nephrectomy and complete metastasectomy was attempted, including 64% of the patients the metastatic process was in a single site.[35] Complete excision of all identifiable lesions was accomplished in 88%. 3-year survival was 59% and 5-year survival was 31%, suggesting that a long-term benefit may be realized by an aggressive surgical approach in carefully selected patients.

The subset of patients that may benefit most from nephrectomy and aggressive metastasectomy are those with solitary pulmonary lesions.[29,36] In a series by Kavoulius and colleagues in which 94 patients with solitary metastases were managed with nephrectomy and metastasectomy, patients with pulmonary only metastases were found to have the most favorable prognosis.[37] Five-year survival rates for patients with pulmonary only metastases were 54% compared to 44% for the group as a whole and 18% for patients with solitary CNS metastases.

Although it is clear that the majority of patients with resectable metastases will manifest other signs of metastases over a period of time and die of metastatic RCC, nephrectomy and excision of minimal metastatic disease, particularly when confined to the lungs, may substantially benefit a small number of patients.

CYTOREDUCTIVE NEPHRECTOMY

A brief overview of the immunobiology of RCC is germaine in any discussion of cytoreductive nephrectomy because much of today's approach to cytoreductive nephrectomy is closely tied to adjuvant immune-based therapies.

The introduction of interferon therapy represents one of the first breakthroughs in immunotherapy for metastatic RCC, and interferon is still the only agent that has been tested along with cytoreductive nephrectomy in a randomized, prospective fashion.[38] After binding to the cell membrane, interferons initiate a complex sequence of intracellular events leading to suppression of cellular proliferation, and a variety of other potentially beneficial immunomodulatory effects, including the enhancement of specific lymphocyte cytotoxicity for target cells, increased natural killer (NK) cell activity, and the upregulation of MHC antigen expression. Monotherapy trials of interferon-alpha, using a variety of dosage schedules, have yielded response rates anywhere between 0 and 33%, with a mean of approximately 15%.[1]

Interluekin-2 also forms an integral component of current immunotherapy armamentarium. IL-2 leads to the generation and proliferation of lymphokine activated killer cells (LAK cells) as well as cytotoxic tumor infiltrating T lymphocytes (TIL cells). An overall response rate of 15–20% with complete response rate of 5–7% was noted. Importantly, the very durable responses noted in the complete responder group led to its FDA approval for use in metastatic RCC.[1,2] Significant toxicity is associated with the use of high dose IL-2 therapy. This fact has led investigators to alter the schedule of administration of IL-2 alone, as well as to evaluate the use of combination IL-2/IFN-alpha regimens and protocols combining cytotoxic agents and immunotherapy.

Over time, a number of fundamental observations of the immunobiology of RCC have suggested a potential benefit to cytoreductive nephrectomy. For example, Freed speculated that the lung, with its rich supply of macrophages and lymphocytes, might restrain the disease via host immune mechanisms and speculated that this might explain most cases of spontaneous regression of metastatic RCC have occurred in patients with lung only metastastes.[26] He cited animal data showing that cell-mediated cytotoxicity was diminished with progressive growth of the primary tumor. Other authors have described the primary tumor as an "immunologic sink," which is capable of monopolizing the efforts of circulating lymphocytes while sequestering antibodies targeted to the tumor, and preventing an effective response against distant metastases.[39] RCC can also actively suppress immunological responses by modulating key signal transduction pathways within lymphocytes and through secretion of high levels of immunosuppressive cytokines such as IL-10 or TGF-β.[40,41,42] Theoretically, therefore, cytoreductive nephrectomy might enhance responses to adjuvant systemic immunotherapies. Another potential advantage of early cytoreductive nephrectomy is that further seeding of the blood stream with cancer cells by the primary tumor is promptly eliminated. Local control is also optimized, reducing the risk of developing renal hemorrhage and chronic flank pain.[31,43]

Clinically, several studies have noted longer survival in patients that have undergone nephrectomy than in those with their primary tumor in-situ, leading some investigators to argue that cytoreductive nephrectomy may enhance the efficacy of systemic immunotherapy.[1,2,17,19,22,44] In some series, the value of prior nephrectomy has been independent of other well-recognized prognostic factors including performance status and site or burden of disease. In the 1980's several trials using interferon therapy suggested an advantage for cytoreductive nephrectomy. Muss and associates reported an 8% response rate for patients with primary intact, metastatic RCC treated with interferon-α, compared to patients with prior nephrectomy and a lack of bone metastases who experienced a much higher 23% response rate.[44] In another, large multicenter study of 371 patients in Japan, Umeda and Niijma also demonstrated significantly higher response rates with systemic interferon therapy for patients who had undergone prior radical or palliative nephrectomy.[45] Similarly, patients with metastatic RCC treated with IL-2 and LAK cells have demonstrated improved response rates when the primary tumor had been removed. Fisher and colleagues reported only one objective response in 14 patients with an intact renal primary (7% response rate) compared to a 26% response rate for all patients in the series.[46] All of the above reports were retrospective, non-randomized, studies with relatively liberal selection criteria. Hence, the main concern in interpreting these results has been selection bias.

A number of more recent reports have detailing an experience with cytoreductive nephrectomy as summarized in Table 5. The largest series is from the National Cancer Institute, which comprised 195 patients treated with cytoreductive nephrectomy in preparation for IL-2 immunotherapy.[47] Surgery consisted of removal of the primary tumor as well as contiguous or adjacent metastases. The overall response rate in this series was 18%, which included 4% complete responses and 14% partial responses, and was not significantly different than the results of systemic immunotherapy alone. Thirty-eight percent of patients in that series were unable to

Table 5. Cytoreductive nephrectomy in preparation for immunotherapy: retrospective studies.

Author	No. of patients	Surgical Mortality (%)	Unable to Receive Postoperative BMR therapy (%)	Overall Response (%)[§]	Complete Response (%)	Partial Response (%)
Rackley et al (1994)[42]	37	1 (2.7)	8 (21.6)	3 (8.1)	0 (0.0)	3 (8.1)
Wolf et al (1994)[80]	23	0 (0.0)	6 (26.1)	3 (13.0)	2 (8.7)	1 (4.3)
Bennett et al (1995)[48]	30	5 (17)	23 (76.6)	4 (13.3)	3 (10.0)	1 (3.3)
Fallick et al (1997)[43]	28	1 (3.6)	2 (7.1)	11 (39.3)	5 (17.9)	6 (21.4)
Walther et al (1997)[47]	195	2 (1.0)	74 (37.9)	19 (17.8)	4 (3.7)	15 (14.0)
Figlin et al (1997)[3]	62	0 (0.0)	7 (11.3)	19 (34.5)	5 (9.1)	14 (25.5)
Levy et al (1998)[81]	66	2 (3.0)	12 (18.1)	—	—	—
Total	441	11/441 (**2.5**)	132/441 (**29.9**)	59/375 (**15.7**)	19/375 (**5.1**)	40/375 (**10.7**)

[§] Values as reported in each study. The calculations, however, are not always based on intent-to-treat analysis and may be overestimations of true response rates.

receive systemic immunotherapy due to rapid tumor progression or postoperative complications or debilitated state. As seen in Table 5, the response rates reported in these trials vary widely. Patient selection, including the distribution of patients with good vs. poor performance status, limited vs. extensive metastases, and long vs. short metastasis free intervals, may account for these divergent results. In addition, many of these series calculated their response rates based on only those patients who received adjuvant immunotherapy after nephrectomy, effectively overestimating response rates. Employment of *intention-to-treat analysis* (the ratio of responders to *all* patients who enter a study including those that do not qualify for adjuvant therapy) would more accurately reflect the response rate to therapy.

One of the major concerns about cytoreductive nephrectomy is the risk of postoperative morbidity that may delay or obviate the delivery of systemic therapy. The incidence of post-surgical complications has ranged from 7–77% (Table 5), with most series reporting lower incidence rates. Overall, 70.2% of patients in these series were able to proceed on to systemic therapy. Poor patient selection is particularly evident in the Bennett series, in which almost one third of the patients had brain metastases, 43% had osseous lesions, 37% had hepatic metastases, and performance status was suboptimal or poor in a high percentage of patients.[48] Another concern about cytoreductive nephrectomy is perioperative mortality, which has been reported in 2.5% of patients in these retrospective series (Table 5).

In an attempt to reduce the perioperative morbidity and mortality of cytoreductive nephrectomy, Walther and colleagues have investigated the use of minimally

Table 6. Survival analysis of nephrectomy followed by interferon-alpha 2b.

		Median Survival (months)		P value (logrank)
		No Surgery	Surgery	
Not Stratified		8.1	11.1	.0012
Not Stratified by Disease Measurability		7.8	10.3	.010
Stratified by Disease Measurability		11.2	16.4	
Stratified by Performance Status	"0"	11.7	17.4	.080
	"1"	4.8	6.9	
Stratified by Type of Metastases	Lung Only	10.3	14.3	.008
	Other	6.3	10.2	

Adopted from Flanigan R.C, Salmon S, Blumenstien BA, et al: Nephrectomy plus interferon alfa-2b versus interferon alfa-2b alone for renal cell cancer. N Engl J Med, Vol. 345, No. 23. 1655–1659, 2001.

invasive techniques.[49] In comparing 3 treatment groups: open nephrectomy, laparoscopic assisted nephrectomy (primarily performed laparoscopically with a small incision made to finish the dissection and deliver the specimen intact), and pure laparoscopic nephrectomy with tissue morcellation, a median of 67 days (range of 50–151 days) elapsed after open surgery before IL-2 could be administered compared to a median of 60 days (range 47–63) for the laparoscopic assisted patients. The greatest benefit was seen in those who had undergone pure laparoscopic surgery with morcellation as they proceeded to systemic therapy within a median of 37 days (range of 37–57). In these series, minimally invasive surgery was performed with morbidity that was comparable to the traditional open procedure and tumor morcellation was feasible even for large tumors. The authors concluded that laparoscopic cytoreduction offered a number of distinct advantages for cytoreduction in preparation for systemic therapy.

In a follow-up study, however, the same group reported on 31 attempted laparoscopic cytoreductive nephrectomies at their institution.[50] Eleven cases required conversion to open nephrectomy, and blood loss was relatively high (750–3000 cc). Only 18 patients (58%) were eligible to proceed to immunotherapy postoperatively. This data suggests that these cases are technically challenging and that the true benefits of minimally invasive surgery in this setting are unclear.

The Southwest Oncology Group (SWOG) and EORTC recently reported data from randomized, prospective trials that studied the role of cytoreductive nephrectomy followed by systemic Intron A (interferon alfa-2b) therapy vs. Intron A alone in patients with metastatic RCC.[38,51,82,83] In SWOG trial 8949, 246 patients were enrolled and 21 were declared ineligible primarily due to incorrect interpretation of the pathology or inadequate documentation at presentation. Fourteen of the 120 patients randomized to the nephrectomy plus interferon arm did not undergo surgery, and 1 of 121 patients randomized to the interferon only arm refused treatment. Analysis was performed in an *intention-to-treat* manner (Table 6). Overall, the survival advantage for the nephrectomy plus interferon arm was approximately 50% (median survival of 11.1 months vs. 8.1 months), and this persisted across all of the pre-study stratifications including of performance status (0 vs. 1), site of metastasis (pulmonary only vs. other) and measurable disease (present vs. absent). This study also demonstrated minimal surgical morbidity (grade III and IV toxicity included 2 cardiac events, 2 infections, and 1 patient with hypotension), with no perioperative complications in 79.2%. The combined operative and perioperative mortality rate was 1%. 98% if the patients were able to proceed to interferon therapy after nephrectomy. Patients with good performance status demonstrated the largest benefit from cytoreductive nephrectomy with median survival of 17.4 months compared to 11.7 months in the interferon alone group. In the nephrectomy arm there were only 3 partial responders and 0 complete responders, and in the interferon alone arm there were 2 partial responders and one complete responder. In summary, SWOG 8949 demonstrated a clear-cut survival advantage for cytoreductive nephrectomy within the context of interferon-based systemic immunotherapy.

The EORTC study 30947 adopted the SWOG protocol design and essentially echoed these findings of SWOG 8949, although there were a few unique and interesting findings that should be highlighted.[51] This study comprised 85 patients with 42 in the cytoreduction arm and 43 in the interferon alone arm. 86% of the patients undergoing nephrectomy experienced no perioperative complications, and 40/41 were able to proceed on to receive systemic immunotherapy. The response rates were higher in EORTC 30947 than SWOG 8949. There were 5 complete responders in the nephrectomy arm compared to only one in the interferon only arm, while partial responders and patients with stable disease were similarly distributed between the treatment arms. *Time to progression* and duration of *survival* both in favored the cytoreductive nephrectomy. Moreover, median survival improved from 7 months in the interferon alone arm to 17 months in the cytoreductive nephrectomy arm. The congruence of results between these two independent trials provides the most compelling data in favor of cytoreductive nephrectomy to date.

While this data supports the role of cytoreductive nephrectomy in the management of patients with metastatic RCC, one must emphasize that this procedure should not be performed indiscriminately. Slaton reported that patients with metastatic RCC involving multiple organs, particularly the liver, spine, or brain, are at high risk for dying in the first 6 months after cytoreductive nephrectomy and are less likely to achieve palliation after surgery.[52] Similarly, Wood found that high grade tumors, particularly sarcomatoid variants, have a poor prognosis after cytoreductive nephrectomy, and have suggested that tumor biopsy may be useful prior to considering surgery in this patient population.[53] They also reported that patients with an elevated white blood count, which may reflect a paraneoplastic phenomenon, or an abnormal PTT, which may reflect hepatic involvement or dysfunction, are less likely to benefit from cytoreductive surgery. Fallick and colleagues have proposed the following criteria for cytoreductive nephrectomy: 1) the ability to perform >75% tumor debulking; 2) no CNS, bone, or liver metastases; 3) adequate pulmonary and cardiac reserve; 4) ECOG performance status of 0 or 1; and 5) predominately clear cell histology.[43] Some of these criteria remain controversial and many would consider them relative rather than absolute. In general, however, these recommendations are in accord with SWOG trial 8949 that showed that relatively healthy patients with good performance status, and preferably with pulmonary only metastases, are the most likely to benefit from cytoreductive nephrectomy.

A recently published retrospective analysis of RCC cases emphasized the diverse nature of this group of patients. Thirty-four percent (94/268) patients were found to have metastatic RCC, and 40% (38/94) of these cases were judged to be inoperable. Furthermore, only 20 of the remaining 56 patients (36%) had a performance status sufficient to undergo cytoreductive nephrectomy. Thus, only 7% of all the patients in this series, and only 21% (20/94) of patients presenting with metastatic RCC, were candidates for cytoreductive nephrectomy based on standard patient selection criteria.[84] *Patient selection is the key to the management of this group of patients and selecting the appropriate candidates who will benefit from cytoreductive nephrectomy.*

NEPHRECTOMY OR METASTASECTOMY TO CONSOLIDATE THERAPY AFTER SYSTEMIC IMMUNOTHERAPY

Some investigators favor treating patients initially with systemic immunotherapy, reserving cytoreductive surgery for those who demonstrate a favorable response in their metastatic foci. Advocates of this approach argue that surgery has significant morbidity, mortality, cost, and it should therefore be reserved for those who demonstrate a favorable response to systemic therapy. One major concern about cytoreductive nephrectomy relates to the potential for perioperative morbidity that can preclude administration of systemic therapy. Extensive evidence also suggests that surgery itself may have detrimental effects on the immune system, and might theoretically diminish the efficacy of adjuvant systemic immunotherapy. In an elegant animal study examining the effects of laparotomy on intraperitoneal tumor growth, Eggermont demonstrated how surgical trauma could inhibit the effects of IL-2 and LAK cells on the tumor cells and thus enhance tumor propagation.[49] They speculate that peptide growth factors that are released during the inflammatory response to surgical trauma, such as TGF-α, TGF-β, and PDGF, may enhance tumor growth. By promoting the growth of natural tissues and wound healing, these factors may augment tumor cell proliferation and invasion same time suppressing the immune system and hindering the host's natural antitumor responses.

Finally, the phenomenon of rapid tumor progression at metastatic sites following removal of the primary tumor has been reported in up to 33% of cases.[47,48] Potential mechanisms to account for this phenomenon include a debilitated immune system after surgery and the removal of a source of systemic antineoplastic modulators. In animal models, primary tumors that elaborate high levels of anti-angiogenic substances such as angiostatin have been described, such that, removal of the primary tumor allows rapid neovascularization and progressive growth of the metastatic foci.[54] It is likely that human counterparts may be found.

In 1991 Fleischmann reported on 10 patients with advanced RCC treated with IL-2 based immunotherapy, 3 of which had complete regression of disease outside of the abdomen. Two of the latter were rendered disease-free after surgical excision of the renal primary or a retroperitoneal recurrence, and remained disease-free for 9 and 18 months respectively after surgery.

Several more recent studies have suggested that surgical consolidation after initial immunotherapy may provide a benefit. A review of 14 separate clinical trials comprising 399 patients treated with IL-2 based therapy with or without LAK cells, identified 62 patients (15.5%) with an objective response.[57] 11 of these 62 patients (18%) underwent resection of residual disease within the lung, kidney, retroperitoneum, or pelvis to become disease-free. All 11 patients remained alive and without evidence of disease with median follow-up of 21 months. Similarly, Krisnamurthi reported 14 patients treated with adjuvant surgery following biological response modifier therapy, 9 of with a partial response and 5 with stable disease.[58] All were then rendered disease-free by surgical excision of residual metastatic lesions and nephrectomy. Cancer-specific survival at 3 years was 82%, with 7 patients (50%) alive and disease-free with mean follow-up of 41 months. 3 patients were also alive with recurrent disease with mean follow-up of 48.3 months. Sella and colleagues reported similar results for surgery after interferon-based therapy.[59] *Such studies suggest that adjuvant surgery can extend the survival of selected patients with metastatic RCC that exhibit a response or stabilization of disease with systemic therapy.*

Other studies have not demonstrated favorable response rates in patients treated with immunotherapy first. In 51 patients with metastatic RCC treated at the National Cancer Institute (NCI) with various immunotherapy regimens, including IL-2 and IFN-α, an overall response rate of only 6% was reported.[56] No responses were observed in the primary tumor itself. Of 3 patients who demonstrated an objective response in their metastatic lesions and underwent nephrectomy, 2 had a continued partial response for 4 and 11 months before progressing, while one patient experienced a durable complete response for more than 88 months. Median survival for all the patients in this study was 13 months. This study highlights the major concern about administering systemic immunotherapy upfront—the lack of response in the primary tumor that has been a common finding in this setting, and overall response rates that appear to be lower than what can be achieved after cytoreduction.

NEPHRECTOMY AS A COMPONENT OF ADOPTIVE IMMUNOTHERAPY

Nephrectomy has been used as a vital component of adoptive immunotherapy protocols for the management of metastatic RCC. In these protocols tumor infiltrating lymphocytes (TIL cells) were harvested from the nephrectomy specimen, expanded in vitro, and reinfused along with IL-2 in an attempt to treat the remaining metastases. Many patients also received preoperative cytokines to improve the yield of TILs and in some cases CD8+ cytotoxic lymphocytes were enriched to enhance responses. In 1997 Figlin et al. reported 55 patients treated in this manner with an overall response rate of 34.6% (9.1% complete response and 25.5% partial) and with a median duration of response of 14 months. Response rates were 43.5% in the 23 patients receiving CD8+ enriched TIL's compared to 28.2% in the remaining 32 patients that received standard TIL's.[3] There were no perioperative deaths and 89% of the patients were able to proceed to immunotherapy without significant delay. Based on these promising results a prospective, phase III, multicenter trial was undertaken for patients with metastatic RCC randomized to receive either low dose IL-2 monotherapy or combination CD8+ TILs with low dose IL-2 after nephrectomy.[60] Unfortunately, neither objective response rates nor 1-year survival rates were significantly different between the two groups (9.9% vs. 11.4%, and 55% vs. 47%, respectively), and this trial was closed early after an interim analysis failed to demonstrate a potential advantage to TIL therapy. Difficulty in reliably preparing the CD8+ TILs was encountered during this study and may have been related to the need for transport of the nephrectomy specimens. This, combined with patient selection issues, may account for the divergent results reported in these studies.

While enthusiasm for TIL therapy has diminished, there are a number of novel and promising approaches to adoptive immunotherapy that should be investigated in future trials, including the use of dendritic cells, heatshock protein vaccination, or gene therapy that may further enhance immunologic responses and may finally provide the breakthrough that is so greatly needed for the treatment of patients with metastatic RCC. Hence, adoptive immunotherapy protocols will continue to remain a viable indication for nephrectomy in patients with metastatic RCC, but only within the context clinical trials performed primarily at tertiary care centers that are capable of supporting these highly technical protocols.

CONCLUSIONS

When is surgery justified in the face of metastatic RCC? Current data supports a survival benefit for cytoreductive nephrectomy in patients with favorable prognostic parameters, but not for patients with poor performance status or extensive burden of disease. Another valid indication for nephrectomy in this patient population is as a part of adoptive immunotherapy protocols, but only in the setting of well constructed clinical trials. In contrast, nephrectomy with intent to induce spontaneous regression is no longer justified, and palliative nephrectomy is now only required in exceptional circumstances. After initial immunotherapy, resection of metastases (or locally recurrent RCC) can be performed for palliative or curative purposes. It is clear that patients with metastatic ural cancer should be counseled and managed on an individual basis. In general, patients with good performance status, a prolonged metastasis-free interval, and limited burden of disease are most likely to benefit from an aggressive surgical approach.

REFERENCES

1. Flanigan RC: Role of Surgery in Patients With Metastatic Renal Cell Carcinoma. Seminars in Urologic Oncology, Vol. 14(4):227–229, 1996.
2. Motzer R and Russo P: Systemic therapy for renal cell carcinoma. J Urol 163:408–417, 2000.
3. Figlin RA, Pierce WC, Kaboo R: Treatment of metastatic renal cell carcinoma with nephrectomy, interleukin-2 and cytokine-primed or CD8(+) selected tumor infiltrating lymphocytes from primary tumor. J Urol 158(3):740, 1997.
4. Greenlee RA, Murray T, Bolden S, et al: Cancer Statistics, 2000. CA Cancer J Clin 50:7–33, 2000.

5. Thrasher JB and Paulson DF: Prognostic Factors in Renal Cancer, Urologic Clinics of North America, 20, No. 2:247, 1993.
6. Libertino, long term results of resection of renal cell cancer with extension into inferior vena cava. J Urol 137:21, 1987.
7. Bassil B, Dosoretz DE, Prout GR Jr.: Validation of the tumor, nodes, and metastasis classification of renal cell carcinoma. J Urol 134:450, 1985.
8. Frank I, Blute M, Weaver A, et al: TNM Staging alone is inadequate for predicting cancer-specific survival following radical nephrectomy for unilateral renal cell carcinoma. J Urol 165(5; Supplement): 185, 2001.
9. Fuhrman et al, Am J Surg Path 6:655, 1982.
10. Tsui KH, Shvarts O, Smith RB, et al: Prognostic indicators for renal cell carcinoma: a multivariate analysis of 643 patients using the revised TNM staging criteria. J Urol 163(4):1090–1095, 2000.
11. Zambrano NR, Lubensky IA, Merino MJ, et al: Histopathology and molecular genetics of renal tumors: Toward unification of a classification system. J Urol 162:1246–1258, 1999.
12. Störkel S, Eble JN, Adlakha K, et al: Classification of renal cell carcioma. Cancer 80(5):987–989, 1997.
13. Renshaw AA and Richie JP: Subtypes of renal cell carcinoma. Different onset and sites of metastatic disease. Am J of Clin Path 111(4):539–543, 1999.
14. Renshaw AA, Henske EP, Loughlin KR, et al: Aggressive variants of chromophobe renal cell carcinoma. Cancer 78(8):1756–1761,1996.
15. Crotty TB, Farrow GM, Lieber MM, et al: Chromophobe cell renal cell carcinoma: Clinicopathological features of 50 cases. J Urol 154:946–967, 1995.
16. Renshaw AA, Zhang H, Corless CL, et al: Solid variants of papillary (chromophil) renal cell carcinoma: clinicopathologic and genetic features. Am J Surg Path 21(10):1203–1209, 1997.
17. Mani S, Todd MB, Katz K, et al: Prognostic factors for survival in patients with metastatic renal cancer treated with biological response modifiers. J Urol 154:34–40, 1995.
18. Canobbio L, Rubagotti A, Loredana M, et al: Prognostic factors for survival in patients with advanced renal cell carcinoma treated with interleukin-2 and interferon-α. J Cancer Res Clin Oncol 121:753–756, 1995.
19. Motzer RJ, Mazumdar M, Bacik J, et al: Survival and prognostic stratification of 670 patients with advanced renal cell carcinoma. J Clin Oncol 17(8):2530–2540, 1999.
20. Elson PJ, Witte RS, Trump DL: Prognostic factors for survival in patients with recurrent or metastatic renal cell carcinoma. Cancer Res 48:7310–7313, 1988.
21. Palmer PA, Vinke J, Philip T, et al: Prognostic factors for survival in patients with advanced renal cell carcinoma treated with recombinant interleukin-2. Ann Oncol 3:475–580, 1992.
22. Elson PJ: Prognostic factors in metastatic renal cell carcinoma. In *Current Clinical Oncology*: Renal Cell Carcinoma: *Molecular Biology, Immunology and Clinical Management*. Bukowski RM and Novick AC (eds.), Humana Press, Totowa, NJ, 2000.
23. Johnson DE, Kaesler KE, Samuels ML: Is nephrectomy justified in patients with metastatic renal carcinoma? J Urol 114:27, 1975.
24. Elson PR, Witte RS, Trump DL: Prognostic factors for survival in patients with recurrent or metastatic renal cell carcinoma. Cancer Res 48:7310–7313, 1988.
25. Negrier S, Escudier B, Lasset C: Recombinant human interleukin-2, recombinant human interferon alfa-2a, or both in metastatic renal cell carcinoma. New Eng J Med 338:1272, 1998.
26. Freed S: Nephrectomy for renal cell carcinoma with metastases. Urology, IX, Number 6:613, 1977.
27. Montie JE, Stewart, BH, Straffon, RA: The role of adjunctive nephrectomy in patients with metastatic renal cell carcinoma. J Urol 117:272, 1977.
28. Walther MM, Patel B, Choyke PL: Hypercalcemia in patients with metastatic renal cell carcinoma: Effect of nephrectomy and metabolic evaluation. J Urol 158(3):733, 1997.
29. deKernion JB and Lindner A: Treatment of Advanced Renal Cell Carcinoma. Renal Tumors: Proceedings of the First International Symposium on Kidney Tumors: 641, 1982.
30. Couillard DR and deVere White RW: Surgery of Renal Cell Carcinoma. Urol Clin North Am 20(2):263–275, 1993.
31. Walther MM, Alexander RB, Weiss GH: Cytoreductive surgery prior to interleukin-2-based therpay in patients with metastatic renal cell carcinoma. Urology 42(3):250, 1993.
32. Swanson D, Johnson D, von Eschenbach, AC: Angioinfarction plus nephrectomy for metastatic renal cell carcinoma—an update. J Urol 130:449, 1983.
33. Kurth KH, Cinqualbre J, Oliver RTD, et al: Embolization and subsequent nephrectomy in metastatic renal cell carcinoma. World J Urol: 122–126, 1986.

34. Gottesman JE, Crawford ED, Grossman HS, et al. Infarction—Nephrectomy for metastatic renal cell carcinoma. Urology 25:248, 1985.
35. Kierney PC, van Heerden JA, Segura JW, et al: Surgeon's role in the management of solitary renal cell carcinoma metastases occurring subsequent to initial curative nephrectomy: An institutional review. Ann Surg Onc 1:345–352, 1994.
36. Tolia BM, Whitmore WF Jr: Solitary metastasis from renal cell carcinoma. J Urol 114:836–838, 1975.
37. Kavolius DP, Mastorakos C, Pavlovich P, et al: Resection of Metastatic Renal Cell Carcinoma. J Clin Onc 16(6):2261–2266, 1998.
38. Flanigan RC, Blumenstien BA, Salmon S, et al: Cytoreduction nephrectomy in metastatic renal cancer: The result of Southwest Oncology Group Trial 8949. J Urol 163(4; Supplement): 154, 2000.
39. Spencer WF, Linehan, WM, McClellan, MW: Immunotherapy with interleukin-2 and interferon in patients with metastatic renal cell cancer in situ primary cancers: A pilot study. J Urol 147:24, 1992.
40. Figlin RA: Renal cell carcinoma: Management of advanced disease. J Urol 161(2):381, 1999.
41. Robertson, CN, Linehan, WM, Pass HI: Preparative cytoreductive surgery in patients with metastatic renal cell carcinoma treated with adoptive immunotherapy with interleukin-2 or interleukin-2 plus lymphokine activated killer cells. J Urol 144:614, 1990.
42. Rackley R, Novick A, Klein E: The impact of adjuvant nephrectomy on mutlimodality treatment of metastatic renal cell carcinoma. J Urol 152:1399, 1994.
43. Fallick ML and McDermott DF: Nephrectomy before interleukin-2 therapy for patients with metastatic renal cell carcinoma. J Urol 158(5):1691, 1997.
44. Muss H, Constanzi JJ, et al: Recombinant alpha interferon in renal cell carcinoma: Randomized trial of two routes of adminstration. J Clin Oncol 5:286–291, 1987.
45. Umeda T, Niijma T: Phase II study of alpha interferon on renal cell carcinoma. Cancer 58:1231–1235, 1986.
46. Fisher RI, Coltman CA, Doroshaw JH, et al: Metastatic renal cancer treated with interleukin-2 and lymphokine-activated killer cells. Ann Intern Med 108:518–523, 1988.
47. Walther MM, Yang JC, Pass HI: Cytoreductive surgery before high dose interleukin-2 based therapy in patients with metastatic renal cell carcinoma. J Urol 158:158, 1997.
48. Bennett RT, Lerner SE, Taub HC: Cytoreductive surgery for stage IV renal cell carcinoma. J Urol 154(1):32, 1995.
49. Walther MM, Lyne JC, Libutti SK, et al. Laparoscopic Cytoreductive Nephrectomy as Preparation for Administration of Systemic Interleukin-2 in the Treatment of Metastatic Renal Cell Carcinoma: A Pilot Study. Urology 53(3):496–500, 1999.
50. Paulter SE, Choyke PL, Philips, et al: Laparoscopic cytoreductive radical nephrectomy for metastatic renal cell carcinoma: A feasibility study. J Urol 165 (5, Supplement): 185, 2001.
51. Mickisch GH, Garin A, Madej M, et al: Tumor nephrectomy plu interefon α is superior to interferon α alone in metastatic renal cell carcinoma. J Urol 163(4; Supplement): 176, 2000.
52. Slaton JW, Perrotte P, Balbay MD, et al: Reassessment of the selection criteria for cytoreductive nephrectomy in patients with metastatic renal cell carcinoma. J Urol 163(4, Supplement): 179, 2000.
53. Wood CG, Huber N, Madsen L, et al: Clinical variables that predict survival following cytoreductive nephrectomy for metastatic renal cell carcinoma. J Urol 165(5, Supplement): 184, 2001.
54. O'Reilly MS, Holmgren L, Shing Y: Angiostatin: A novel angiogenesis inhibitor that mediates the suppresion of metastases by a Lewis lung carcinoma. Cell 2:315, 1994.
55. Fleischmann JD and Kim B: Interleukin-2 immunotherapy followed by resection of residual renal cell carcinoma. J Urol 145:938, 1991.
56. Wagner, JR, McClellan M, Linehan WM: Interleukin-2 based immunotherapy for metastatic renal cell carcinoma with the kidney in place. J Urol 162(1):43, 1999.
57. Kim B and Louie AC: Surgical resection following interleukin 2 therapy for metastatic renal cell carcinoma prolongs remission. Arch. Surg 127:1343, 1992.
58. Krishnamurthis V, Novick AC, Bukowski RM, et al: Efficacy of multimodality therapy in advanced renal cell carcinoma. Urology 51(6):933–937, 1998.
59. Sella A, Swanson DA, Ro JY: Surgery following response to interferon-based therapy for residual renal cell carcinoma. J Urol., 149:19, 1993.
60. Figlin RA, Thompson JA, Bukowski RM, et al: Multicenter, Randomized, Phase III Trial of CD8+ Tumor-Infiltrating Lymphocytes in Combination with Recombinant Interleukin-2 in Metastatic Renal Cell Carcinoma. J Clin Onc 17(8):2521–2529, 1999.
61. Eggermont, AM, Steller EP, Sugarbaker PH: Laparotomy enhances intraperitoneal tumor growth and abrogates the antitumor effects of interleukin-2 and lymphokine-activated killer. Surgery 102(1):71, 1987.

62. Riches EW, Griffiths IH, Thrackray AC: New Growths of the Kidney and Ureter. Br J Urol 23:297–356, 1951.
63. Middleton RG: Surgery for renal cell carcinoma. J Urol 97:973, 1967.
64. Skinner DG, Colvin RV, Vermillion CD, et al: Diagnosis and management of renal cell carcinoma: A Clinical and pathological study of 309 cases. Cancer 28:1165–1177, 1971.
65. Thompson IM, Shannon H, Ross G Jr, et al: An analysis of factors affecting survival in 150 patients with renal carcinoma. J Urol 117:272–275, 1997.
66. Klugo RC, Detmers M, Stiles RE, et al: Aggressive versus conservative management of Stage IV renal cell carcinoma. J Urol 118:244–246, 1977.
67. Dekernion JB, Ramming KP, Smith RB. The natural history of metastatic renal cell carcinoma: a computer analysis. J Urol 120(2):148–152, 1978.
68. McNichols DW, Segura JW, DeWeerd JH: Renal cell carcinoma: Long term survival and alter recurrence. J Urol 126:17–23, 1981.
69. Golimbu M, Al-Askari S, Tessler A, et al: Aggressive treatment of metastatic renal cancer. J Urol 136:805–807, 1986.
70. Giuliani L, Giberti C, Martorana G, et al: Radical extensive surgery for renal cell carcinoma: Long term results and progostic factors. J Urol 143(3):468–473, 1990.
71. Rafla S: Renal cell carcinoma: Natural history and results of treatment. Cancer 25:26–40, 1970.
72. Wagle DG and Seal DR: Renal cell carcinoma: A review of 256 cases. J Surg Oncol 2:23, 1970.
73. Bottinger LE: Prognosis in renal cell carcinoma. Cancer 26:780–787,1970.
74. Mims MM, Christenson B, Schlumberger FC, et al: A ten year evaluation of nephrectomy for extensive renal cell carcinoma. J Urol 95:10, 1966.
75. Cokich IL and Harrison JH: Renal cell carcinoma: Natural history and chemotherapeutic experience. J Urol 114:371–374,1975.
76. O'Dea MJ, Zincke H, Utz DC, et al: The treatment of renal cell carcinoma with solitary metastasis. J Urol 120:540–542, 1978.
77. Jett JR, Hollinger CG, Zinmeister AR, et al: Pulmonary resection of metastatic renal cell carcinoma. Chest 84:442–445, 1983.
78. Dernevik L, Bergggren H, Larson S, et al: Surgical removal of pulmonary metastases from renal cell carcinoma. Scan J Urol Nephrol 19:133–137, 1985.
79. Dinney CPN, Slaton JW, Perrotte PC, et al: The effect of organ site on survival after resection of a solitary renal cell carcinoma (RCC) metastasis. J Urol 161(4, Supplement): 193, 1999.
80. Wolf JS, Aaronson FR, Small EF, et al: Nephrectomy for metastatic renal cell carcinoma: A component of systemic treatment regimens. J Surg Onc 5:7–13, 1994.
81. Levy DA, Swanson DA, Slaton JW: Timely delivery of biological therapy after cytoreductive nephrectomy in carefully selected patients with metastatic renal cell carcinoma. J Urol 159(4):1168, 1998.
82. Flanigan RC, Salmon SE, Blumenstein BA, et al. Nephrectomy followed by interferon-alpha-2b compared with interfereon alfa-2b alone for metastatic renal cell cancer. N Engl J Med; 345:1655–1659, 2001.
83. Mickisch GHJ, Garin A, van Poppel H, de Prijck L, Sylvester R, EORTC Group: Radical Nephrectomy plus interferon-alfa-based immunotherapy compared with interferon-alfa alone in metastatic renal-cell carcinoma: a randomized trial. The Lancet 358:966–970, 2001.
84. Bromwich E, Hendry D, Aitchison M: Cytoreductive nephrectomy: is it a realistic option in patients with renal cancer? BJU International; 89:523–525, 2002.
85. Symbas NP, Townsend MF, El-Galley R, Keane TE, Graham SD, Petros JA: Poor prognosis associated with throbocytosis in patients with renal cell carcinoma. BJU International; 86:203–207, 2000.

III. METASTATIC RENAL CELL CARCINOMA: CURRENT AND FUTURE APPROACHES

8. PROGNOSTIC FACTORS FOR METASTATIC KIDNEY CANCER

BEVERLY J. DRUCKER, M.D., Ph.D., MADHU MAZUMDAR, Ph.D., AND ROBERT J. MOTZER, M.D.

Memorial Sloan Kettering Cancer Center, New York, NY 10021

INTRODUCTION

Metastatic renal cell carcinoma is associated with a poor prognosis, a result of the lack of effective systemic therapy.[1] Conventional cytotoxic chemotherapy and hormone therapy lack significant antitumor effect in the treatment of metastatic RCC. Response rates to standard cytotoxic chemotherapies are less than 10%,[2] and hormonal therapy is inactive (antiandrogens, antiestrogens, androgens, progestins), with response rates of 1–2%. The rare but consistent incidence of spontaneous tumor regression,[3,4] plus the naturally occurring phenomenon of lymphocytic infiltration in the renal tumors of untreated patients,[5] instigated the study of immunotherapy against renal cell cancer.

Interferon-α and interleukin-2 (IL-2) are two cytokines used in the biologic therapy of RCC. Increased T-lymphocyte and natural killer cell activity, as well as the induction of specific antigen expression, have been cited as potential anti-neoplastic effects of interferon-α.[5,6] IL-2 is produced by activated T and NK cells and plays a pivotal role in the regulation of lymphocyte activation and proliferation.[7] Cytokine therapy with either interleukin-2 or interferon-α achieves responses in 10–20% of patients, with occasional long-term survivors.[8] These therapies may be associated with significant toxicity yet few long-term survivors. High dose IL-2 therapy requires inpatient administration due to the induction of capillary leak syndrome and severe hypotension. Subcutaneous interferon-α has less severe side effects, but still induces flu-like symptoms, including fever, chills, decreased appetite, muscle aches, fatigue, diarrhea, generalized malaise, and depression.

R.A. Figlin (ed.). KIDNEY CANCER. Copyright © 2003. Kluwer Academic Publishers. Boston. All rights reserved.

Cytokines used in treating renal cell carcinoma frequently have responses that may not become evident until 3 months or more after the initiation of therapy.[9] Response rates to interferon-α, IL-2 or combinations vary considerably among phase II trials,[10] implying that patient selection is an important factor in achieving a favorable treatment outcome. Given the low percentage of patients who respond to immunotherapy, and the significant side effects, it would be helpful to identify a sub-population of patients with metastatic RCC who are more likely to respond or achieve longer survival following therapy. Identification of appropriate prognostic factors that predict the likelihood of survival prior to commencement of immunotherapy would allow for the selection of individuals who would benefit from cytokine-based treatment and minimize the number of patients who would suffer needless toxicity without therapeutic benefit.

Determining prognostic factors of survival for patients with advanced RCC is also valuable in directing therapy and interpreting the results of clinical trials of new agents. The ability to assess prognosis across patient groups allows for the comparison of treatment results among different clinical trials. Although the majority of patients with metastatic RCC have rapidly progressive disease with a median survival of less than one year, there is a small proportion of patients with indolent disease whose long-term survival can be in excess of five years. The ability to define such patients in advance can aid in the planning and interpretation of phase II clinical trials. Prognostic factors leading to improved survival could also define patient populations for Phase II trials. Clinical trials that include patient survival as an endpoint must account for prognostic factors to assure that treatment groups are comparable. Factors that have been examined include performance status at diagnosis, time from diagnosis to metastasis, location and number of metastases, weight loss, nephrectomy status and laboratory parameters. Earlier prognostic models focused on factors predicting survival only. More recently, models stratified patients based on the likelihood of survival while receiving cytokine therapies. Prognostic models are now used in the stratification of patients in phase 3 trials, making possible the identification of subgroups that may have a greater likelihood of responding to therapy.

PROGNOSTIC FACTORS IN RENAL CELL CANCER

Univariate Analysis

A number of different clinical factors have been reported to correlate with survival in patients with metastatic renal cell cancer. These features were identified in univariate analyses, and were later applied to multivariate analyses. One of the earliest analyses of prognostic factors in metastatic renal cell carcinoma was performed by Maldazys and deKernion.[11] They analyzed 181 cases of metastatic renal cell carcinoma treated from 1973 to 1982. Survival was assessed from the date of the first known metastasis and analyzed with respect to patient age, sex, interval free of disease, performance status (PS), site of metastasis and nephrectomy. Metastatic sites were defined as lung-only, single site other than lung, or multiple sites. The effect of treatment on survival was not examined. Age and sex was not found to influence survival, but improved survival was associated with a long interval between initial nephrectomy and discovery of metastases, normal performance status, metastases limited to the lung parenchyma, and removal of the primary tumor. The effect of nephrectomy on survival was not separable from effects of patient selection, as only patients with good performances status were likely to be chosen for nephrectomy. Patients with favorable characteristics had a relatively favorable prognosis with 50% surviving at three years and a median survival time of 24 months.

Multivariate Analysis

Factors identified by univariate analysis may be interdependent. To assess redundancy, multivariate analysis is performed to identify factors that are independently associated with prognosis. Variables identified by multivariate analysis to have independent prognostic significance have included patient performance status, prior nephrectomy, weight loss, number of metastatic sites, and interval between diagnosis and treatment, to name a few. Once identified, these factors can be used to stratify patients into subgroups that can be analyzed for survival, leading to the development of prognostic survival models. Several groups have developed prognostic models that can be used to predict both survival and likelihood of response to therapy. Models differ based on the number of patients used in generating the model, parameters included in the model, patient stage, and number of prognostic groups. Major points are compared in Table 1.

Prognostic Models for Survival

ECOG Model

Elson et al[12] proposed a prognostic model using the clinical factors identified as prognostic factors in their survival analysis of 610 patients with metastatic RCC treated with chemotherapy. All patients entered into ECOG Phase II protocols for advanced RCC between 1975 and 1984 were considered for inclusion. None of the agents used showed antitumor activity. Factors that were identified as independently associated with poor prognosis included low performance status, time from diagnosis to clinical trial entry of ≤ 1 year, weight loss, prior nephrectomy, prior cytotoxic chemotherapy, and clinically evident hepatic, osseous and brain metastases. Gender, race, age, associated chronic disease, and prior radiotherapy did not affect prognosis. Prognostic factors that were used in the model included baseline ECOG PS, time from diagnosis to enrollment in clinical trial, number of metastatic sites, prior chemotherapy and a history of weight loss. Five distinct risk groups were identified using these factors, with the most favorable group having no or one risk factor. The other groups were composed of patients with two, three, four, or more risk factors. Median survival for the groups was 12.8, 7.7, 6.3, 3.4 and 2.1 months from best to worst subgroup.

Institut Gustave-Roussy Model

De Forges et al[13] also devised a prognostic model for survival in metastatic renal cell carcinoma, based on a group of 134 patients treated from 1971 to 1986 at the

Table 1.

Investigator	Year	# of Patients	Therapy Examined	Prognostic Factors Incorporated into Model
Maldazys et al (UCLA)	1986	181	Chemotherapy	Performance Status, Disease Free Interval, Nephrectomy Status Age, Sex, Metastatic Site
Elson et al (ECOG)	1988	610	Unspecified	Performance Status, Time from Diagnosis to Treatment, Nephrectomy status, Prior chemotherapy, Number of Metastatic Sites
DeForges et al (InstitutGustave Roussy)	1988	134	Unspecified	Disease Free Interval, Presence of Liver Metastasis, # and size of lung Lesions, ESR/weight loss
Palmer et al (CETUS)	1992	327	Interleukin-2	Performance Status, Time from Diagnosis to Treatment, Number of metastatic sites
Fossa et al (Multi-Institution)	1994	295	Interferon vs Chemotherapy	Performance Status, ESR, ≤10% weight loss
Motzer et al (MSKCC)	1999	640	Chemotherapy or Cytokines	Performance Status, Nephrectomy Status, LDH, Hemoglobin, Corrected Calcium
Motzer et al (MSKCC)	2002	463	Interferon	Performance Status, Time from Diagnosis to start of therapy, LDH, Hemoglobin, Corrected Calcium
Negrier et al (Group Francais d'Immunotherapie)	2002	782	Cytokines	Performance Status, # of Metastatic Sites, Disease-Free Interval, Signs of Inflammation, Hemoglobin

Institut Gustave-Roussy. Patients received various hormonal and chemotherapeutic regimens. Analysis was performed on 17 variables, with nine identified by univariate analysis to be significantly related to 1-year survival and relative risk of death. Multivariate analysis identified only four of these clinical features to be independently significant: 1) a variable based on weight loss and sedimentation rate, 2) presence of hepatic metastasis 3) size and number of lung metastases, and 4) disease free interval between diagnosis and metastatic disease. A mathematical model was then generated that was predictive of survival rates based on these variables. Each variable was assigned a mathematic coefficient in a survival equation generated by the cox regression model. This in turn created six prognostic subgroups that stratified patients according to survival projections.

Multi-Institution Model

Researchers at two European centers collaborated in their attempt to define whether immunotherapy was beneficial in all patients or only in certain subgroups.[14] They analyzed prognostic factors and survival in 295 patients with metastatic renal cell carcinoma treated with either chemotherapy or interferon. At the Institute Gustave Roussy, 159 patients were treated with various cytotoxic agents and drug combinations between 1975 and 1990. During the same time period 136 patients were treated with interferon-α given three times weekly at the Norwegian Radium Hospital. The subsequent analysis revealed that the three-year survival rate was significantly better in the group treated with interferon-α than the chemotherapy group, with 24% versus 8% of patients alive at three years, respectively. Improved survival was correlated with the following factors in the univariate analysis: 1) age ≤60, 2) prior nephrectomy, 3) >1 year between diagnosis and treatment, 4) ECOG performance status 0 or 1, 5) absence of liver metastases, 6) low ESR and/or ≤10% of weight loss (WL) within the past 6 months. Cox regression analysis indicated that a low ESR, good performance status and lack of >10% weight loss (WL) were independent prognostic factors for survival. Using these variables, the investigators formed an equation that created an index of prognosis (Index = 0.01*ESR + 0.40*WL + 0.40PS) that could categorize patients into one of three prognostic groups: poor, intermediate and good. The regression coefficient of ESR was a gradient associated with its own level, whereas the coefficients for weight loss and ECOG PS of 0,1 were 0 or 1 depending on the absence or presence of this discrete variable. After the final calculation, patients with scores of <0.5 were classified as good risk, those with score >=1 were poor risk and those in between were intermediate risk. In the poor and intermediate risk groups, no significant survival difference was observed between patients treated with chemotherapy versus interferon. In good risk patients, however, there was a significant improvement in survival of patients treated with interferon, with a 48% 3-year survival rate versus a 15% 3-year survival rate in patients treated with chemotherapy. Interferon may therefore increase survival in good risk patients, but is as ineffective as chemotherapy in poor risk patients.

Cetus Model

Palmer et al[15] studied the relationship between pretreatment clinical features and survival of patients with advanced renal cell carcinoma who were treated with continuous infusion IL-2. A database of 327 patients who received IL-2 therapy was analyzed to identify pretreatment features that could predict survival. Thirteen clinical characteristics were examined, and six factors were associated with improved survival: ECOG PS (0 or 1), time from diagnosis to treatment of >24 months, prior nephrectomy, presence of lung metastasis, bone metastasis and other metastases. Multivariate analysis identified three factors that were independently related to prognosis as important predictors for survival: baseline performance status (ECOG 0 vs 1), time from diagnosis to treatment (>24 months vs < or = 24 months), and the number of metastatic sites (1 vs 2 or more). These factors were then used to create a model in which patients were classified into 4 subgroups based on the number of risk factors present. Median survival for each group was 28, 17 10 and 5 months. The model was validated with an independent group of 125 patients with RCC who were treated with subcutaneous IL-2, and survival was predicted accurately.

Memorial Sloan Kettering Cancer Center (MSKCC) Model

A model was devised at our center predictive of survival in patients with metastatic renal cell cancer. Factors related to survival in 670 patients with advanced RCC treated in 24 consecutive clinical trials from September 1975 to July 1996 were analyzed.[16] All patients had histologically confirmed RCC and stage IV disease, with measurable lesions. The number and sites of metastases (lung, bone liver, mediastinum, and/or retroperitoneum), Karnofsky performance status, prior treatment (radiation, chemotherapy, and immunotherapy) prior nephrectomy, and time interval from diagnosis to the start of treatment were recorded. Biochemical features were also recorded and included hemoglobin, serum albumin, alkaline phosphatase, lactate dehydrogenase, and corrected calcium concentrations. Clinical features were first examined by univariate analysis. Factors associated with an adverse prognosis in univariate analysis included the presence of hepatic metastasis, two or more sites of metastases, a Karnofsky performance status of less than 80%, prior radiation or chemotherapy, lack of prior nephrectomy, and a time interval from disease diagnosis to treatment of less than one year. Biochemical parameters found to be significant for an adverse prognosis in univariate analysis included low serum albumin, elevated serum alkaline phosphatase, low hemoglobin, an elevated serum lactate dehydrogenase, and a high corrected serum calcium level.

Seven variables identified in the univariate analysis were analyzed by multivariate analysis to determine whether they had an independent relation to survival. These included hemoglobin, serum lactate dehydrogenase, corrected calcium, prior nephrectomy, Karnofsky performance status, hepatic metastases, and the interval from diagnosis to treatment. Pretreatment features associated with a shorter survival that maintained independent significance after the multivariate analysis were: low Karnofsky performance status (<80%), high serum lactate dehydrogenase (>1.5 times upper limit of normal), low hemoglobin (below the lower limit of normal), high "corrected" serum calcium (>10 mg/dL), and absence of prior nephrectomy.

These five prognostic factors were then used to categorize patients with metastatic RCC into three different risk groups (see Figure 1). Median survival times of the risk groups were separated by 6 months or more. Patients were divided based on their number of negative prognostic factors: those with zero risk factors (favorable-risk), those with one or two (intermediate risk), and those with three or more (poor-risk). The median survival time of all patients was 10 months (95% confidence interval, 9–11 months). The median time to death in the 25% of patients with zero risk factors (favorable-risk) was 20 months. Fifty three percent of the patients had one or two risk factors (intermediate risk) and the median survival time in this group was 10 months. Patients with three or more risk factors (poor-risk) who comprise 22% of the patients had a median survival time of 4 months.

The predictive performance of the model was internally validated through a two-step nonparametric bootstrapping process.[17] The model was also applied to an external data set from ECOG composed of 175 patients treated in a randomized trial of interferon-α with or without 13-cis-retinoic acid. In this group, the median survival

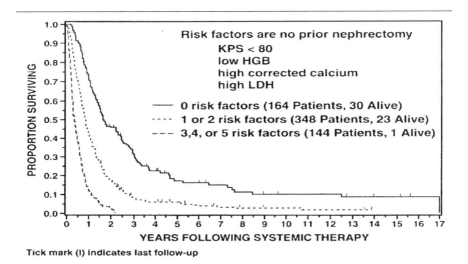

Figure 1. Renal cell carcinoma survival by risk group.

times of favorable, intermediate, and poor risk patients treated with interferon-α were 29, 14, and 4 months, respectively.

The relationship between treatment with cytokine therapy or chemotherapy was a significant predictor of survival and was accounted for in the analysis of the 670 patients to define prognostic factors. Treatment was categorized as cytokine (containing interferon-α and/or interleukin-2) in 396 patients and chemotherapy (cytotoxic or hormonal therapy) in 274 (41%). Patients treated with cytokine therapy had a longer survival time than did those treated with chemotherapy, regardless of how long after diagnosis treatment was started or the risk category of the patient based on pretreatment features (Figure 2). Using the same risk model as defined previously, median survival times for favorable, intermediate, and poor risk patients were 27, 12 and 6 months for those treated with cytokines and 15, 7 and 3 months for those treated with chemotherapy, respectively (Table 2). The magnitude of difference was greater in the favorable and intermediate risk groups. The median survival time was less than 6 months in the poor risk groups for both therapies. In this retrospective study, patients treated with cytokine therapy experienced longer survival compared with patients treated with chemotherapy. When survival after therapy was considered according to pretreatment risk status, the difference in median survival between interferon and chemotherapy was greatest in the group with more favorable prognostic features. In contrast, survival for patients with poor risk features was less than 6 months regardless of treatment type. These observations suggest that patients with favorable prognostic features as described by this model experienced longer survival following treatment with cytokine therapy, and that novel treatment strategies should be considered first-line for patients with unfavorable prognostic features.

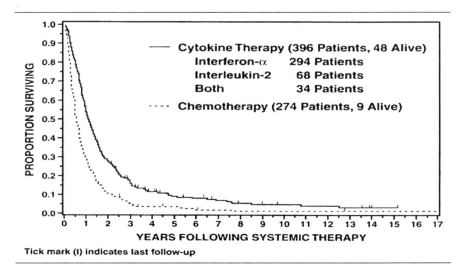

Figure 2. Renal cell carcinoma survival by treatment.

Table 2. Renal Cell Carcinoma
Survival by Treatment and Risk Group.

Risk Group	Agent	Pts	Median Surv (Mo)
Favorable	Cytokine	114	27
(0)	Chemo	134	15
Intermediate	Cytokine	214	12
(1, 2)	Chemo	134	7
Poor	Cytokine	59	6
(3, 4, 5)	Chemo	85	3

Since the development of the original MSKCC prognostic model,[8] the role of cytoreductive nephrectomy in the metastatic setting in patients with good performance status was established.[18] In light of this development, prognostic variables were reassessed[19] based on the assumption that patients with metastatic disease would now be considered for cytoreductive nephrectomy prior to cytokine treatment. An analysis was performed on a group of 463 patients who had received interferon-alpha therapy as first-line systemic therapy.[19] As a group without regard to prognostic features, the median survival time of all patients with interferon-α was 13 months, with the median time to progression of 4.7 months. Patients were then divided into three risk categories for survival on the basis of the five pretreatment clinical features that had been determined in the previous multivariate analysis:[8] low Karnofsky performance status (<80%), high LDH (1.5× normal), low serum hemoglobin, high corrected serum calcium and time from initial RCC diagnosis to start of interferon-α therapy of less than one year.[19] Those patients with zero risk factors were consid-

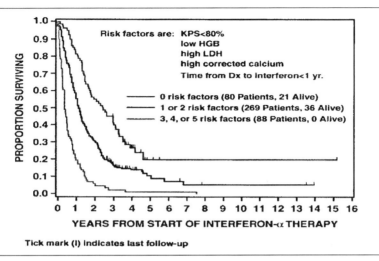

Figure 3. Interferon as a comparative therapy in survival by risk following interferon-α.

ered to have favorable risk, those with one or two were considered to have intermediate risk, and those with three or more risk factors had poor risk. Median time to death in patients with favorable risk was 30 months, with the intermediate risk group and poor risk groups having median survival times of 14 months and 5 months respectively. (Figure 3) This survival data derived from patients receiving interferon as first line therapy can by used as a standard against which novel therapies can be compared in phase II and III trials.

French Model

The Group Francais d'Immunotherapie recently completed an analysis of prognostic factors of survival and rapid progression in patients with metastatic renal cell carcinoma treated by cytokines.[33] Over a six year period, they enrolled 782 patients in 5 successive multicenter trials using cytokine regimens containing interferon-α interleukin-2 or both. Univariate and multivariate analyses were performed to identify prognostic factors associated with survival. Nine parameters were identified as independent prognostic factors: signs of inflammation as detected by sedimentation rate or C-reactive protein, time interval from renal tumor to metastases, number of circulating neutrophils, presence of liver metastases, presence of bone metastases, ECOG performance status, number of metastatic sites, elevated level of alkaline phosphatase, and hemoglobin level. They then compared the factors they identified to those in previous published prognostic models, and identified five that were validated through repeated identification in multiple models: performance status, number of metastatic sites, disease-free interval, biological signs of inflammation and hemoglobin level. They also identified four independent factors that were predictive of rapid disease progression while receiving cytokine therapy: presence of hepatic metastases, less than one year interval from renal tumor to metastases, more than 1 metastatic site, and elevated neutrophil counts. They determined that patients who had 3 or more of these factors had greater than an 80% probability of rapid progression within 3 months despite treatment, and recommended that these patients be considered for novel therapies rather than cytokine regimens.

UCLA Model

Prognostic indicators were analyzed for patients with renal cell cancer undergoing nephrectomy at initial diagnosis.[20] This series of 643 patients included mostly patients with tumors localized to the kidney, but some had known metastatic disease. Patients were evaluated for preoperative functional status, TNM stage, tumor stage, and disease grade. The 5 year cancer specific survival rate based on TNM stage was 91%, 74%, 67%, 32% for stages I, II, III, and IV tumors respectively. Survival rates for stages T1, T2, T3 and T4 were 83%, 57%, 42%, and 28% respectively. Tumor grade also correlated with survival. Multivariate analysis revealed that the overall TNM stage and grade of disease were the most important prognostic indicators, with ECOG classification prior to surgery and tumor stage less significant, although this may reflect a bias in patient selection, as patients with poor ECOG performance status would be unlikely to be taken to surgery.

Data from the 477 patients undergoing nephrectomy was used to derive a mathematical model to predict individual survival and thus guide decisions regarding surgery.[21] A database containing 292 nonmetastatic RCC patients and 262 metastatic RCC patients who underwent either radical or partial nephrectomy was reviewed, with time to death being the primary endpoint. Metastatic and nonmetastatic patients were analyzed separately. For nonmetastatic patients, the significant factors predicting survival were Furhman's grade of the tumor and ECOG performance status. For metastatic patients, the significant factors predicting survival were 1997 classification T stage, number of symptoms, nodal involvement and immunotherapy. These variables were then implanted into an exponential Nadas equation to derive a mathematical model to predict survival, with separate equations for non-metastatic and metastatic patients. This model, when used in devising a treatment plan, can help to predict which patients will benefit from nephrectomy.

PROGNOSTIC VALUE OF HISTOLOGY

Prognostic models have focused on clinical and laboratory parameters, and have not fully accounted for tumor pathology and the underlying genetics. Recent progress in understanding the genetic features of RCC has facilitated classification into clear cell and non-clear cell subtypes such as papillary, chromophobe, and collecting duct histology. The responsiveness of these cell types to immunotherapy remains to be defined. The majority (60–62%) of renal cell cancers are considered conventional (or clear cell) carcinomas.[22] The remainder of cases consist of papillary RCC, chromophobic RCC, collecting duct carcinoma and medullary carcinoma. When confined to the kidney, papillary RCC and chromophobic RCC generally have a better prognosis than the conventional type, with a smaller likelihood of developing micrometastatic disease. Collecting duct tumors and medullary carcinomas generally have a poor prognosis. In addition, regardless of the pathologic classification, tumors containing a sarcomatous pattern have been reported to have a worsen prognosis.[22]

The outcome data was a in patients with metastatic renal cell carcinoma with histologies other than clear cell type has been reviewed.[23] Sixty-four patients with metastatic, non-clear cell RCC were reviewed retrospectively. The prevalent histology was collecting duct tumor, present in 26 of the 64 patients (41%). The remainder included chromophobe tumors (19%), papillary tumors (28%) and unclassifiable tumors (12%). Of the original 64 patients, only 42 were treated with systemic therapy. In all, 86 systemic therapies were attempted, with 37 of them including cytokines. Only two patients (5%) were observed to have a partial response. The median overall survival time was 9.4 months. Survival was longer for patients with chromophobe tumors compared to collecting duct or papillary histology. Overall, metastatic RCC of non-clear cell histology appear resistant to systemic therapies, with a lower response rate to interferon than documented in previous studies, which suggests that histology may be considered in guiding treatment decisions.

BIOLOGIC INVESTIGATIONAL PROGNOSTIC MARKERS

Many laboratories and clinical investigators are examining novel biologic markers related to oncogenesis and angiogenesis to see if they can predict progression or prognosis in renal cell cancer. At present, there is no convincing data to justify the common use of these variables in evaluating patients with renal cell cancer, but the hope is that with increased study these investigational markers may not only predict prognosis and response to cytokine therapy but ultimately suggest new therapeutic possibilities. These markers have generally fallen into one of two groups, those related to the angiogenic/metastatic potential of the tumor and those related to the immune system of the host.

Markers of Increased Angiogenesis

Markers of increased angiogenesis, such as basic fibroblast growth factor and vascular endothelial growth factor, have been reported to be both overexpressed in tumor tissue and elevated in the serum of affected patients.[24,25] When VEGF serum levels were measured in 164 patients with RCC before nephrectomy, these levels were significantly increased in patients with RCC when compared to healthy controls. In addition, VEGF levels in serum correlated to both clinical stage and histo-pathological grade, with levels higher in metastatic disease compared to non-metastatic disease.[24,25] Patients with VEGF levels below the median value had significantly longer survival time than patients with higher levels.[26]

Increased expression of factors associated with tissue invasion and metastasis has also been linked to prognosis. Loss of the cell adhesion marker E-cadherin was correlated with RCC disease progression.[27] Urokinase plasminogen activator (U-PA) is believed to play a critical role in invasion and metastasis and has been suggested to be an independent prognostic factor for early relapse and overall survival in renal cell cancer.[28] The role of these markers in prognosis of metastatic renal cell carcinoma remains to be determined, and their study is particularly relevant to the evaluation of anti-angiogenesis agents in clinical trials.

Markers of Immune Parameters

The ability to predict responsiveness of patients to immunotherapy by means of serum or cellular assays would be useful in directing cytokine therapy. A prospective study by Lauerova et al[29] explored several non-specific and specific immune parameters in 78 RCC patients prior to nephrectomy. Preoperative values were then related to disease outcome and the response of patients to cytokine-based immunotherapy during a 3-year followup. Cytokine treated patients who relapsed within the 3 year follow-up had significantly reduced proportions of CCD80+ and CD10/80+ lymphocytes at the time of in initial diagnosis as compared to those patients surviving for 3 years disease free. No such relationship was seen in untreated patients who relapsed within three years, suggesting a relationship between decreased numbers of this lymphocytes population and an "incorrect" response to cytokine therapy rather than a marker of overall poor prognosis.

Interleukin 10 is produced by type 2 helper T-lymphocytes[30] and acts as a cytokine synthesis inhibitory factor. It has a direct effect on IL-2 production by T cells and blocks the development of pre-dendritic cells into mature dendritic cells *in vitro*.[31] IL-10 mediated immunosuppression could therefore be an important escape mechanism for tumors. Wittke et al[32] used a highly sensitive enzyme linked immunosorbent assay (ELISA) to measure pretreatment serum concentrations of IL-10 in 80 consecutive patients with metastatic renal cell carcinoma. Patients received systemic immunotherapy with subcutaneous IL-2 and interferon-α which was continued until disease progression. Elevated serum levels of IL-10 (>1 pm/ml) were detected in 21 of 80 RCC patients and were associated with an unfavorable outcome. Median survival in these patients was 11+ months, and opposed to patients with low IL-10 levels (<= 1 pg/ml, n = 59) who had a median survival of 27+ months, with the difference being statistically significant. In this study, an elevated pretreatment serum level of IL-10 was a statistically independent predictor of poorer response to cytokines. These markers of immune function are considered interesting from research point only, and are not used in patient management.

RISK DIRECTED THERAPY

The multiple prognostic models discussed in this chapter provide guidance is determining which patients will derive benefit from medical or surgical interventions. The UCLA model[20] defines which patients will derive benefit from nephrectomy, and spares patients unlikely to benefit an unnecessary surgery. Several other models investigated the impact that prognostic factors have in response to medical therapies. The Multi-Institution model generated by Fossa et al[13] demonstrated a significant improvement in three-year survival (48% vs 15%) in good risk patients treated with interferon compared to a similar group treated with chemotherapy. No such benefit of interferon over chemotherapy was seen in poor risk patients, suggesting that both therapies were ineffective in that group. In the development of the MSKCC model,[8] patients were also initially grouped according to whether they had treatment with cytokine therapy or chemotherapy, while later analysis concentrated on patients treated with interferon only.[19] Patients treated with cytokine therapy had a longer survival compared to patients treated with chemotherapy, regardless of the year of treatment or risk category based on pretreatment features,[8] but the magnitude of difference in median survival was greater in the favorable-risk and intermediate-risk groups. Similarly, patients in the favorable-risk group treated with interferon had a significant survival benefit, with median survival of 30 months, whereas those in the poor-risk group treated with interferon received no benefit.[19] Focusing on a slightly different perspective, the Group Francais d'Immunotherapie used their model[33] to identify patients most likely to progress quickly on cytokine therapy, finding that patients with three or more poor risk features were likely to progress within three months of cytokine therapy. These models strongly suggest that patients with favorable prognostic features may derive therapeutic benefit from cytokine therapy, whereas patients with poor prognostic features are unlikely to benefit from cytokine therapy and should be offered supportive care, or, if their performance status permits, experimental therapies.

CONCLUSION

Metastatic renal cell carcinoma is a tumor highly refractory to treatment with systemic therapy. Only a minority of patients respond to or achieve prolonged survival on immunotherapy with interferon and/or IL-2. This emphasizes the need for clinical investigation to identify more effective therapies. Prognostic models based on pretreatment clinical and laboratory variables can help define patients more likely to benefit from standard therapies, as well as assist in the interpretation of drug effectiveness in phase II clinical trials. Investigations into new prognostic factors based on the biology of the cancer and pathology of patient immune response are useful in that they may lead to new therapeutic strategies in the future.

REFERENCES

1. Motzer RJ, Russo P, Nanus DM, Berg WJ. Renal cell carcinoma. *Curr Probl Cancer*. 1997;21(4): 185–232.
2. Motzer RJ, Bander NH, Nanus DM. Renal-cell carcinoma. *N Engl J Med*. 1996;335(12):865–75.
3. Fairlamb DJ. Spontaneous regression of metastases of renal cancer: A report of two cases including the first recorded regression following irradiation of a dominant metastasis and review of the world literature. *Cancer*. 1981;47(8):2102–6.
4. Marcus SG, Choyke PL, Reiter R, et al. Regression of metastatic renal cell carcinoma after cytoreductive nephrectomy. *J Urol*. 1993;150(2 Pt 1):463–6.
5. Balch CM, Riley LB, Bae YJ, et al. Patterns of human tumor-infiltrating lymphocytes in 120 human cancers. *Arch Surg*. 1990;125(2):200–5.
6. Holan V, Kohno K, Minowada J. Natural human interferon-alpha augments interleukin-2 production by a direct action on the activated IL-2-producing T cells. *J Interferon Res*. 1991;11(6): 319–25.

7. Trinchieri G, Matsumoto-Kobayashi M, Clark SC, Seehra J, London L, Perussia B. Response of resting human peripheral blood natural killer cells to interleukin 2. *J Exp Med*. 1984;160(4):1147–69.
8. Motzer RJ, Mazumdar M, Bacik J, Russo P, Berg WJ, Metz EM. Effect of cytokine therapy on survival for patients with advanced renal cell carcinoma. *J Clin Oncol*. 2000;18(9):1928–35.
9. Wirth MP. Immunotherapy for metastatic renal cell carcinoma. *Urol Clin North Am*. 1993; 20(2):283–95.
10. Vogelzang NJ, Lipton A, Figlin RA. Subcutaneous interleukin-2 plus interferon alfa-2a in metastatic renal cancer: an outpatient multicenter trial. *J Clin Oncol*. 1993;11(9):1809–16.
11. Maldazys JD, deKernion JB. Prognostic factors in metastatic renal carcinoma. *J Urol*. 1986;136(2): 376–9.
12. Elson PJ, Witte RS, Trump DL. Prognostic factors for survival in patients with recurrent or metastatic renal cell carcinoma. *Cancer Res*. 1988;48(24 Pt 1):7310–3.
13. De Forges A, Rey A, Klink M, Ghosn M, Kramar A, Droz J. Prognostic Factors of Adult Metastatic Renral Carcinoma: A Multivariate Analysis. *Seminars in Surgical Oncology*. 1988;4:149–54.
14. Fossa SD, Kramar A, Droz JP. Prognostic factors and survival in patients with metastatic renal cell carcinoma treated with chemotherapy or interferon-alpha. *Eur J Cancer*. 1994;9(4):1310–4.
15. Palmer PA, Vinke J, Philip T, et al. Prognostic Factors for Survival in Patients with Advanced Renal Ccell Carcinoma Treated with Recombinant Interleukin-2. *Annals of Oncology*. 1992;3:475–80.
16. Motzer RJ, Mazumdar M, Bacik J, Berg W, Amsterdam A, Ferrara J. Survival and Prognostic Stratification of 670 Patients with Advanced Renal Cell Carcinoma. *Journal of Clinical Oncology*. 1999; 17(8):2530–40.
17. Chen C, George S. The Bootstrap and Identification of Prognostic Factors via Cox's Proportional Hazards Regression Model. *Statistical Medicine*. 1985;11:39–46.
18. Flanigan RC, Yonover PM. The role of radical nephrectomy in metastatic renal cell carcinoma. *Semin Urol Oncol*. 2001;19(2):98–102.
19. Motzer RJ, Bacik J, Murphy BA, Russo P, Mazumdar M. Interferon-alfa as a comparative treatment for clinical trials of new therapies against advanced renal cell carcinoma. *J Clin Oncol*. 2002;20(1): 289–96.
20. Tsui KH, Shvarts O, Smith RB, Figlin RA, deKernion JB, Belldegrun A. Prognostic indicators for renal cell carcinoma: a multivariate analysis of 643 patients using the revised 1997 TNM staging criteria. *J Urol*. 2000;163(4):1090–5; quiz 1295.
21. Zisman A, Pantuck AJ, Dorey F, et al. Mathematical model to predict individual survival for patients with renal cell carcinoma. *J Clin Oncol*. 2002;20(5):1368–74.
22. Reuter VE, Presti JC, Jr. Contemporary approach to the classification of renal epithelial tumors. *Semin Oncol*. 2000;27(2):124–37.
23. Motzer RJ, Bacik J, Mariani T, Russo P, Mazumdar M, Reuter V. Treatment outcome and survival associated with metastatic renal cell carcinoma of non-clear-cell histology. *J Clin Oncol*. 2002;20(9):2376–81.
24. Sato K, Tsuchiya N, Sasaki R, et al. Increased serum levels of vascular endothelial growth factor in patients with renal cell carcinoma. *Jpn J Cancer Res*. 1999;90(8):874–9.
25. Dosquet C, Coudert MC, Lepage E, Cabane J, Richard F. Are angiogenic factors, cytokines, and soluble adhesion molecules prognostic factors in patients with renal cell carcinoma? *Clin Cancer Res*. 1997;3(12 Pt 1):2451–8.
26. Jacobsen J, Rasmuson T, Grankvist K, Ljungberg B. Vascular endothelial growth factor as prognostic factor in renal cell carcinoma. *J Urol*. 2000;163(1):343–7.
27. Fisher RI, Coltman CA, Jr., Doroshow JH, et al. Metastatic renal cancer treated with interleukin-2 and lymphokine-activated killer cells. A phase II clinical trial. *Ann Intern Med*. 1988;108(4):518–23.
28. Kamel D, Turpeenniemi-Hujanen T, Vahakangas K, Paakko P, Soini Y. Proliferating cell nuclear antigen but not p53 or human papillomavirus DNA correlates with advanced clinical stage in renal cell carcinoma. *Histopathology*. 1994;25(4):339–47.
29. Lauerova L, Dusek L, Spurny V, et al. Relation of prenephrectomy CD profiles and serum cytokines to the disease outcome and response to IFN-alpha/IL-2 therapy in renal cell carcinoma patients. *Oncol Rep*. 2001;8(3):685–92.
30. Fiorentino DF, Bond MW, Mosmann TR. Two types of mouse T helper cell. IV. Th2 clones secrete a factor that inhibits cytokine production by Th1 clones. *J Exp Med*. 1989;170(6):2081–95.
31. Buelens C, Verhasselt V, De Groote D, Thielemans K, Goldman M, Willems F. Interleukin-10 prevents the generation of dendritic cells from human peripheral blood mononuclear cells cultured with interleukin-4 and granulocyte/macrophage-colony-stimulating factor. *Eur J Immunol*. 1997; 27(3):756–62.

32. Wittke F, Hoffmann R, Buer J, et al. Interleukin 10 (IL-10): an immunosuppressive factor and independent predictor in patients with metastatic renal cell carcinoma. *Br J Cancer.* 1999;79(7–8): 1182–4.
33. Negrier S, Escudier B, Gomez F, Douillard JY, Ravaud A, Chevreau C, Buclon M, Perol D, Lasset C. Prognostic factors of survival and rapid progression in 782 patients with metastatic renal carcinomas treated by cytokines: a report from the Groupe Francais d'Immunotherapie. *Ann Oncol.* 2002 Sep;13(9):1460–8.

9. INTERLEUKIN-2 BASED THERAPY FOR KIDNEY CANCER

JANICE P. DUTCHER, M.D.

Our Lady of Mercy Cancer Center, New York Medical College

INTRODUCTION

Interleukin-2 (IL-2) is a 15 kDa glycoprotein, originally characterized as T-cell growth factor,[1] and is produced in response to T-cell activation. Interleukin-2 binds to cells through T-cell receptors which are up-regulated with activation, and through these receptors, signals clonal expansion of T-cells, with specific and non-specific immunity, and expansion of natural killer (NK) cells, all with cytotoxic activity.[2] In addition, secondary cytokines are released, such as interferon-gamma, tumor necrosis factor, and interleukin-1, among others.[3] Recombinant DNA technology has allowed the production of IL-2 in large quantities, allowing for clinical investigation of this agent.[4] The most generally used formulation is that produced by Chiron, Proleukin®. Subsequent to this, clinical trials have demonstrated efficacy in the treatment of metastatic renal cell cancer and melanoma, and IL-2 was approved for these indications. The initial approval was for therapy with high dose IL-2, to be described below, which remains the gold standard for IL-2 administration in renal cell causes and melanoma. This approval is based on the durability of the responses that are produced. However, due to the toxicity and the need for patient selectivity with high dose IL-2, a variety of regimens exploring lower doses and different schedules and combinations have been investigated. These will be summarized.

R.A. Figlin (ed.). KIDNEY CANCER. Copyright © 2003. Kluwer Academic Publishers. Boston. All rights reserved.

HIGH DOSE IL-2 TREATMENT OF METASTATIC RENAL CELL CANCER

United States High Dose Bolus Regimens (Table 1)

The high dose IL-2 regimen that is the FDA-approved regimen in the United States was developed based on animal model data in which short, bolus infusions were administered at frequent intervals. In the animal studies, there appeared to be a dose-response relationship for tumor eradication using the combination of IL-2 and lymphokine activated killer (LAK) cells.[5] Based on these animal studies, a clinical regimen for humans was devised, utilizing high dose IL-2, and initially in conjunction with activated killer lymphocytes (LAK cells).[6,7] Studies were initially conducted at the National Cancer Institute utilizing the high dose bolus regimen described below, as well as a high dose continuous infusion regimen and both demonstrated clinical responses.[6,7] Subsequently, the National Cancer Institute contracted to other Cancer Centers to evaluate this high dose regimen and as the treatment approach became more generalizable, other centers conducted trials.[8-10] Eventually it became apparent that outcome of treatment utilizing high dose IL-2 is not enhanced by administration of ex vivo activated killer cells and that cumbersome procedure was removed from the treatment protocol.[11-14]

The current high dose regimen consists of bolus intravenous doses of IL-2, either 600,000 U/kg or 720,000 U/kg, administered every 8–12 hours as toxicity allows, for 5 days, followed by a 9 day rest, followed by another 5 days of treatment. This regimen, at the 720,000 U/kg dose was that initially explored at the National Cancer Institute (NCI),[6,13] and the regimen at 600,000 U/kg is utilized by the Cytokine Working Group (CWG).[8-10] Despite the difference in individual doses, the total amount of IL-2 administered by these two research groups is essentially the same, 10.6×10^6 IU/kg for those receiving 720,000 IU/kg and 11.6×10^6 IU/kg for those receiving 600,000 IU/kg.[6,8-14] With both of these regimens, a small subset of patients have demonstrated major clinical responses, including complete responses that have been durable for more than 10 years.[6-14]

In a summary of results of 255 patients with metastatic renal cell cancer treated with either of these two regimens of high dose recombinant IL-2, the overall response rate was 15% (90% confidence interval 10% to 19%), with 17 complete and 20 partial responses.[13,14] The median duration of response for all responders was 54 months, but the median duration of response for complete responders has not been reached (range 7 to 107+ months at the last report).[13,14] The median duration of partial responses was 20.0 months (range 3 to 97+ months at the last report). In addition, some partial responders underwent resection of residual disease, rendering them disease-free. Several of these have remained ongoing surgical complete responders.

All patients entered into these trials were of good performance status with adequate cardiac, pulmonary and renal function. They had multiple disease sites, however, and site of disease did not appear to determine response. In this summary of data, the only predictor of response was good performance status. Among those with ECOG performance status 0, there were 11 of the 12 complete responses.

Table 1. High Dose IL2 Studies, Bolus and Continuous
Infusion, with and without LAK Cells in Patients with Renal Cancer.

Study/Yr (Ref)	# Patients	Response CR/PR (%)	Response Duration (Months)
BOLUS IL-2 TRIALS*			
Fisher (1988)[8]	35	2/3 (16%)	PR's 4, 15+, 16+
IL-2 + LAK			CR's 9+, 12+
Rosenberg (1989)[12]	72	8/17 (35%)	PR med 6.5;
IL-2 + LAK			(R 1–36+)
			CR med 14;
			(R 6–30+)
Fyfe (1995)[13]	255	17/20 (15%)	PR med 20;
Fisher (1997)[14]			(R 3–97+)
Summary of 7 trials			CR med not reached
IL-2 alone[9–12,17,19]			
Yang (1994,97)[15,16]	65	2/11 (20%)	NA
IL-2 alone			
Gitlitz (2001)[17]	124	7/11 (14.5%)	Med OR 18+
IL-2 alone			(CR + PR)
Atkins (1993)[18]	71	5/7 (17%)	med OR 53+
IL-2 alone			(R 4–84+)
McDermott (2001)[19]	99	8/17 (25%)	med OR 10+
IL-2 alone			
CONTINUOUS INFUSION IL-2 TRIALS**			
West (1987)[7]	6	0/3 (50%)	PR: 2, 2, 2
Weiss (1992)[20]	94	5/11 (17%)	PR med 12
IL2 IVCI + LAK			(R 3–24+)
IL2 Bolus + LAK			CR med not reached
			(R 10+–23+)
Negrier (1989)[21]	95	7/13 (21%)	Med OR 6+
			(R 3–12+)
			(CR + PR)
Shulman (1996)[22]	17	0/1 (6%)	NA
1 wk high dose			
1 wk low dose			
Escudier (1994)[23]	104	4/16 (18%)	NA
48 hr very high dose			
weekly × 5 wks			

* Bolus every 8 hours, 5 days on, 1 wk off, 5 days on, unless otherwise stated.
** Continuous infusion, 5 days on, 1 wk off, 5 days on, unless otherwise stated.
LAK = Lymphokine activated killer cells; PR = partial response; CR = complete response; OR = overall response; med = median; R = range.

Other factors that were not predictive of response included site of disease, time from diagnosis to treatment, prior nephrectomy or disease limited to the lung.

Subsequent to the initial reports of activity of high dose bolus IL-2 from the NCI and the CWG, a number of investigators have explored its activity and have demonstrated similar response rates for high dose bolus IL-2.[15–19] These include studies of continuous infusion IL-2, and bolus IL-2 and alternative schedules. Several of these are described below. Additional later studies also demonstrate lesser toxicity with the regimen, as the learning curve of its administration becomes better managed.

Continuous Infusion Regimens of High Dose IL-2 (Table 1)

As a result of the report by West et al, utilizing the continuous infusion schedule of IL2,[7] this was also evaluated as a potentially less toxic approach to high dose IL-2. This was initially administered in conjunction with LAK cells.[7,20] The CWG conducted one such study, at a dose of $1 mg/m^2/day$ (equivalent to $18 MIU/m^2/day$), administered as a continuous intravenous infusion for 5 days, followed by a 6 day break for collection of LAK cells, then another 5 days of IL2 at a dose of $1.25 mg/m^2/day$, with LAK cell administration. At this dose and schedule, there was no less toxicity than with the bolus schedule, and there was an increase in infectious complications in the continuous infusion approach in a CWG study.[20] Clinical activity was observed, with a 15% objective response rate, including 2 durable complete responses (more than 1 year and more than 2 years at the time of report). However, since there was no increase in activity with this schedule, the CWG continued to explore the bolus administration regimen. A large European multi-center study, reported by Negrier, et al, utilized interleukin-2 with or without LAK cells utilized high dose IL-2, $18 MIU/m^2/day$, as an IVCI.[21] Clinical activity, including partial and complete responses were observed, with an overall response rate of 19%. Toxicity was considered manageable and reversible. This is consistent with the other trials described above using IL-2 at this dose and schedule.

Shulman reported a modification of this regimen, in which high dose continuous infusion IL-2 ($18 MU/m^2/day$ for 5 days) was administered week 1, with a 6 day break, followed by lower dose continuous infusion of IL-2 ($10 MU/m^2/day$ for 5 days) during the second week. This regimen had limited activity (one partial response) and was considered to have substantial toxicity not warranting further evaluation.[22] Others have evaluated lower doses given during 5-day monthly infusions and prolonged infusions and this will be discussed in the section on lower dose IL-2.

In a more recent study of an alternative schedule of IVCI high dose IL-2, Escudier has reported a schedule of a 48 hour infusion weekly for 5 consecutive weeks. The dose employed is a daily dose of $24 MIU/m^2/day$ for 48 hours.[23] Grade 3-4 hypotension was observed in 58% of patients and a response rate of 20% was observed in 104 patients treated, including 4 complete responses.[23] Durability of response was not reported.

In general, the standard high dose regimen in the United States remains the high dose bolus regimen, administered in the schedule originally designed. In Europe, the continuous infusion regimen is more frequently utilized when high dose IL-2 is given, and the regimen described by Escudier is provacative.

As a result of the summation of all of these evaluations, and repeated outcome of a response rate of approximately 20%, albeit with very long-lived responses and survivals, attempts have been made to enhance the activity of high dose and lower dose IL-2 regimens. Described below are some of these efforts.

Combinations to Enhance High Dose Bolus IL-2

In attempts to enhance the response rate and to improve the therapeutic ratio of this treatment modality in metastatic renal cell cancer, the NCI, CWG and many other investigators have designed trials to augment immune activation and antigen recognition. Although initial studies were conducted with the addition of ex vivo activated killer cells administered with IL-2, this was eventually not found to be synergistic in terms of response or outcome.[6–14]

High Dose IL-2 plus Interferon-alpha

Subsequent studies explored the possible combination of cytokines to enhance immune activation and response. The combination of IL-2 and IFN-α was developed clinically, based on very promising animal data demonstrating synergy for this combination.[24–26] The synergy was believed to result from enhancement of expression of class I HLA antigens and tumor associated antigens under the influence of IFN, followed by activation of cytotoxic cells by IL2.[27–28] This led to a series of studies in humans with varying doses of IL-2 and IFN.

Initial studies at the NCI attempted to combine escalating does of IL-2 with interferon, followed by escalation of the dose of IFN.[29,30] Both were initially administered every 8 hours in the same schedule as the high dose IL-2 studies. The starting does were IFN-α 3 MU/m^2/dose and IL-2 2.6 MU/m^2. The IL-2 was increased to 11.7 MU/m^2. IFN was then escalated, but at the higher doses, the interferon was given only once daily due to toxicity. Seventy-five renal cell carcinoma patients were included in these studies. Nine had long-lasting responses, 57+–74+ months. At the highest dose of IFN administered 3 times daily, there was a higher response rate than with the lower doses or with historical data for IL-2 alone.[30] However, with longer follow-up, it was determined that there was significantly greater toxicity and no long term survival benefit over IL-2 alone.[30]

The CWG also conducted studies to combine high dose IL-2 with increasing doses of IFN-alpha. Initially a phase II trial combining the NCI schedule of IL-2 plus IFN-α2a with LAK cells was performed.[31] However, this combination was exceedingly toxic. Although there was clinical activity, with 3 responses (1 CR/ 2 PR), there were 3 deaths among 25 patients treated. This was cause for re-evaluation.

A subsequent phase I trial of Il-2 plus IFN-α2b was initiated, omitting LAK cells.[32] The dose of IL-2 was initially low (0.4 mg/m^2/dose) and was escalated to 0.8 mg/m^2/dose and 1.2 mg/m^2/dose and the IFN-α2b was kept at the same dose of 3 MU/m^2/dose. Both agents were administered every 8 hours on days 1–5 and 15–19, again, for a maximum of 28 doses. In this study, there were 3 responses among 24 patients, including 14 with renal cell cancer. The second dose level (0.8 mg/m^2) was accepted for a phase II evaluation.[32]

Because of the considerable synergy noted in preclinical studies, and the higher response rate noted in the NCI study on early evaluation, further evaluation of the combination of maximally tolerated IL-2 (0.8 mg/m^2) with interferon (3 MU/m^2), both given every 8 hours, appeared to be warranted. This was evaluated in a randomized phase II trial, in which the control arm was IL-2 alone, $1.33\,mg/m^2/dose$, in the same schedule.[18,33] The study was designed such that the endpoint required that the response rate of the combination be double that of IL-2 alone. A required interim analysis showed that this goal could not be met, and the combination arm was closed with only 28 patients enrolled. There were 3 partial responses in that arm (11%) and 12 responses among 71 patients in the IL-2 alone arm (17%) including 5 CR and 7 PR.[33] Toxicities were similar between the two arms, and there were no treatment-related deaths. The median progression-free survival at 3 years was 13% for high dose IL-2, and 3% for the combination.[33] The conclusion was that the combination was no better, and more toxic at higher doses, and perhaps that limiting the dose of IL-2 to allow combination with IFN-α in this schedule impacted negatively.

Another agent evaluated by the CWG in combination with high dose IL-2 in renal cell cancer was OKT3. OKT3 is a monoclonal antibody that binds to CD3, the major T-cell antigen. T-cells are activated by low doses of OKT3, but are suppressed by higher doses.[34] It was hypothesized that enhancing T-cell activity more specifically would enhance anti-tumor effect without increasing toxicity, based on substantial preclinical data.[35] A phase I trial was initiated in patients with metastatic renal cell cancer, evaluating the combination of high dose IL-2 with OKT3.[36] OKT3 was escalated from doses of 75–$600\,\mu gm/m^2$ on day 1, followed by IL-2, at an initial dose of $0.45\,mg/m^2$, then followed by $1.33\,mg/m^2$ every 8 hours on days 2–6 and 16–20.[36] Fourteen patients received high dose IL-2 alone as a control group. Circulating T-cells were evaluated as a biologic marker of response. The outcome showed to correlation between OKT3 administration and the level of increase in T-cell activation, which was seen equivalently in those patients receiving IL-2 alone. There were 5 responders among a total of 43 patients, with 1 CR and 4 PR. Two responders received IL-2 alone. Therefore, it was concluded that OKT3, in the doses and schedule evaluated did not increase the number or level of patients with T-cell activation nor did it enhance clinical response.[36]

Combinations with More Specific Killer Cells

Other investigators have focused on improving cellular cytotoxicity and exploration of the cellular means of tumor killing. The initial cellular studies utilized activation of mononuclear cells obtained from the peripheral blood, which, when activated, demonstrated a broad range of cytotoxicity against tumor and tumor cell line targets. These cells were termed lymphokine-activated killer cells.[5,37] The NCI and subsequently others demonstrated in vitro killing of human tumor cells by these activated cells.[37] As stated above, there were attempts to in vivo activate more specific cellular immunity, but others have attempted to expand more tumor-specific cytotoxic cellular populations. However, attempts to make these cells more tumor-specific have been hampered by the lack of identifiable tumor targets in renal cell cancer.

Other cells observed adjacent to the tumors in vivo and initially thought to be important in an anti-tumor response were the tumor-infiltrating lymphocytes (TILs) identified during histologic examination of the nephrectomy specimen. It was postulated that these cells played a role in tumor containment, and that further activation of these cells would enhance anti-tumor activity. Several studies have demonstrated the ability to extract these cells and then activate them with IL-2 in vitro.[38,39] Subsequently, these were administered to patients in the setting of IL-2 administration.[38,39] These studies have many technical difficulties, in terms of obtaining adequate numbers of cells, and the details of ex vivo growth and expansion of the cells.[39] Clinical trials were conducted, however, and demonstrated no enhanced anti-tumor effect with the addition of activated TILs compared to IL-2 alone.[38-40] Additionally, in vitro studies of activated TIL demonstrated a somewhat lower rate of cytotoxicity than was initially expected.[38] Subsequent immunologic investigation of these cells has suggested that there is a tumor-induced dysfunction of the infiltrating T-cells, with reduction in local IL-2 production, and thus these cells have limited capacity to develop an anti-tumor response.[41-43]

Toxicity and Management of High Dose IL-2

The toxicity of high dose IL-2 therapy has been considered a barrier to the wide usage of the initial NCI or CWG regimen. Toxicities are significant, but are also predictable and manageable. Most centers with experience in the use of high dose IL-2 can accomplish this outside of the intensive care unit,[17] while smaller institutions still utilize the support and monitoring available in intensive care units. Toxicity from IL-2 is dose-dependent, and increases in intensity and severity with increasing doses and duration of IL-2 therapy. Thus, the level of toxicity noted in the package insert for IL-2 utilizes results from studies performed in the 1980's.[13,14,15,18,46] Acute toxicities associated with administration of IL-2 include multi-organ system effects, including hypotension requiring pressor support in at least half of patients, capillary leak syndrome, tachyarrhythmias, renal and hepatic dysfunction, cytopenias, rash and intense pruritis, and susceptibility to intravenous line infections. In less than 10% of patients there can be acute neuro-psychiatric toxicity requiring medication. All toxicities resolve with cessation of the drug administration, and many can be modulated during treatment by withholding doses or increasing the interval between doses.[44-46] It has been noted that the numbers of doses of high dose IL-2 administered has been reduced over time, as the learning curve for safe administration has been maximized.[46] In a recent review of toxicity from the NCI, the number of doses administered during the first week of treatment has been reduced from 13 to 7, over a period of 10 years, with no reduction in overall response rate in patients with renal cell cancer.[46] In the experience of the CWG, a recent study demonstrated the total number of doses for the two week cycle to be a median of 20 doses,[19] down from a median of 22 in our previous studies.[14,18,20] There has been no reduction in either response rate or complete response and the responses appear to be durable.[19] With experience, the toxicity of high dose IL-2 is quite manageable and predictable and experienced nursing and medical staffs can reliably conduct this treatment. In addition, several groups have produced guidelines for management of the expected toxicities.[44–46]

Nevertheless, the above considerations regarding high dose IL-2 therapy have led to exploration of lower dose regimens and combinations with other cytokines, again at lower doses.

LOWER DOSE REGIMENS OF IL-2 BASED THERAPY FOR RENAL CANCER

Continuous Infusion IL-2 (Table 2)

Early in the development of IL-2, more chronic, lower doses of IL-2 were evaluated for their ability to stimulate activated killer cells and generate an immune-mediated anti-tumor response. Both intravenous continuous infusions and bolus subcutaneous administration schedules were evaluated, some with more prolonged administration. An initial study of this approach by Thompson et al utilized a low dose of IL-2 at $6\,MU/m^2/day$ continuous infusion for days 1–5 followed by collection of LAK cells during days 7–9.[47] This was followed by re-infusion of LAK cells with additional IL2 at the same dose on days 12–16 (part A). In the second part of the protocol, the maintenance IL-2 was administered days 10–20, but at a lower dose of $2\,MU/m^2/day$ (part B).[47] In the initial group, there were 2 CR and 3 PR (5/20–25%) and in part B, there was 1 CR and 7 PR out of 22 patients

Table 2. Moderate Dose Continuous Infusion IL-2 +/− Other.

Study/Yr (Ref)	# Patients	Response CR/PR (%)	Response Duration (Months)
Thompson (1992)[47]			
a) IVCI + LAK	20	2/3 (25%)	★CR: 36+, 18+, 18+
b) IVCI + LAK, lower Dose IL2 2nd wk	22	2/7 (41%)	★CR: 14+, 9+, 6+,5+
Palmer (1993)[48]			
IVCI IL2 alone	225	9/25 (15%)	NA
Figlin (1992)[49] IL2 2MU/m2/d IVCI, D 1–4; IFN 6MU/m2 D1 and 4; daily × 4, wkly × 4 2wk break; continue	30	0/9 (30%)	Median 12+ mo
Ilson (1992)[50] IVCI IL2 + SC IFN 4 days/wk, wkly × 3 lower dose maint × 3wk monthly × 6mo.	34	1/3 (12%)	★★CR 8+, 7+, 4+
Negrier (1998)[51]			1yr event free survival
a) IL-2 IVCI	138	6.5%	15%
b) IFN SC	147	7.5%	12%
c) IL-2 IVCI + IFN SC	140	18.6%	20%

★ 1 PR in A and 2 PR in B surgically converted to CR.
★★ 2 PR converted surgically to CR.

(41%). Three partial responders were converted to CR by surgery. CR durations were prolonged (36+, 18+, 18+ 14+, 9+, 6+, 5+), and the toxicity was less with the lower dose of maintenance IL-2 (part B).

Others have evaluated a variety of continuous moderate-low dose regimens of IL-2 alone or in combination with interferon.[48–50] Palmer et al evaluated IL-2 alone in 225 patients and achieved a 15% overall response rate, with 4% complete responders, but response duration is not available. Figlin et al initiated studies of continuous infusion IL-2 plus subcutaneous interferon.[49] He noted a partial response rate of 30% in 30 patients. Ilson et al evaluated a similar dose and schedule of IVCI IL-2 with interferon, given weekly for 4 days, for 3 weeks on, 1 week off, for as many as 6 cycles and found an overall response rate of 12%, but with one complete responder and 2 surgical CR's.[50]

Negrier et al conducted a randomized study in which 425 patients were entered. They were randomized to IVCI IL-2 alone, IFN-α alone, or to IVCI IL-2 plus IFNα.[51] In this study, there was an enhanced response rate for the combination (18.6%) compared to IL-2 alone (6.5%) or IFNα alone (7.5%) and there was prolonged event-free survival at one year (20% for the combination versus 15% for IL-2 alone and 12% for IFNα alone).[51] Subsequent follow-up of this study has showed that the long-term survival of the IL-2 alone group is now similar to that of the combination group.[52] They noted that some disease characteristics also impact on long-term survival (fewer sites of metastatic disease, better performance status). However, the ability to achieve a complete response to IVCI IL-2 had a significant impact on long-term survival, with 60% of complete responders alive at 5 years compared to 18% of partial responders and 1% of those with progressive disease.[52]

Low Dose IL-2 plus TIL

Additionally, there have been evaluations of moderate-low dose IVCI combined with activated tumor infiltrating lymphocytes.[53–57] The numbers of patients treated in these studies range from 7 to 56, and responses have been observed in those with sufficient numbers to evaluate the regimen.[56,57] The schedule was for days of CIV IL-2, weekly. In these larger studies, both PR and CR were observed, with response rates of 3/33 (9%)[57] and 19/56 (34%).[56] In the latter study, IFNα was added to IL2 plus TIL.[56] Again, with the evolution in understanding of the biology of TIL, these results are consistent with the outcome of studies of IL-2 alone.

Low Dose Intravenous Bolus IL-2 as a Single Agent (Table 3)

Several studies have evaluated moderate dose or intermittent schedules of IL-2 using intravenous administration. The concern of this approach is the short half-life of IL-2 whereas the pharmacokinetics of subcutaneous administration is similar to intravenous continuous infusion. Bukowski et al evaluated a higher dose, but intermittent (three times weekly) schedule of IL2 in 41 patients and obtained a response rate of 15% (1 CR/ 5 PR).[58] The median duration of response was 5 months and median survival 10 months. Yang et al have evaluated a lower dose IL-2, 72,000 U/kg every 8 hours on the same schedule as the NCI high dose IL2 protocol.[16] The response

Table 3. Low Dose Bolus IL-2 Alone Trials.

Study/Yr (Ref)	# Patients	Response CR/PR (%)	Response Duration (Months)
INTRAVENOUS BOLUS IL-2			
Bukowski (1990)[58]	41	1/5 (15%)	med 5 mo
60 MU/m2 tiw			
Yang (1997)[16]	112	5/6 (10%)	3–61+
72,000 U/kg IV q8 hr			
SUBCUTANEOUS BOLUS IL-2			
Sleijfer (1992)[59]	27	2/4 (23%)	CR: 35+, 29+
Buter (1993)[60]			
18 MU d 1–2; 9 MU d 3–5			
6 wks; 3 wk break, repeat			
Yang (1997)[16]	53	3/3 (11%)	NA

tiw = three times per week.

rate in this study is 10% (5 CR/6 PR of 112 patients). Response duration ranges from 3–61+ months.

Bolus Subcutaneous IL-2 as a Single Agent (Table 3)

At the same time, others evaluated IL-2 as a single agent administered via a subcutaneous injection. This route of administration leads to a somewhat prolonged effect due to the slow release of the injected IL-2 into the systemic circulation. Although this approach has the benefit of simplicity of administration, there are very few published data on IL-2 alone in this schedule. The most cited study is that of Sleijfer et al[59] and the update by Buter et al[60] in which IL-2 was administered at a dose of 18 MU/day for the first 2 days of a 5 day cycle, and on days 3–5, IL-2 at a dose of 9 MU was administered. This was repeated for 6 weeks with a 3-week rest period, and then repeated. The initial report described a 23% response rate with 2 complete responders.[59] The update of this study reported the two complete responders as durable, 29 and 35 plus months.[60] Variations of this approach have been utilized in smaller studies and ad hoc, but there are no other published data.

Yang et al have used an arm of bolus subcutaneous IL-2 in their study comparing various doses of IL-2.[16] These consist of 3 arms: high dose bolus (720,000 U/kg) to moderate dose bolus (72,000 U/kg) to subcutaneous IL2 at 250,000 U/kg/day, days 1–5, followed by 125,000 U/kg/day, 5 days per week, weeks 2 through 6. Preliminary response data suggests a response rate of 11% for the subcutaneous IL-2 alone arm.[16]

Combination of Subcutaneous IL-2 with Interferon–alpha (IFN–α) (Table 4)

Although the combination of IL-2 with IFN-α was too toxic in the high dose regimens,[30–31] it has been successfully utilized as a regimen at lower doses. As described above, subcutaneous IFN has been combined with IVCI IL-2 demonstrated activity and tolerability (Table 2).[49–52] More recently, both agents have been administered

Table 4. Subcutaneous IL-2 plus Subcutaneous IFN-α.

Study/Yr (Ref)	# Patients	Response CR/PR (%)	Response Duration (Months)
Palmer (1993)[48]	200	8/32 (20%)	NA
Vogelzang (1992)[61] IL-2 4.5 MU/m2 wkly × 4 wks, 2 wk break; cont. IFN—7.5 MU/m2 tiw	42	1/4 (12%)	NA
Atzpodien (1990)[62] IL-2 18 MU/m2 d1–2 3.6 MU/m2/D IVCI 6 wks IFN 6 MU tiw	40	4/6 (25%)	NA
Negrier (2000)[80] IL-2 9 MU/d × 6 d, IFN 6 MU/d tiw Both wks 1, 3, 5, 7	70	0/1	2.5
Atzpodien (1995)[63] IL-2 5 MU/m2 q 8 hr × 3 d1 IL-2 5 MU/m2/d daily d2–5, Then 5 MU/m2 d 1–5 × 3 wks 2 wk break, then continue IFN 5 MU/m2/dose tiw × 4 wk	152	9/26 (25%)	2–39+; med 12 mo
Dutcher (1993, 1995, 1997)[64–66] same dose and schedule as Atzpodien (1995)	47	2/6 (17%)	1–49+; med 12 mo CR: 15, 49+ mo
McDermott (2001)[19] Same dose and schedule As Dutcher (1997)	94	2/10 (12%)	med 7 mo (R 2–28+)

Tiw = three times per week; med = median; CR = complete response; PR = partial response.

by the subcutaneous route, again at lower doses. At the lower doses, there is considerably better tolerability and this has produced a regimen that can be administered in the outpatient setting. The combination regimens overall have yielded results that suggest activity in the same range as that of high dose IL-2, with a response rate of approximately 20% when all studies are evaluated (Table 4). The study by Negrier et al suggests that the combination at lower doses is more active than either agent alone.[51] However, the question has remained as to whether the outpatient dose and schedule can yield the same durable responses that are observed with high dose IL-2 therapy.

This question led the CWG to embark on a large randomized trial of high dose IL-2 alone compared to outpatient subcutaneous injection IL-2 and IFN-α.[19] The regimens used were those previously studied by the CWG.[18,64–66] In the randomized trial, 194 patients were entered, and 94 received IL-2/IFN and 99 received high dose IL-2. The randomized design ensured that all patients entered would meet eligibility to receive high dose IL-2. The response rate to high dose IL-2 is 25% (95% CI 17.1–35.0) with 8 complete and 17 partial responses. The response rate for IL-2/IFN is 12% (95% CI 6.8–21.2) with 2 complete and 10 partial responses.

Table 5. Subcutaneous IL-2, IFN-α and 5-FU.

Study/Yr (Ref)	# Patients	Response CR/PR (%)	Median Survival (Months)
SIMULTANEOUS COMBINATION			
Hofmockel (1996)[74]	34	3/10 (38%)	12.6
Ellerhorst (1997)[75]	55	4/12 (31%)	22.9
Tourani (1998)[76]	62	1/11 (19.3%)	16
Ravaud (1998)[77]	105	0/2 (1.8%)	11.9
Savage (1996)[78]	24	1/3 (17%)	NA
Joffe (1996)[79]	38	0/9 (23.6%)	11.9
Negrier (2000)[80]	61	0/5 (8.2%)	13
SEQUENTIAL COMBINATION			
Atzpodien (2001)[81]	41	7/9 (39%)	24
Lopez Hannimen (1996)[82]	120	13/34 (39%)	NA
Kirchner (1998)[83]	246	26/54 (32.6%)	21
Dutcher (1997, 2000)[84,85]	50	2/7 (18%)	17.5

The preliminary conclusion is that there is a statistically significantly better response and complete response rate with high dose IL-2, but as yet there is no survival advantage. Long-term follow-up is ongoing. A recent update suggests that patients with disease involving liver have even greater benefit from high dose IL-2, whereas those with lung disease benefit from either.[67]

Thus, both high dose IL-2 and IL-2/IFN can produce complete responses in patients with metastatic renal cell cancer, and the appropriate regimen in large part depends upon other clinical factors defined by the patient. Judgment as to which regimen is best tolerated will decide the treatment plan. Nevertheless, for otherwise healthy, young patients, it seems that the high dose regimen may provide some advantage with a satisfactory risk/benefit ratio.

Combination of Subcutaneous IL-2, IFNα and 5-Fluorouracil (5FU) (Table 5)

Data have suggested synergy between IFN-α and 5FU in preclinical evaluation demonstrating biochemical modulation.[68] In a study utilizing this combination in the RENCA renal cell tumor model, there also appeared to be a synergistic interaction.[69] Therefore studies of IFN plus 5FU were conducted in patients with metastatic renal cell cancer with variable results.[70-73] This led to studies of the combination of IL-2, IFN-α and 5FU in the outpatient setting. Studies were conducted with simultaneous administration[74-80] and with sequential administration.[81-85]

Early reports with this combination were quite promising, and initially suggested an improvement in results with response rates of 31–38% for the simultaneously administered regimen[74,75] and of 33–39% for the sequentially administered combination.[81-83] However, the median survival did not appear to be extended by this enhanced response rate. Subsequent evaluations of these regimens have not yielded as dramatic results, and in fact this regimen appears to be similar in outcome to IL2/IFN but with the addition of myelosuppression. Recently, a randomized study was performed by the Groupe Francais D'Immunotherapie, comparing IL2/IFN to IL2/IFN simultaneously with continuous infusion of 5-fluorouracil.[80] There was no difference in progression-free or overall survival and the response rate in both arms was low in the dose and schedule utilized. The CWG recommendation for optimal outpatient treatment, in patients who can tolerate the regimen, is the intensive out-patient regimen of IL2 plus IFN-α utilized by the CWG.[84,85]

Other Combinations with Subcutaneous IL-2

Additional combinations that have been studied with IL-2 ± IFNα include cis-retinoic acid, vinblastine, and granulocyte-macrophage colony stimulating factor (GM-CSF).[86–89] Response rates to these combinations remain within the 95% confidence intervals of studies with IL-2 plus interferon in combination. Therefore, it does not appear that these molecules greatly enhance the activity of outpatient sub-cutaneous IL-2.

Other Formulations of IL-2

New formulations of IL-2 have been developed in attempts to improve the therapeutic window, and provide a more active agent and perhaps less toxicity. The earliest modification was the development of polyethylene glycolated IL-2 (PEG-IL-2). This formulation produced are prolongation of the half-life, similar to a continuous infusion.[90,91] Initial studies attempted to determine the maximally tolerated dose in the outpatient setting, where it could be administered on a weekly basis.[92] This formulation appeared to have toxicity similar to IL-2 administered on a more continuous basis, but perhaps of lesser degree. However, drug availability has been curtailed so that a full clinical evaluation has not been possible.

Bayer corporation has developed a new formulation of IL-2 which is a mutein with a single amino acid change.[93] This molecule more selectively activates T-cells, and in animal studies exhibits more potent anti-tumor effect.[93] It has entered clinical trials with the goal to define an maximally tolerated dose, as well as to define a dose that allows continuous bolus dosing, not necessitating re-evaluation with each dose. The hope is to produce a product with the activity of standard IL-2 but with reduced and more manageable toxicity. Initial findings suggest that there is activity at lower doses, but the toxicity appears to be similar to IL-2 and the complete responses occur at higher doses.[94]

Finally a liposomal preparation has been developed but has not yet entered clinical trials.[95,96]

SUMMARY

In summary, IL-2 based therapy remains the basis for treatment of metastatic renal cell cancer. Un-answered questions remain in the development of regimens that exceed a mean response rate of 20%.

Additionally, there may be differences among the histologic subtypes of renal cell cancer that predispose to response or lack there of to immunotherapy, and this is being further explored. As can be noted from the studies presented in this paper, there are numerous variations on the regimens for IL-2 based therapy. Current recommendations are to use the simplest and most feasible in a given institution. Certainly high dose IL-2 remains the standard regimen to which all others are measured.

REFERENCES

1. Morgan, DA, Ruscetti FW, Gallo R: Selective in vitro growth of T-lymphocytes from normal human bone marrows. Science 1976; 192:1007–1009.
2. Baker PE, Gillis S, Ferm MM, Smith KA: The effect of T-cell growth factor on the generation of cytolytic T-cells. J Immunol 1978; 121:2168–2172.
3. Mier J, Vachino G, Vander Meer J, et al: Induction of circulating tumor necrosis factor as the mechanism for the febrile response to interleukin-2. J Clin Immunol 1988; 8:426–431.
4. Taniguchi T, Matsui H, Fujita T, et al: Structure and expression of a cloned cDNA for human interleukin-2. Nature 1983; 302:305–310.
5. Mule JJ, Shu S, Schwarz SL, Rosenberg SA: Adoptive immunotherapy of established pulmonary metastases with LAK cells and recombinant interleukin-2. Science 1984; 225:1487–1489.
6. Rosenberg SA, Lotze MT, Muul LM, et al: Observations on the systemic administration of autologous lymphokine-activated killer cells and recombinant interleukin-2 to patients with metastatic cancer. N Engl J Med 1985; 313:1485–1492.
7. West WH, Tauer KW, Yanelli JR, et al: Constant infusion recombinant interleukin-2 in adoptive immunotherapy of advanced cancer. N Engl J Med 1987; 316:898–905.
8. Fisher RI, Coltman CA, Doroshow JH, et al: Metastatic renal cancer treated with interleukin-2 and lymphokine-activated killer cells. Ann Intern Med 1988; 108:518–523.
9. McCabe MS, Stablein D, Hawkins MJ: The modified Group C experience-Phase III randomized trials of IL-2 vs IL-2/LAK in advanced renal cell carcinoma and advanced melanoma. Proc Am Soc Clin Oncol 1991; 10:213 (abst).
10. Abrams JS, Raynor AA, Wiernik PH, et al: High dose recombinant interleukin-2 alone: A regimen with limited activity in the treatment of advanced renal cell carcinoma. N Jatl Cancer Insti 1990; 82:1202–1206.
11. Rosenberg SA, Lotze MT, Yang JC, et al: Prospective randomized trial of high-dose interleukin-2 alone or in conjunction with lymphokine-activated killer cells for the treatment of patients with advanced cancer. J Natl Cancer Inst 1993; 85:622–632.
12. Rosenberg SA, Lotze MT, Yang JC, et al: Experience with the use of high-dose interleukin-2 in the treatment of 652 cancer patients. Ann Surg 1989; 210:474–485.
13. Fyfe G, Fisher RI, Rosenberg SA, et al: Results of treatment with 255 patients with metastatic renal cell carcinoma who received high-dose recombinant interleukin-2 therapy. J Clin Oncol 1995; 13: 688–696.
14. Fisher RI, Rosenberg SA, Sznol M, Parkinson DR, Fyfe G: High does Aldesleukin in renal cell carcinoma: Long-term survival update. Cancer J Sci Amer 1997; 3(Supple 1):S2–S4.
15. Yang JC, Topalian SL, Parkinson D, et al: Randomized comparison of high-dose and low-dose intravenous interleukin-2 for the therapy of metastatic renal cell carcinoma: An interim report. J Clin Oncol 1994; 12:1572–1576.
16. Yang JC, Rosenberg SA: An ongoing prospective randomized comparison of interleukin-2 regimens for the treatment of metastatic renal cell cancer. Cancer J Sci Amer 1997; 3:S79–S84.
17. Gitlitz BJ, Hoffman DM, Moldawer N, et al: Treatment of metastatic renal cell carcinoma with high-dose bolus interleukin-2 in a non-intensive care unit: an analysis of 124 consecutively treated patients. Cancer J Sci Am 2001: 7:112–120.
18. Atkins MB, Sparano J, Fisher RI, et al: Randomized phase II trial of high dose IL-2 either alone or in combination with interferon alfa 2b in advanced renal cell carcinoma. J Clin Oncol 1993; 11: 661–670.
19. McDermott D, Flaherty L, Clark J, et al: A randomized phase III trial of high-dose interleukin-2 versus subcutaneous IL2/Interferon in patients with metastatic renal cell carcinoma. Proc Am Soc Clin Oncol 2001; 20:172a.
20. Weiss GR, Margolin KA, Aronson FR, et al: A randomized phase II trial of continuous infusion interleukin-2 or bolus injection interleukin-2 plus lymphokine-activated killer cells for advanced renal cell carcinoma. J Clin Oncol 1992; 10:275–281.

21. Negrier S, Philip T, Stoter G, et al: Interleukin-2 with or without LAK cells in metastatic renal cell carcinoma: A report of a European multicentre study. Eur J Cancer Clin Oncol 1989; 25 (Suppl 3): S21–S28.
22. Shulman KL, Stadler WM,, Vogelzang NJ: High dose continuous intravenous infusion of interleukin-2 therapy for metastatic renal cell carcinoma: the University of Chicago experience. Urology 1996; 47:194–197.
23. Escudier B, Ravaud A, Fabbro M, et al: High-dose interleukin-2 two days a week for metastatic renal cell carcinoma: A FNCLCC multicenter study. J Immunother Emphasis Tumor Immunol 1994; 15:306–312.
24. Iigo M, Sakurai M, Tamura T et al: In vivo anti-tumor activity of multiple injections of recombinant interleukin-2 alone and in combination with three different types of recombinant interferon, on various syngeneic murine tumors. Cancer Res 1988; 48:260–264.
25. Brunda MJ, Bellantoni D, Sulich V: In vivo anti-tumor activity of combinations of interferon-alpha and interleukin-2 in a murine model: Correlation of efficacy with the induction of cytotoxic cells resembling natural killer cells. Int J Cancer 1987; 40:365–371.
26. Cameron RB, McIntosh JK, Rosenberg SA: Synergistic anti-tumor effects of combination immunotherapy with recombinant interleukin-2 and a recombinant hybrid alpha-interferon in the treatment of established murine hepatic metastases. Cancer Res 1988; 48:5810–5817.
27. Weber JS, Rosenberg SA: Modulation of murine tumor major histocompatibility antigens by cytokines in vivo and in vitro. Cancer Res 1988; 48:5818–5824.
28. Guadagni F, Schlom J, Johnston WW, et al: Selective interferon-induced enhancement of tumor-associated antigens on a spectrum of freshly isolated human adenocarcinoma cells. J Natl Cancer Inst 1989; 81:502–511.
29. Rosenberg SA, Lotze MT, Yang JC, et al: Combination therapy with interleukin-2 and alpha-interferon for the treatment of patients with advanced cancer. J Clin Oncol 1989; 7:1863–1874.
30. Marincola FM, White DE, Wise AP, Rosenberg SA: Combination therapy with interferon alfa-2a and interleukin-2 for the treatment of metastatic cancer. J Clin Oncol 1995; 13:1110–1122.
31. Aronson FR, Sznol M, Atkins MB, et al: A phase II trial of interleukin-2, interferon-alpha, and lymphokine activated killer cells for advanced renal cell carcinoma. Proc Am Soc Clin Oncol 1990; 9: 182.
32. Sznol M, Mier J, Sparano J, et al: A phase I study of high dose interleukin-2 in combination with interferon-alfa 2B. J Biol Resp Modifers 1990; 9:529–537.
33. Atkins MB, Dutcher JP, Weiss G, et al: Kidney Cancer: The Cytokine Working Group Experience (1986–2001). Part I: IL-2 based clinical trials. Med Oncol 2001; 18:197–207.
34. Hirsch R, Eckhuar M, Auchincloss, et al: Effects of in vivo administration of anti-CD3 monoclonal antibody on T cell function in mice: I. Immunosuppression or transplantation responses. J Immunol 1988; 140:3766–3772.
35. Hirsch R, Gress RE, Pluznik DH, et al: Effects of in vivo administration of anti-CD3 monoclonal antibody on T cell function in mice: II. In vivo activation of T cells. J Immunol 1989; 142:737–740.
36. Sosman JA, Weiss GR, margolin KA, et al: A phase IB clinical trial of anti-CD3 (OKT3) followed by high dose bolus IL-2 in patients with metastatic melanoma and advanced renal cell carcinoma: clinical and immunological effects. J Clin Oncol 1993; 11:1496–1505.
37. Grimm EA, Mazumder A, Zhang HZ, Rosenberg SA: Lymphokine-activated killer cell phenomenon. Lysis of natural killer-resistant fresh solid tumor cells by interleukin-2 activated autologous human peripheral blood lymphocytes. J Exp Med 1982; 155:1823–1841.
38. Topalian SL, Solomon D, Avis FP, et al: Immunotherapy of patients with advanced cancer using tumor-infiltrating lymphocytes and recombinant interleukin-2: A pilot study. J Clin Oncol 1988; 6: 839–853.
39. Figlin RA, Thompson JA, Bukowski RM, et al: Multicenter, randomized, phase III trial of CD8 (+) tumor-infiltrating lymphocytes in combination with recombinant interleukin-2 in metastatic renal cell carcinoma. J Clin Oncol 1999; 17:2521–2529.
40. Bukowski RM, Sharfman W, Murthy S, et al: Clinical results and characterization of tumor-infiltrating lymphocytes with or without recombinant interleukin-2 in human metastatic renal cell carcinoma. Cancer Res 1991; 51:4199–4205.
41. Rayman P, Uzzo RG, Kolenko V, et al: Tumor-induced dysfunction in interleukin-2 production and interleukin-2 receptor signaling: A mechanism of immune escape. Cancer J Sci Amer 2000; 6 (Suppl 1): S81–S87.

42. Alexander JP, Kudoh S, Melsop KA et al: T-cells infiltrating renal cell carcinoma display a poor proliferative response even though they can produce interleukin-2 and express interleukin-2 receptors. Cancer Res 1993; 53:1380–1387.

43. Miescher S, Stoeck M, Qiao L et al: Proliferative and cytolytic potentials of purified human tumor-infiltrating T lymphocytes. Impaired response to mitogen-driven stimulation despite T-cell receptor expression. Int J Cancer 1988; 42:659–666.

44. Margolin KA, Rayner AA, Hawkins MJ, et al: Interleukin-2 and lymphokine-activated killer cell therapy of solid tumors: Analysis of toxicity and management guidelines. J Clin Oncol 1989; 4: 486–498.

45. Dutcher JP, Atkins MB, Margolin K, et al: Kidney Cancer: The Cytokine Working Group Experience (1986–2001). Part II. Management of IL-2 toxicity and studies with other cytokines. Med Oncol 2001; 18:209–219.

46. Kammula US, White DE, Rosenberg SA: Trends in the safety of high dose bolus interleukin-2 administration in patients with metastatic cancer. Cancer 1998; 83:797–805.

47. Thompson JA, Shulman KL, Benyunes MC, et al: Prolonged continuous intravenous infusion interleukin-2 and lymphokine-activated killer-cell therapy for metastatic renal cell carcinoma. J Clin Oncol 1992; 10:960–968.

48. Palmer PA, Atzpodien J, Philip T, et al: A comparison of 2 modes of administration of recombinant interleukin-2: continuous intravenous infusion alone versus subcutaneous administration plus interferon alpha in patients with advanced renal cell carcinoma. Cancer Biother 1993; 8:123–136.

49. Figlin RA, Belldegrun A, Moldawer N, et al: Concomitant administration of recombinant human interleukin-2 and recombinant interfreron alfa-2A: An active outpatient regimen in metastatic renal cell carcinoma. J Clin Oncol 1992; 10:414–421.

50. Ilson DH, Motzer RJ, Kradin RL, et al: A phase II trial of interleukin-2 and interferon-alfa-2a in patients with advanced renal cell carcinoma. J Clin Oncol 1992; 10:1124–1130.

51. Negrier S, Escudier B, Lasset C, et al: Recombinant human interleukin-2, recombinant human interferon alfa-2a, or both in metastatic renal cell carcinoma. N Engl J Med 1998; 338:1272–1278.

52. Negrier S, Maral J, Drevon M, et al: Long-term follow-up of patients with metastatic renal cell carcinoma treated with intravenous recombinant interleukin-2 in Europe. Cancer J Sci Amer 2000; 6 (Suppl 1): S93–S98.

53. Kraden RL, Lazarus DS, Dubinette SM, et al: Tumor-infiltrating lymphocytes and interleukin-2 in treatement of advanced cancer. Lancet 1989; 1:577–580.

54. Hayakawa K, Salmeron MA, Parkinson DA, et al: Study of tumor-infiltrating lymphocytes for adoptive therapy of renal cell carcinoma (RCC) and metastatic melanoma: Sequential proliferation of cytotoxic natural killer and non-cytotoxic T-cells in RCC. J Immunother 1991; 10:313–325.

55. Oldham RK, Dillman RO, Yannelli JR, et al: Continous infusion interleukin-2 and tumor-derived activated cells as treatment of advanced solid tumors: A National Biotherapy Study Group Trial. Mol Biother 1991; 3:68–73.

56. Figlin R, Gitlitz B, Franklin J, et al: Interleukin-2 based immunotherapy for the treatment of metastatic renal cell carcinoma: An analysis of 203 consecutively treated patients. Cancer J Sci Amer 1997; 3:S92–S97.

57. Bukowski RM, Sharfman W, Murthy S etal: Clinical results and characteristics of tumor-infiltrating lymphocytes with or without recombinant interleukin-2 in human metastatic renal cell carcinoma. Cancer Res 1991; 51:4199–4205.

58. Bukowski RM, Goodman P, Crawford ED, et al: Phase II trial of high-dose intermittent interleukin-2 in metastatic renal cell cancer: A Southwest Oncology Group Study. J Natl Cancer Inst 1990; 82:143–146.

59. Sleijfer DT, Jannsen RAJ, Buter J, et al: Phase II study of subcutaneous interleukin-2 in unselected patients with advanced renal cell cancer on an outpatient basis. J Clin Oncol 1992; 10:1119–1123.

60. Buter J, Sleijfer DT, vanderGraaf WTA, et al: A progress report on the outpatient treatment of patients with advanced renal carcinoma using subcutaneous recombinant interleukin-2. Semin Oncol 1993; 20:16–21.

61. Vogelzang NJ, Lipton A, Figlin RA: Subcutaneous interleukin-2 plus interferon alfa-2a in metastatic renal cancer: An outpatient multicenter trial. J Clin Oncol 1993; 11:1809–1816.

62. Atzpodien J, Korfer A, Franks C, et al: Home therapy with recombinant interleukin-2 and interferon α2b in advanced human malignancies. Lancet 1990; 335:1509–1512.

63. Atzpodien J, Hanninen EL, Kirchner H, et al: Multi-institutional home therapy trial of recombinant human IL-2 and IFN-alpha-2 in progressive metastatic renal cell carcinoma. J Clin Oncol 1995; 13:497–501.

64. Dutcher JP, Fisher RI, Weiss G, et al: An outpatient regimen of subcutaneous interleukin-2 plus alpha-interferon in metastatic renal cell cancer. Proc Am Soc Clin Oncol 1993; 12:248.
65. Dutcher JP, Fisher R, Weiss G, et al: Outpatient subcutaneous interleukin-2 plus alpha-interferon in metastatic renal cell cancer: 3 year follow-up of the Cytokine Working Group study. Proc Am Soc Clin Oncol 1995; 14:332.
66. Dutcher JP, Fisher RI, Weiss G, et al: Outpatient subcutaneous interleukin-2 plus alpha-interferon in metastatic renal cell cancer: Five-year follow-up of the Cytokine Working Group study. Cancer J Sci Amer 1997; 3:157–162.
67. McDermott D, Flaherty L, Clark J, et al: A randomized phase III trial of high-dose interleukin-2 versus subcutaneous IL2/Interferon in patients with metastatic renal cell carcinoma. J Immunotherapy 2001; 24:S15.
68. Schwartz EL, Hoffman M, O'Connor C, Wadler S: Stimulation of 5-fluorouracil metabolic activation by interferon-α in human colon carcinoma cells. Biochem Biophys Res Commun 1991; 182:1232–1239.
69. Marumo K, Oya M, Murai M: Biochemical modulation of 5-fluorouracil with murine interferon-α/β against murine renal cell carcinoma. Int J Urol 1997; 4:163–168.
70. Hanninen EL, Poliwoda H, Atzpodien J: Interferon-α/5-fluorouracil: a novel outpatient chemo/Immunotherapy for progressive metastatic renal cell carcinoma. Cancer Biother 1995; 10: 21–24.
71. Sparano JA, Dutcher JP, Wiernik PH, et al: A phase II trial of low-dose continuous infusion 5-fluorouracil plus interferon-α in patients with advanced renal cell carcinoma. Proc Soc Biol Therapy 1993.
72. Gebrosky NP, Koukol S, Nseyo UO, et al: Treatment of renal cell carcinoma with 5-fluorouracil and α-interferon. Urology 1997; 50:863–868.
73. Elias L, Blumenstein BA, Kish J, et al: A phase II trial of interferon-α and 5-fluorouracil in patients with advanced renal cell carcinoma. A Southwest Oncology Group study. Cancer 1996; 78: 1085–1088.
74. Hofmockel G, Langer W, Theiss M, et al: Immunochemotherapy for metsatatic renal cell carcinoma using a regimen of interleukin-2, interferon-α, and 5-fluorouracil. J Urol 1996; 156:18–21.
75. Ellerhorst JA, Sella A, Amato RJ, et al: Phase II trial of 5-fluorouracil, interferon-α and continuous infusion interleukin-2 for patients with metastatic renal cell carcinoma. Cancer 1997; 80:2128–2132.
76. Tourani J-M, Pfister C, Berdah J-F, et al: Outpatient treatment with subcutaneous interleukin-2 and interferon-α administration in combination with fluorouracil in patients with metastatic renal cell carcinoma: results of a sequential nonrandomized phase II study. J Clin Oncol 1998; 16:2505–2513.
77. Ravaud A, Audhuy B, Gomez F, et al: Subcutaneous interleukin-2, interferon-α2a, and continuous infusion of fluorouracil in metastatic renal cell carcinoma: a mutlicenter phase II trial. J Clin Oncol 1998; 16: 2728–2732.
78. Savage P, Costelna D, Moore J, Gore ME: A phase II study of continuous infusional 5-fluorouracil and subcutaneous interleukin-2 in metastatic renal cell cancer. Eur J Cancer 1996; 33:1149–1151.
79. Joffe JK, Banks RE, Forbes MA, et al: A phase II study of interferon-α, interleukin-2 and 5-fluorouracil in advanced renal carcinoma: Clinical data and laboratory evidence of protease activation. Br J Urol 1996; 77:638–649.
80. Negrier S, Caty A, Lesimple T, et al: Treatment of patients with metastatic renal carcinoma with a combination of subcutaneous interleukin-2 and interferon alfa with or without fluorouracil. J Clin Oncol 2000; 18:4009–4015.
81. Atzpodien J, Kirchner H, Illiger HJ, et al: IL-2 in combination with interferon-alpha and 5-FU versus tamoxifen in metastatic renal cell carcinoma: long-term results of a controlled randomized clinical trial. Br J Cancer 2001; 85:1130–1136.
82. Hanninen EL, Kirchner H, Atzpodien J: Interleukin-2 based home therapy of metastatic renal cell carcinoma: risks and benefits in 215 consecutive single institution patients. J Urol 1996; 155:19–25.
83. Kirchner H, Buere J, Probst-Kepper M, et al: Risk and longer-term outcome in metastatic renal cell carcinoma patients receiving SC interleukin-2, SC interferon-αf 2A, and IV 5-fluorouracil. Proc Am Soc Clin Oncol 1998; 17:310.
84. Dutcher JP, Atkins M, Fisher R, et al: Interleukin-2 based therapy for metastatic renal cell cancer: The Cytokine Working Group Experience, 1989–1997. Cancer J Sci Amer 1997; 3(Suppl 1): S73–S78.
85. Dutcher JP, Logan T, Gordon M, et al: Phase II trial of interleukin-2, interferon -α, and 5-fluorouracil in metastatic renal cell cancer: A Cytokine Working Group Study. Clin Cancer Res 2000; 6:3442–3450.

86. Atzpodien J, Kirchner H, Duensing S, et al: Biochemotherapy of advanced metastatic renal cell carcinoma; results of the combination of interleukin-2, α-interferon, 5-fluorouracinl, vinblastine, and 13-*cis*-retinoic acid. World J Urol 1995; 13:174–177.

87. Stadler WM, Kuzel T,Dumas M, Vogelzang NJ: Multi-center phase II trial of interleukin-2, interferon-alpha, and 13-cis-retinoic acid in patients with metastatic renal-cell carcinoma. J Clin Oncol 1998; 16:1820–1825.

88. Dutcher JP, Caliendo G, Novik Y, et al: Phase II study of moderate dose bolus or continuous infusion IL-2 plus GM-CSF in metastatic renal cell cancer. Proc Am Soc Clin Oncol 1999; 18:451a (abst 1740).

89. Ryan CW, Vogelzang NJ, Dumas MC, et al; Granulocyte-macrophage colony-stimulating factor in combination immunotherapy for patients with metastatic renal cell carcinoma: Results of two phase II clinical trials. Cancer 2000; 88:1317–1324.

90. Abuchowski A, McCoy JR, Palczuk NC, et al: Effect of covalent attachment of polyethylene glycol on immunogenicity and circulating life of bovine liver catalase. J Biol Chem 1977; 252:3582–3586.

91. Davis S, Abuchowski A, Park YK, Davis FF: Alteration of the circulating life and antigenic properties of bovine adenosine deaminase in mice by attachment of polyethylene glycol. Clin Exp Immunol 1981; 46:649–652.

92. Yang JC, Topalian S, Schwartzentruber DJ et al: The use of polyethylene glycol-modified interleukin-2 (PEG-IL-2) in the treatment of patients with metastatic renal cell carcinoma and melanoma. A phase I study and a randomized prospective study comparing IL-2 alone versus IL-2 combined with PEG-IL-2. Cancer 1995; 687–694.

93. Shanafelt AB , Lin Y, Shanafelt M-C, et al: A T-cell selective interleukin-2 mutein exhibits potent antitumor activity and is well tolerated in vivo. Nature Biotechnol 2000; 18:1197–1202.

94. Margolin KA, Atkins MB, Weber J, Dutcher JP, et al: Phase I study of interleukin-2 selective angoist BAY-50–4798 (BAY) in patients with advanced melanoma and renal cell cancer. Proc Am Soc Clin Oncol 2002; 12:10a (abst 46).

95. Neville ME, Boni LT, Pflug LE, et al: Biopharmaceutics of liposomal interleukin-2, oncolipin. Cytokine 2000; 12:1691–1701.

96. Kedar E, Gur H, Babai I, et al: Delivery of cytokines by liposomes: hematopoietic and immunomodulatory activity of interleuin-2 encapsulated in conventional liposomes and I long-circulating liposomes. J Immunother 2000; 23:131–145.

10. THE ROLE OF SYSTEMIC CHEMOTHERAPY IN THE TREATMENT OF KIDNEY CANCER

CHRISTOPHER M. GEORGE, M.D.

Clinical Associate, Section of Hematology/Oncology, University of Chicago Medical Center, 5841 South Maryland Ave, MC 2115, Chicago, IL 60637-1470, E-mail: cgeorge@wideopenwest.com

WALTER M. STADLER, M.D., F.A.C.P.

Associate Professor, Sections of Hematology/Oncology and Urology, Departments of Medicine and Surgery, University of Chicago Medical Center, 5841 South Maryland Ave, MC 2115, Chicago, IL 60637-1470, E-mail: wstadler@medicine.bsd.uchicago.edu

The prognosis for patients with metastatic renal cell carcinoma (RCC) is poor. The median overall survival time of patients with advanced disease is approximately 10 months with a 3-year survival rate of about 10%.[1] RCC is typically described as chemotherapy (and radiation therapy) resistant. Most authors agree that biologic response modifiers (i.e. immunotherapy) represent standard first-line treatment for advanced RCC.

To date, no cytotoxic agent or combination of cytotoxic agents has reproducibly demonstrated response rates greater than 10%. Thus, no chemotherapeutic regimen can be considered standard treatment at any stage of the current treatment paradigm.

Efforts to develop new agents and strategies in the treatment of RCC are complicated by this tumor's unusual behavior. Although the median survival time is less than one year, the range of outcomes is wide. Prolonged stable disease is often observed in the absence of treatment and spontaneous regression of advanced renal cell carcinoma has been well documented.[2-4] These observations complicate the results of small phase II trials. The rate of tumor regression with placebo alone has been reported as high as 7%.[5]

Table 1. Efficacy of Selected Cytotoxic Agents in Renal Cell Carcinoma.

Agent	Year and Reference	N	Response Rate (%)
2-Deoxycoformycin (Pentostatin)	1991[63]	18	0
	1992[64]	25	0
5-Fluorouracil	1989[65]	14	0
	1991[66]	27	7
	1993[67]	35	11
	1994[20]	61	5
Bleomycin	1975[68]	15	0
	1976[69]	8	37
	1977[70]	7	0
Carboplatin	1988[71]	19	0
	1990[72]	18	0
Cisplatin	1978[73]	23	0
	1979[74]	10	0
Cyclophosphamide	1975[75]	10	0
	1979[76]	44	4
	1980[77]	12	0
Dactinomycin	1981[78]	61	2
Docetaxel	1994[79]	18	0
Doxorubicin	1977[80]	38	5
Epirubicin	1982[81]	20	0
	1983[82]	19	0
Estramustine	1981[83]	16	0
Etoposide	1979[76]	43	2
Floxuridine/FUDR	1990[21]	68	20
	1990[23]	42	14
	1991[24]	14	0
	1991[22]	40	10

HORMONE THERAPY

Based on provocative laboratory and animal data, hormonal agents have been studied in the treatment of RCC. Although early clinical data suggested agents such as medroxyprogesterone (Megace) were active in a fraction of patients, more recent studies with more rigorous response criteria have shown a response rate closer to 2%.[6] Published data using anti-estrogens have generally shown response rates of less than 10%.[7] One recent unpublished study, however, suggested activity using high-dose toremifene (an anti-estrogen).[8] If these data were confirmed, further evaluation of high-dose anti-estrogen therapy may be warranted.

SINGLE AGENT CHEMOTHERAPY

Since the 1970's, investigators have been struggling to find cytotoxic agents with reproducible activity against RCC. A number of comprehensive reviews have been published.[3,9–11] One particularly inclusive review looked at published series using 72 different cytotoxic agents in 3502 patients. The objective response rate was 5.6%.[12] Selected single agent efficacy data for commonly used cytotoxic agents is presented in Table 1.

Table 1 (continued)

Agent	Year and Reference	N	Response Rate (%)
	1991[25]	15	0
	1991[26]	29	0
	1992[27]	26	8
	1993[28]	28	14
Fludarabine	1987[84]	30	0
	1989[85]	15	0
Gemcitabine	1992[29]	30	10
	1993[30]	18	6
	1996[86]	37	8
Hydroxyurea	1981[87]	19	5
Ifosfamide	1980[88]	11	9
	1981[89]	10	20
	1987[90]	16	0
	1988[91]	9	0
Liposomal encapsulated doxorubicin	1994[92]	14	0
Melphalan	1993[93]	8	0
Methotrexate	1980[94]	8	25
Mitomycin	1987[95]	12	25
Mitotane	1981[96]	12	0
Mitoxantrone	1984[97]	20	0
	1984[98]	49	0
	1984[99]	29	0
	1986[100]	48	0
Paclitaxel	1982[101]	15	0
	1991[102]	18	0
Suramin	1991[103]	10	0
	1992[104]	26	4
Temazolamide	2002[105]	12	0
Thiotepa	1977[70]	7	14
Topotecan	1994[106]	14	0
Vinblastine	1977[70]	10	0
	1984[13]	19	16
	1984[15]	10	0
	1985[16]	14	0
	1987[17]	21	9
	1988[18]	35	9
	1992[14]	26	4
Vindesine	1977[107]	17	0
	1983[108]	24	0
Vinorelbine	1991[109]	14	0
	1993[110]	24	4

Two agents deserve particular attention. Vinblastine is frequently cited as one of the few agents with single agent activity. One 1984 study reported a 16% response rate[13] No subsequent study has shown a response rate greater than 10% although several have been performed.[14–18] Perhaps the best insight into the activity of vinblastine comes from a phase III comparison of vinblastine to vinblastine/IFN. The response rate was only 2.5% in the 81 patients treated with vinblastine alone.[19]

5 FU and related agents have had consistent, but low activity, with phase II studies reporting objective response rates generally in the 10% range. However, recent data from the Southwest Oncology Group demonstrated a response rate of 5.2% in 61 patients with advanced RCC.[20] Similarly, continuous infusion FUDR has also had impressive phase II data published. Hrushesky et al. treated 68 patients with continuous infusion FUDR. Of these, 63 were felt to have assessable disease and 56 of those received the study treatment. The overall response rate was 20 %.[21] Subsequent trials using this agent, however, have struggled to duplicate these data.[22–28] Interestingly, other nucleoside analogs may also have low level activity with 2 reports using gemcitabine reporting 6 and 10% objective response rates[29,30] and one study with the novel analog troxacitabine reporting a 6% objective response rate.[31]

COMBINATION CHEMOTHERAPY

Given the marginal success of single agent cytotoxic therapy, it is perhaps not surprising that there has been limited success with combination chemotherapy. Numerous trials have shown minimal, if any, activity.[32–39] One recently published trial warrants mention. Rini, et al.[40] reported on weekly gemcitabine with continuous infusion 5-fluorouracil (5-FU) in RCC. The regimen appears to be modestly active. Of 39 patients treated, there was a 17% objective response rate and the median progression-free survival for the entire group was 29 weeks.[40] This compares favorably to other reported phase II studies. Subsequent analysis of this regimen suggests a response rate closer to 11%, with evidence of a prolonged survival compared to historical controls.[41] Randomized trials will be required to determine if this level of activity is significantly greater than that observed with 5 FU and other nucleoside analogs alone.

COMBINED CHEMOIMMUNOTHERAPY

After the discovery that biologic response modifiers had activity in RCC, interest arose in combination cytotoxic and biologic therapy. Several of these studies have been performed with different combinations. These trials have been reviewed elsewhere.[42] Note is made that the response rate correlates inversely with year of publication, dampening enthusiasm for this approach. Furthermore, two randomized trials have failed to show a survival benefit for IFN + vinblastine compared to IFN alone.[14,43] Although there is great interest in combining novel agents with biologic response modifiers, there is no current evidence that these biologic agents have enhanced efficacy when combined with "traditional" cytotoxic drugs.

MECHANISMS OF RESISTANCE

The vast majority of RCC's arise from cells of the proximal tubule. These cells have been shown to express high levels of RNA coding for the multidrug resistance gene (mdr1).[44] This mdr1 RNA has also been found in high levels in RCC tissue.[45]

One study looked at expression of p-glycoprotein (the mdr1 gene product) on renal cell carcinoma cells via immunocytochemistry in patients with local disease treated by nephrectomy. The clinical course [measured by progression free survival (PFS)] correlated with the immunocytochemistry results: patients having less than 1% positive tumor cells had longer PFS than those patients with greater than 1%.[46] Drug efflux mediated by p-glycoprotein likely explains, at least in part, this tumor's resistance to various natural product chemotherapeutics.

The glutathione redox cycle has also been postulated to contribute to chemotherapy resistance. One group found that *in vitro* carboplatin and doxorubicin resistance correlated to elevated glutathione levels in renal cancer tumor cells.[47]

A number of strategies have been espoused to overcome RCC chemotherapy resistance, most directed at inhibition of p-glycoprotein. Several agents have shown the ability to sensitize RCC cell *in vitro* including verapamil[45] and quinidine,[44] which were studied with vinblastine. In human RCC patients, phase II studies of vinblastine with cyclosporine (another putative inhibitor of p-glycoprotein) failed to show any improvement in tumor response [48,49] and treatment was poorly tolerated.[49] Other agents used clinically in an attempt to reverse p-glycoprotein mediated chemotherapy resistance include nifedipine,[50] dipyridamole,[51] dexverapamil,[52] quinidine,[53] and tamoxifen.[48] Agents developed specifically to inhibit p-glycoprotein-mediated resistance are now in clinical trials. For example, PSC-833 is a second-generation p-glycoprotein antagonist currently in development for a variety of cancers.[54] Further clinical trials will be necessary to determine if these newer p-glycoprotein inhibitors can overcome RCC resistance to natural products. However, it must be recognized that chemotherapy resistance may be due to a number of factors, besides overexpression of p-glycoprotein.

FUTURE DIRECTIONS

New agents are badly needed for the treatment of RCC and all eligible patients should be given the option of novel therapy on a clinical trial to hasten the development of promising compounds. Although new cytotoxics continue to be investigated, most investigators agree that a major breakthrough using these agents is unlikely. There has thus been increasing emphasis placed on investigating agents that work through novel mechanisms of action, especially agents that target specific known molecularly altered pathways in this disease.

Along these lines, it is now recognized that clear cell carcinomas of the kidney typically have an inactivated or mutated VHL gene. This leads to upregulation of several key molecules likely critical to the RCC phenotype including hypoxia inducible factor (HIF1α and HIF1β), vascular endothelial growth factor (VEGF), and platelet derived growth factor (PDGF). Similarly, papillary renal cell cancers may be characterized by activation of the met receptor tyrosine kinase.

Upregulation of VEGF, PDGF and other factors likely leads to this tumor's highly vascular pathology and has lead to the hypothesis that the tumor vasculature should be considered a valuable target in RCC. In fact a recent study using the anti-VEGF antibody bevacizumab suggested that this agent leads to a 10% objective response and can delay time to progression in clear cell carcinoma patients who have failed standard IL2 based therapy.[55] In addition, several studies suggest that thalidomide, a drug with many putative mechanisms of action including antiangiogenic mechanisms, may have a low level of activity as well.[56,57] Interestingly, interferon-α, whose mechanism of action in renal cell carcinoma is typically thought of as being immunologic, may inhibit basic fibroblast growth factor (bFGF) mediated angiogenesis as well, especially at low doses.[58] This raises the issue as to whether the modest survival advantage seen with this agent, despite the low objective response rate, is due to its effects on the tumor vasculature.

Finally, in terms of other signaling pathway inhibitors, it is interesting to note that an inhibitor of the mTOR signaling pathway, CCI-779, has modest activity in renal cell cancer.[59] PTEN mutations, which have been suggested to be predictive of response to mTOR inhibitors,[60] have been found in 7% of renal cancers.[61] These results suggest that further investigation of mTOR pathway inhibitors and correlation with PTEN mutations should be undertaken.

Preclinical data, as well as the limited clinical data to date, suggest that anti-angiogenic agents and many signal transduction inhibitors, if effective, will only slow disease progression when used as single agents and will be most effective when used in combination with each other or with cytotoxic therapies. Given the multiple putative antiangiogenic agents under development, the almost infinite number of combinations possible, and the difficulty in determining whether lack of growth in an individual patient represents drug effect or simply natural history complicates drug development in this area. It is thus likely that newer clinical trial designs will be necessary for evaluating antiangiogenic and other cytostatic agents.[62]

SUMMARY

Traditional cytotoxic chemotherapy has been considered to be ineffective in renal cell carcinoma, likely due to multiple mechanisms of high-level drug resistance proteins such as p-glycoprotein expressed by these cancers. Nonetheless, low level activity of several nucleoside analogues and the elucidation of critical molecular pathways and targets in this disease, such as the angiogenic pathway, provide hope that important advances can and will be made.

REFERENCES

1. Motzer RJ, Mazumdar M, Bacik J, et al. Survival and prognostic stratification of 670 patients with advanced renal cell carcinoma. J Clin Oncol 17: 2530–2540, 1999.
2. Vogelzang NJ, Priest ER, Borden L. Spontaneous regression of histologically proved pulmonary metastases from renal cell carcinoma: a case with 5-year followup. J Urol 148: 1247–1248, 1992.
3. Motzer RJ, Russo P. Systemic therapy for renal cell carcinoma. J Urol 163: 408–417, 2000.
4. Oliver RT, Nethersell AB, Bottomley JM. Unexplained spontaneous regression and alpha-interferon as treatment for metastatic renal carcinoma. Br J Urol 63: 128–131, 1989.
5. Gleave ME, Elhilali M, Fradet Y, et al. Interferon gamma-1b compared with placebo in metastatic renal-cell carcinoma. Canadian Urologic Oncology Group. N Engl J Med 338: 1265–1271, 1998.
6. Hrushesky WJ, Murphy GP. Current status of the therapy of advanced renal carcinoma. J Surg Oncol 9: 277–288, 1977.
7. Henriksson R, Nilsson G, Colleen S. Survival in renal cell carcinoma—a randomized evaluation of tamoxifen vs. interleukin-2, alpha-interferon (leucocyte) and tamoxifen. Br J Cancer 77: 1211, 1998.

8. Gershanovich MM, Gorelov AI, Hajba A, et al. High-dose toremifene (HDT) for the treatment of locally advanced and metastatic renal cell carcinoma. Proc Amer Soc of Clin Oncol 21:19a (abstract 757): 757, 2002.

9. Amato RJ. Chemotherapy for renal cell carcinoma. Semin Oncol 27: 177–186, 2000.

10. Harris DT. Hormonal therapy and chemotherapy of renal-cell carcinoma. Semin Oncol 10: 422–430, 1983.

11. Yagoda A, Abi-Rached B, Petrylak D. Chemotherapy for advanced renal-cell carcinoma: 1983–1993. Semin Oncol 22: 42–60, 1995.

12. Yagoda A, Petrylak D, Thompson S. Cytotoxic chemotherapy for advanced renal cell carcinoma. Urol Clin North Am 20: 303–321, 1993.

13. Kuebler JP, Hogan TF, Trump DL, et al. Phase II study of continuous 5-day vinblastine infusion in renal adenocarcinoma. Cancer Treat Rep 68: 925–926, 1984.

14. Fossa SD, Droz JP, Pavone-Macaluso MM, et al. Vinblastine in metastatic renal cell carcinoma: EORTC phase II trial 30882. The EORTC Genitourinary Group. Eur J Cancer: 878–880, 1992.

15. Zeffren J, Yagoda A, Kelsen D, et al. Phase I-II trial of a 5-day continuous infusion of vinblastine sulfate. Anticancer Res 4: 411–413, 1984.

16. Tannock IF, Evans WK. Failure of 5-day vinblastine infusion in the treatment of patients with renal cell carcinoma. Cancer Treat Rep 69: 227–228, 1985.

17. Crivellari D, Tumolo S, Frustaci S, et al. Phase II study of five-day continuous infusion of vinblastine in patients with metastatic renal-cell carcinoma. Am J Clin Oncol 10: 231–233, 1987.

18. Elson PJ, Kvols LK, Vogl SE, et al. Phase II trials of 5-day vinblastine infusion (NSC 49842), L-alanosine (NSC 153353), acivicin (NSC 163501), and aminothiadiazole (NSC 4728) in patients with recurrent or metastatic renal cell carcinoma. Invest New Drugs 6: 97–103, 1988.

19. Pyrhonen S, Salminen E, Ruutu M, et al. Prospective randomized trial of interferon alfa-2a plus vinblastine versus vinblastine alone in patients with advanced renal cell cancer. J Clin Oncol 17: 2859–2867, 1999.

20. Kish JA, Wolf M, Crawford ED, et al. Evaluation of low dose continuous infusion 5-fluorouracil in patients with advanced and recurrent renal cell carcinoma. A Southwest Oncology Group Study. Cancer 74: 916–919, 1994.

21. Hrushesky WJ, von Roemeling R, Lanning RM, et al. Circadian-shaped infusions of floxuridine for progressive metastatic renal cell carcinoma. J Clin Oncol 8: 1504–1513, 1990.

22. Dexeus FH, Logothetis CJ, Sella A, et al. Circadian infusion of floxuridine in patients with metastatic renal cell carcinoma. J Urol 146: 709–713, 1991.

23. Damascelli B, Marchiano A, Spreafico C, et al. Circadian continuous chemotherapy of renal cell carcinoma with an implantable, programmable infusion pump. Cancer 66: 237–241, 1990.

24. Merrouche Y, Negrier S, FL, et al. Phase II study of continous circadian infusion FUDR in metastatic renal cell cancer (RCC). Eur J Cancer Clin Oncol 27: 1991.

25. Dimopoulous MA, Dexeus FH, Jones E, et al. Evidence for additive anti-tumor activity and toxicity for the combination of FUDR and interferon alpha2B in patients (pts) with metastatic renal cell carcinoma (RCC). Proc Am Assoc Cancer Res 32: 186, 1991.

26. Richards F, Cooper MR, Jackson DV, et al. Continuous 5-day (D) intravenous (IV) FUDR infusion for renal cell carcinoma (RCC): A phase I-II trial of the Piedmont Oncology Association. Proc Am Soc Clin Oncol 10: 170, 1991.

27. Budd GT, Murthy S, Klein E, et al. Time-modified infusion of floxuridine in metastatic renal cell carcinoma (mRCC). Proc Am Assoc Cancer Res 33: 220, 1992.

28. Conroy T, Geoffrois L, Guillemin F, et al. Simplified chronomodulated continuous infusion of floxuridine in patients with metastatic renal cell carcinoma. Cancer 72: 2190–2197, 1993.

29. Weissbach L, de Mulder P, Osieka R, et al. Phase II study of gemcitabine in renal cancer. Proc Am Soc Clin Oncol 11: 219, 1992.

30. Mertens WC, Eisenhauer EA, Moore M, et al. Gemcitabine in advanced renal cell carcinoma. A phase II study of the National Cancer Institute of Canada Clinical Trials Group. Ann Oncol 4: 331–332, 1993.

31. Moore MJ, Chi K, Ernst S. A phase II study of troxacitabine in patients with advanced and/or metastatic renal cell carcinoma. NCIC CTG IND.119. Proc Am Soc of Clin Oncol 20:193a (abstract 768): 2001.

32. Dana BW, Alberts DS. Combination chemoimmunotherapy for advanced renal carcinoma with Adriamycin, bleomycin, vincristine, cyclophosphamide, plus BCG. Cancer Clin Trials 4: 205–207, 1981.

33. Droz JP, Theodore C, Ghosn M, et al. Twelve-year experience with chemotherapy in adult metastatic renal cell carcinoma at the Institut Gustave-Roussy. Semin Surg Oncol 4: 97–99, 1988.
34. Wada T, Houjou T, Kubo R, et al. A combined chemo-endocrine treatment with tegafur, adriamycin, methotrexate and tamoxifen for advanced renal cell carcinoma. Anticancer Res 13: 2465–2467, 1993.
35. Katakkar SB, Franks CR. Chemo-hormonal therapy for metastatic renal cell carcinoma with adriamycin, hydroxyurea, vinblastine, and medroxyprogesterone acetate. Cancer Treat Rep 62: 1379–1380, 1978.
36. Jekunen A, Stengard J, Pyrhonen S. Phase II study of vinblastine and doxorubicin in advanced renal cell carcinoma. Eur J Cancer 2: 245, 1994.
37. Sommer HH, Fossa SD, Lien HH. Combination chemotherapy of advanced renal cell cancer with CCNU and vinblastine. Cancer Chemother Pharmacol 14: 277–278, 1985.
38. Merrin C, Mittelman A, Fanous N, et al. Chemotherapy of advanced renal cell carcinoma with vinblastine and CCNU. J Urol 113: 21–23, 1975.
39. Hahn RG, Temkin NR, Savlov ED, et al. Phase II study of vinblastine, methyl-CCNU, and medroxyprogesterone in advanced renal cell cancer. Cancer Treat Rep 62: 1093–1095, 1978.
40. Rini BI, Vogelzang NJ, Dumas MC, et al. Phase II trial of weekly intravenous gemcitabine with continuous infusion fluorouracil in patients with metastatic renal cell cancer. J Clin Oncol 18: 2419–2426, 2000.
41. George GM, Dezheng H, Vogelzang NJ, et al. Pooled analysis of advanced renal cell carcinoma (RCC) patients (pts) treated with gemcitabine (G) and 5-fluorouracil (F). Proc Amer Soc Clin Oncol 21:191a (abstract 762): 2002.
42. Wirth MP. Immunotherapy for metastatic renal cell carcinoma. Urol Clin North Am 20: 283–295, 1993.
43. Neidhart JA, Anderson SA, Harris JE, et al. Vinblastine fails to improve response of enal cancer to interferon alfa-n1: high response rate in patients with pulmonary metastases. J Clin Oncol 9: 832–836, 1991.
44. Fojo AT, Ueda K, Slamon DJ, et al. Expression of a multidrug-resistance gene in human tumors and tissues. Proc Natl Acad Sci USA 84: 265–269, 1987.
45. Fojo AT, Shen DW, Mickley LA, et al. Intrinsic drug resistance in human kidney cancer is associated with expression of a human multidrug-resistance gene. J Clin Oncol 5: 1922–1927, 1987.
46. Duensing S, Dallmann I, Grosse J, et al. Immunocytochemical detection of P-glycoprotein: initial expression correlates with survival in renal cell carcinoma patients. Oncology 51: 309–313, 1994.
47. Mickisch GH, Roehrich K, Koessig J, et al. Mechanisms and modulation of multidrug resistance in primary human renal cell carcinoma. J Urol 144: 755–759, 1990.
48. Samuels BL, Hollis DR, Rosner GL, et al. Modulation of vinblastine resistance in metastatic renal cell carcinoma with cyclosporine A or tamoxifen: a cancer and leukemia group B study. Clin Cancer Res 3: 1977–1984, 1997.
49. Warner E, Tobe SW, Andrulis IL, et al. Phase I-II study of vinblastine and oral cyclosporin A in metastatic renal cell carcinoma. Am J Clin Oncol 18: 251–256, 1995.
50. Schwartsmann G, Medina de Cunha F, Silveira LA, et al. Phase II trial of vinblastine plus nifedipine (VN) in patients with advanced renal cell carcinoma (RCC). Brazilian Oncology Trials Group. Ann Oncol 2: 443, 1991.
51. Murphy BR, Rynard SM, Pennington KL, et al. A phase II trial of vinblastine plus dipyridamole in advanced renal cell carcinoma. A Hoosier Oncology Group Study. Am J Clin Oncol 17: 10–13, 1994.
52. Motzer RJ, Lyn P, Fischer P, et al. Phase I/II trial of dexverapamil plus vinblastine for patients with advanced renal cell carcinoma. J Clin Oncol 13: 1958–1965, 1995.
53. Agarwala SS, Bahnson RR, Wilson JW, et al. Evaluation of the combination of vinblastine and quinidine in patients with metastatic renal cell carcinoma. A phase I study. Am J Clin Oncol 18: 211–215, 1995.
54. Chico I, Kang MH, Bergan R, et al. Phase I study of infusional paclitaxel in combination with the P-glycoprotein antagonist PSC 833. J Clin Oncol 19: 832–842, 2001.
55. Yang JC, Haworth L, Steinberg SM, et al. A randomized double-blind placebo-controlled trial of bevacizumab (anti-VEGF antibody) demonstrating a prolongation in time to progression in patients with metastatic renal cancer. Proc Amer Soc Clin Oncol 21:19a (abstract 15): 2002.
56. Motzer RJ, Bacik J, Mariani T, et al. Treatment outcome and survival associated with metastatic renal cell carcinoma of non-clear-cell histology. J Clin Oncol 20: 2376–2381, 2002.
57. Eisen T Thalidomide in solid malignancies. J Clin Oncol 20: 2607–2609, 2002.

58. Dinney CP, Bielenberg DR, Perrotte P, et al. Inhibition of basic fibroblast growth factor expression, angiogenesis, and growth of human bladder carcinoma in mice by systemic interferon-alpha administration. Cancer Res 58: 808–814, 1998.

59. Atkins MB, Hidalgo M, Stadler W, et al. A randomized double-blinded phase 2 study of intravenous CCI-779 administered weekly to patients with advanced renal cell carcinoma. Proc Amer Soc Clin Oncol 21:10a (abstract 36): 2002.

60. Neshat MS, Mellinghoff IK, Tran C, et al. Enhanced sensitivity of PTEN-deficient tumors to inhibition of FRAP/mTOR. Proc Natl Acad Sci USA 98: 10314–10319, 2001.

61. Kondo K, Yao M, Kobayashi K, et al. PTEN/MMAC1/TEP1 mutations in human primary renal-cell carcinomas and renal carcinoma cell lines. Int J Cancer 91: 219–224, 2001.

62. Stadler WM, Ratain MJ. Development of target-based antineoplastic agents. Invest New Drugs 18: 7–16, 2000.

63. Venner P, Eisenhauer EA, Wierzbicki R, et al. Phase II study of 2'-deoxycoformycin in patients with renal cell carcinoma. A National Cancer Institute of Canada Clinical Trials Group study. Invest New Drugs 9: 273–275, 1991.

64. Witte RS, Walsh C, Fisher H, et al. Evaluation of deoxycoformycin in patients with advanced renal cell carcinoma. An ECOG pilot study. Invest New Drugs 10: 49–50, 1992.

65. Zaniboni A, Simoncini E, Marpicati P, et al. Phase II trial of 5-fluorouracil and high-dose folinic acid in advanced renal cell cancer. J Chemother 1: 350–351, 1989.

66. Schulof R, Lokich J, Wampler G, et al. Phase II trial of protracted infusional 5-FU (PIF) for metastatic renal cell carcinoma. Proc Am Soc Clin Oncol 10: 170, 1991.

67. Ahlgren JD, Lokich J, Auerbach M, et al. Protracted infusional 5FU (PIF): a well tolerated regimen in metastatic renal cell carcinoma (MRC): A Mid-Atlantic Oncology Program (MOAP) study. Proc Am Soc Clin Oncol 12: 244, 1993.

68. Johnson DE, Chalbaud RA, Holoye PY, et al. Clinical trial of bleomycin (NSC-125066) in the treatment of metastatic renal carcinoma. Cancer Chemother Rep 59: 433–435, 1975.

69. Haas CD, Coltman CA, Jr, Gottlieb JA, et al. Phase II evaluation of bleomycin. A Southwest oncology Group study. Cancer 38: 8–12, 1976.

70. Hahn DM, Schimpff SC, Ruckdeschel JC, et al. Single-agent therapy for renal cell carcinoma: CCNU, vinblastine, thioTEPA, or bleomycin. Cancer Treat Rep 61: 1585–1587, 1977.

71. Tait M, Abrams J, Egorin MJ, et al. Phase II carboplatin (CBDCA) for metastatic renal cell cancer with a standard dose (SD) and a calculated dose (CD) according to renal function. Proc Am Soc Clin Oncol 7: 125, 1988.

72. Trump DL, Elson P. Evaluation of carboplatin (NSC 241240) in patients with recurrent or metastatic renal cell carcinoma. Invest New Drugs 8: 201–203, 1990.

73. Rodriguez LH, Johnson DE. Clinical trial of cisplatinum (NSC 119875) in metastatic renal cell carcinoma. Urology 11: 344–346, 1978.

74. Merrin CE. Treatment of genitourinary tumours with cis-dichlorodiammineplatinum(II): experience in 250 patients. Cancer Treat Rep 63: 1579–1584, 1979.

75. Kiruluta G, Morales A, Lott S. Response of renal adenocarcinoma to cyclophosphamide. Urology 6: 557–558, 1975.

76. Hahn RG, Bauer M, Wolter J, et al. Phase II study of single-agent therapy with megestrol acetate, VP-16-213, cyclophosphamide, and dianhydrogalactitol in advanced renal cell cancer. Cancer Treat Rep 63: 513–515, 1979.

77. Wajsman Z, Beckley S, Madajewicz S. High dose cyclophosphamide in metastatic renal cell cancer. Proc Am Soc Clin Oncol 21: 423, 1980.

78. Hahn RG, Begg CB, Davis T. Phase II study of vinblastine-CCNU, triazinate, and dactinomycin in advanced renal cell cancer. Cancer Treat Rep 65: 711–713, 1981.

79. Mertens WC, Eisenhauer EA, Jolivet J, et al. Docetaxel in advanced renal carcinoma. A phase II trial of the National Cancer Institute of Canada Clinical Trials Group. Ann Oncol 5: 185–187, 1994.

80. O'Bryan RM, Baker LH, Gottlieb JE, et al. Dose response evaluation of adriamycin in human neoplasia. Cancer 39: 1940–1948, 1977.

81. Fossa SD, Wik B, Bae E, et al. Phase II study of 4'-epi-doxorubicin in metastatic renal cancer. Cancer Treat Rep 66: 1219–1221, 1982.

82. Benedetto P, Ahmed T, Needles B, et al. Phase II trial of 4'epi-adriamycin for advanced hypernephroma. Am J Clin Oncol 6: 553–554, 1983.

83. Swanson DA, Johnson DE. Estramustine phosphate (Emcyt) as treatment for metastatic renal carcinoma. Urology 17: 344–346, 1981.

84. Balducci L, Blumenstein B, Von Hoff DD, et al. Evaluation of fludarabine phosphate in renal cell carcinoma: a Southwest Oncology Group Study. Cancer Treat Rep 71: 543–544, 1987.
85. Shevrin DH, Lad TE, Kilton LJ, et al. Phase II trial of fludarabine phosphate in advanced renal cell carcinoma: an Illinois Cancer Council Study. Invest New Drugs 7: 251–253, 1989.
86. Rohde D, De Mulder PH, Weissbach L, et al. Experimental and clinical efficacy of $2',2'$-difluorodeoxycytidine (gemcitabine) against renal cell carcinoma. Oncology 53: 476–481, 1996.
87. Stolbach LL, Begg CB, Hall T, et al. Treatment of renal carcinoma: a phase III randomized trial of oral medroxyprogesterone (Provera), hydroxyurea, and nafoxidine. Cancer Treat Rep 65: 689–692, 1981.
88. Fossa SD, Talle K. Treatment of metastatic renal cancer with ifosfamide and mesnum with and without irradiation. Cancer Treat Rep 64: 1103–1108, 1980.
89. Heim ME, Fiene R, Schick E, et al. Central nervous side effects following ifosfamide monotherapy of advanced renal carcinoma. J Cancer Res Clin Oncol 100: 113–116, 1981.
90. De Forges A, Droz JP, Ghosn M, et al. Phase II trial of ifosfamide/mesna in metastatic adult renal carcinoma. Cancer Treat Rep 71: 1103, 1987.
91. Bodrogi I, Baki M, Sinkovics I, et al. Ifosfamide chemotherapy of metastatic renal cell cancer. Semin Surg Oncol 4: 95–96, 1988.
92. Law TM, Mencel P, Motzer RJ. Phase II trial of liposomal encapsulated doxorubicin in patients with advanced renal cell carcinoma. Invest New Drugs 12: 323–325, 1994.
93. Falkson CI. New formulation intravenous melphalan in the treatment of patients with metastatic renal cancer. Invest New Drugs 11: 93, 1993.
94. Baumgartner G, Heinz R, Arbes H, et al. Methotrexate-citrovorum factor used alone and in combination chemotherapy for advanced hypernephromas. Cancer Treat Rep 64: 41–46, 1980.
95. Stewart DJ, Futter N, Irvine A, et al. Mitomycin-C and metronidazole in the treatment of advanced renal-cell carcinoma. Am J Clin Oncol 10: 520–522, 1987.
96. Hogan TF, Citrin DL, Freeberg BL. A preliminary report of mitotane therapy of advanced renal and prostate cancer. Cancer Treat Rep 65: 539–540, 1981.
97. De Jager R, Cappelaere P, Armand JP, et al. An EORTC phase II study of mitoxantrone in solid tumors and lymphomas. Eur J Cancer Clin Oncol 20: 1369–1375, 1984.
98. Taylor SA, Von Hoff DD, Baker LH, et al. Phase II clinical trial of mitoxantrone in patients with advanced renal cell carcinoma: a Southwest Oncology Group study. Cancer Treat Rep 68: 919–920, 1984.
99. van Oosterom AT, Fossa SD, Pizzocaro G, et al. Mitoxantrone in advanced renal cancer: a phase II study in previously untreated patients from the EORTC Genito-Urinary Tract Cancer Cooperative Group. Eur J Cancer Clin Oncol 20: 1239–1241, 1984.
100. Gams RA, Nelson O, Birch R. Phase II evaluation of mitoxantrone in advanced renal cell carcinoma: a Southeastern Cancer Study Group Trial. Cancer Treat Rep 70: 921–922, 1986.
101. Natale RB, Yagoda A, Kelsen DP, et al. Phase II trial of PALA in hypernephroma and urinary bladder cancer. Cancer Treat Rep 66: 2091–2092, 1982.
102. Einzig AI, Gorowski E, Sasloff J, et al. Phase II trial of taxol in patients with metastatic renal cell carcinoma. Cancer Invest 9: 133–136, 1991.
103. La Rocca RV, Stein CA, Danesi R, et al. A pilot study of suramin in the treatment of metastatic renal cell carcinoma. Cancer 67: 1509–1513, 1991.
104. Motzer RJ, Nanus DM, O'Moore P, et al. Phase II trial of suramin in patients with advanced renal cell carcinoma: treatment results, pharmacokinetics, and tumor growth factor expression. Cancer Res 52: 5775–5779, 1992.
105. Park DK, Ryan CW, Dodlan ME, et al. A phase II trial of temozolomide in patients with metastatic renal cell cancer. Cancer Chem Pharm: (in press).
106. Law TM, Ilson DH, Motzer RJ. Phase II trial of topotecan in patients with advanced renal cell carcinoma. Invest New Drugs 12: 143–145, 1994.
107. Wong PP, Yagoda A, Currie VE, et al. Phase II study of vindesine sulfate in the therapy for advanced renal carcinoma. Cancer Treat Rep 61: 1727–1729, 1977.
108. Fossa SD, Denis L, van Oosterom AT, et al. Vindesine in advanced renal cancer. A study of the EORTC Genito-urinary Tract Cancer Cooperative Group. Eur J Cancer Clin Oncol 19: 473–475, 1983.
109. Canobbio L, Boccardo F, Guarneri D, et al. Phase II study of navelbine in advanced renal cell carcinoma. Eur J Cancer 27: 804–805, 1991.
110. Wilding G, Kirkwood J, Clamon G, et al. Phase II trial of navelbine in metastatic renal cancer. Proc Am Soc Clin Oncol 12: 253, 1993.

11. CELL, GENE AND VACCINE BASED STRATEGIES IN KIDNEY CANCER

BARBARA J. GITLITZ, M.D. AND ROBERT A. FIGLIN, M.D.

University of California @ Los Angeles, 10945 Le Conte Avenue, Suite 2333, Los Angeles, CA 90095

CELL BASED THERAPIES

Overview

T lymphocytes are the effector cells of the cellular immune system and recognize antigen via the T cell receptor (TCR), CD3 complex. There are 2 major T cell subsets based upon TCR-restricted recognition of major histocompatability complex (MHC) associated antigens. Antigen presenting cells (APC) such as dendritic cells (DC), macrophages, and tumor cells, continuously process and present both foreign and self antigens in association with MHC molecules. The TCR binds to the antigenic peptide sequence located in a grove formed by the MHC molecule.[1] In general, CD8+ T-cells recognize antigen in association with class I MHC molecules and CD4+ T cells recognize antigen in association with class II MHC molecules. The binding of the TCR/CD3 complex to the MHC-antigen complex is crucial to the generation of effector cell function, including target cell lysis, T-cell clonal expansion, and secretion of cytokines.

Cytokines are proteins produced by mononuclear cells of the immune system. The discovery of the cytokine, interleukin 2 (IL-2), has had an enormous impact on cancer immunology.[2,3] Both CD4+ and CD8+ T cells could be expanded and maintain their in vivo and in vitro activity in the presence of this cytokine growth factor. Interleukin-2 gene expression is initiated by 2 signals; ligation of the (TCR)/CD3 complex, and a "co-stimulatory" or secondary signal provided by an APC expressing B7 (a co stimulatory molecule) which is a ligand for the CD28 or CTLA-4 receptor on the T-cell.[4] When the proper sequence of signals is received, the T-cell produces IL-2, and there is also transcriptional activation of the genes encoding the IL-2 receptor.

The discovery of IL-2 was the key component allowing for in vitro expansion and study of lymphocyte clones responsive to antigen in vivo. Enhanced therapeutic efficacy was observed when cultured immune cells used in adoptive transfer were accompanied by exogenous IL-2 administration.[5,6] This exogenous use of IL-2 was also shown to cause in vivo proliferation and prolonged survival of cells used for adoptive immunotherapy.[7] Based on these observations, exogenous IL-2 is often administered with the adoptive transfer of cultured immune effector cells.

There have been a few well studied lymphocyte populations used in the adoptive immunotherapy of mRCC. These include Lymphokine-Activated Killers cells (LAK), Tumor-Infiltrating Lymphocytes (TIL), and Autolymphocyte Therapy (ALT). Other interesting, adoptively transferred cell populations including Vaccine Primed Lymph Node cells (VPLN) and are discussed below.

Lymphokine Activated Killer Cells

Originally described by Grimm et al,[8,9] LAK are peripherally circulating lymphocytes activated in vitro by exposure to high concentrations of IL-2. These cells lead to non-MHC restricted cytotoxicity of tumor cell targets. When generated from human peripheral blood lymphocytes (PBL), LAK precursors are contained primarily in the large granular lymphocyte (LGL) population containing virtually all active natural killer (NK) cells.[10] The capacity to distinguish between tumor cells and normal cells is a hallmark of LAK activity.

Murine models with experimentally induced metastases demonstrated that the passive transfer of LAK plus IL-2 caused the regression of established metastases from a variety of cancer types.[11,12] In most studies, the combined administration of LAK cells plus IL-2 led to improved efficacy over IL-2 alone.

Initial human clinical trials using activated killer cells alone showed no clinical efficacy, but demonstrated the tolerability of multiple infusions of up to 2×10^{11} cells with minimal side effects.[13,14] In the first reported trial combining LAK plus IL-2, eleven of 25 patients experienced objective tumor response (1 CR and 10 PR).[15] These responses occurred in patients with four histologic tumor types: renal cell, melanoma, lung, and colon carcinoma. This landmark study demonstrated the feasibility of adoptive immunotherapy of human cancers.

Treatment with IL-2 induces lymphopenia, followed by rebound lymphocytosis. To generate LAK cells, patients undergo leukapheresis 48 to 72 hours following the discontinuation of IL-2, at the peak of the rebound lymphocytosis. The PBL are then cultured in vitro in high concentrations of IL-2 (400 to 1000 IU/ml), and approximately 10^{10} to 10^{11} LAK cells are generated. The toxicities of concomitant therapy with LAK cells plus IL-2 are related to the dose of IL-2 used.

Early studies of LAK plus IL-2 generated enthusiasm, with response rates seen in mRCC of up to 35%.[16,17,18] The promise of combined therapy with LAK plus IL-2 is to improve upon the responses to IL-2 alone. To examine this, there have been

3 randomized trials.[19–21] These trials included high dose IL-2 with or without LAK[19] and low dose IL-2 with or without LAK.[21] None of these trials showed superiority of 1 arm over the other thus leading to the pursuit of other therapeutic cell populations for the treatment of mRCC.

Tumor Infiltrating Lymphocytes

Lymphocytes comprise only a small proportion of cells in a neoplastic nodule, some of which contain IL-2 receptors, presumably because of interactions with tumor antigens. Techniques to isolate and expand lymphoid cells infiltrating solid tumors were first described in 1980.[22] Under the influence of IL-2, these lymphocytes can grow in single-cell suspensions of tumor and appear to mediate the destruction of tumor cells, leaving relatively pure cultures of infiltrating lymphocytes. Numerous investigators have successfully established TIL cultures from hundreds of different human tumors, including RCC, melanoma, colon, breast cancer and lymphoma.[23]

Unlike LAK, the anti-tumor activity of TIL is MHC restricted.[24] Murine studies comparing the adoptive transfer of TIL versus LAK (both with accompanying IL-2) demonstrate TIL to be 50 to 100 times more potent on a per cell basis than LAK.[25]

The process of isolating and expanding TIL is as follows.[26] Fresh tumor specimens are obtained and mechanically and enzymatically digested to obtain single cell suspensions containing both viable mononuclear cells and tumor cells. These cells are expanded ex vivo under sterile culture conditions in the presence of low concentration of IL-2 ($20\,U/ml$), supporting a lymphocyte mediated destruction of tumor cells. Following 5 to 6 weeks in culture, 10^8 to 10^9 initial mononuclear cells proliferate to approximately 10^{11} TIL, which are infused into patients together with IL-2.

There have been a few small early phase trials of TIL for patients with advanced cancers including mRCC.[27–33] These trials have varied with respect to their dosing and schedule of administration of IL-2. Some have used concomitant low dose Cyclophosphamide[27,30] and 1 also combined IL-2 with IFN α.[32] They have varied widely in the number of TIL infused, the source of TIL (primary tumor vs. metastatic site) and most importantly in their rates of response; from 0–35%. There has been 1 multi center phase III trial randomizing subjects with mRCC to low dose continuous intravenous infusion (CIV) IL-2 alone vs. low dose CIV IL-2 plus TIL.[34] Unfortunately, this trial was fraught with difficulty especially with regards to the successful preparation of TIL at a centralized facility. Of the subjects randomized to the TIL arm, 41% did not receive these cells due to processing difficulties. After randomization of a total of 160 subjects, intent to treat analysis revealed response rates of 9.9 vs. 11.4% (IL-2 vs, IL-2/TIL). The question of TIL enhancing the response rate or quality of response to IL-2 alone still remains unanswered. The single institution, UCLA experience however, combining TIL with low dose CIV IL-2 plus IFNα demonstrates feasibility of this approach, with an intriguing 35% response rate including durable remissions.[32]

Autolymphocyte Therapy

Autolymphocyte Therapy is adoptive cellular therapy of neoplastic disease using autologous lymphocytes activated ex-vivo by anti-CD3 monoclonal antibody (mAb) and a mixture of previously prepared autologous cytokines. The theoretical basis of ALT relies on the activation of CD44+ memory T lymphocytes.

The preparation of ALT for immunotherapy is a multi-step process.[35] First, patients undergo leukapheresis to obtain PBL which are incubated for 3 days in the presence of anti-CD3 mAb, and the cytokine rich supernatant fluid, called T3CS, is collected. Two weeks after the initial leukapheresis, patients undergo repeat phere-sis for the collection of PBL for activation for 5 days in media containing 25% T3CS, indomethacin, and cimetidine. Following the 5 day incubation, activated cells are irradiated to 50 cGy to reduce the activity of suppressor T lymphocytes, and the cells are then infused into patients. Patients continue to receive oral high dose cime-tidine given to block the activity of suppressor T cell populations that contain the H2 receptor.

In 1990, an initial report of a 90 patient randomized trial of ALT versus high dose cimetidine alone for the treatment of metastatic RCCa was published.[36] Statistically significant findings included a 2.5 fold survival advantage in patients receiving ALT (21 months versus 8.5 months). Unexpected findings in the report included an improved response rate in patients receiving, ALT (21%) but a lack of correlation between response and survival; and males who received ALT had a fourfold survival advantage, whereas females receiving ALT demonstrated no survival advantage.

This initial report has been updated,[37,38] and over 300 patients with mRCC have been accrued into this multi-institutional clinical trial, with a persistent survival advantage being reported in the ALT arm. The early success of ALT in the treat-ment of mRCC led to the establishment of a number of proprietary ALT treat-ment centers.

There has been a small (45 subjects) randomized trial of ALT vs. observation for the adjuvant treatment of RCC.[39] They found a significant difference in favor of ALT over observation for overall median time to progression. This should form the basis for larger confirmatory trials.

Vaccine-Primed Lymph Node Cells (VPLN)

Lymph nodes draining growing tumors presumably harbor pre-effector lymphoid cells that can be activated and expanded ex vivo into competent effector cells via anti-CD3 antibody and low concentrations of IL-2.[40] These VPLN cells can be elicited by the use of a bacterial antigen admixed with irradiated tumor cells and when harvested from a draining lymph node and inoculated in animal studies, showed rejection of poorly immunogenic tumors.[41] Twelve subjects with mRCC participated in an early phase trial of VPLN and high dose bolus IL-2 yielding 2 complete and 2 partial responses.[42] This prompted initiation of a phase II trial of VPLN plus IL-2 for mRCC. Vaccines consisted of autologous tumor cells irradiated and admixed with Tice bacille Calmette-Guerin(BCG). Seven days after vaccine administration, the VPLN cells were harvested from the draining lymph nodes and placed into an anti-CD3/IL-2 activation protocol. These cells were then adoptively transferred with high dose bolus IL-2 (360,000 IU/kg). Of 33 pts evaluable for response there was a promising 24% response rate including durable partial and complete responses.[43] This group is assessing ways of improving their VPLN strategy by using tumor lysate loaded dendritic cell vaccines for the in vivo lymph node priming.[44] Furthermore, in a recent publication using a murine model, it appears that doubly activating the VPLN cells by both anti CD3 and anti CD28 (co-stimulatory signal) yields a more potent tumor reactive effector cell.[45]

T Cell Receptor Activated T cells (TRAC)

T Cell Receptor Activated T cells (TRAC) are manufactured by the ex-vivo stimulation of PBL by anti CD3 mAb and high dose IL-2 (100 IU/ml). They possess both NK and LAK-type cytotoxicity patterns (non-MHC restricted) and produce Th-1 type cytokines.[46] In murine models TRAC were found to be more effective in the reduction of metastases than a similar number of adoptively transferred LAK cells.[47] Clinical trials in advanced cancer patients have been reported.[48,49]

Anti-CD3/Anti-CD28 Coactivated T Cells (COACTS)

While cross-linking of the TCR with anti-CD3 may trigger a stimulatory signaling cascade, other signals are likely needed for optimal activation and avoidance of anergy. These co-stimulatory signals are provided by interaction of the CD28 receptor on T cells by anti-CD28 mAb. Co-stimulation of T-cells lead to enhanced proliferation and stabilization of mRNA for a variety of Th-1 cytokines; enhanced chemokine production[50] and improved resistance to apoptosis.[51] A Phase I trial in patients with refractory cancers showed COACTS to be a feasible and safe approach, and induced immune modulation.[52]

The efficacy of adoptive immunotherapy is dependant on T cells as effector cells. There is growing evidence however of T-cell immune dysfunction associated with a host afflicted with RCC. These include increased T cell sensitivity to tumor induced apoptosis, tumor induced suppression of NFκB related signal transduction pathways,[53,54] and dysfunction in IL-2 production and IL-2 receptor signaling.[55] Adoptive immunotherapy is also limited by the difficulty in isolating and amplifying tumor reactive T-cell clones. Tetramer assays of MHC class I have facilitated the characterization of CD8+ T cells specific for TAA.[56,57] A technique to enrich tumor specific T cell populations for adoptive immunotherapy by their secretion of IFN-γ in response to tumor stimulation has also been described.[58] When adoptively transferred to mice these cells demonstrated potent anti-tumor reactivity. Hopefully this and similar knowledge will aid in the development of improved immune based therapeutic strategies.

VACCINE THERAPIES

The goal of many immunotherapy strategies is to generate tumor specific cytotoxic T lymphocytes (CTL), and T helper cells. Eukaryotic cells are constantly expressing thousands of proteins which have been degraded intracellularly in proteosomes into peptide sequences, enter the endoplasmic reticulum and are then shuttled to the cell surface. The demonstration that tumors can express common peptide antigenic determinants that can be recognized by MHC restricted CTL has led to efforts aimed at identifying these tumor associated antigens (TAA).

Tumor cells evade cellular immune surveillance and destruction by a few key mechanisms. They alter, down regulate, or ineffectively display their TAA. The tumor micro-environment itself is repulsive to cell based immunity via tumor derived immunosuppressive cytokines. Thus, tumor cells are not efficient APC and for the most part fail to elicit an adequate immune response. Many ongoing vaccine trials in RCC and other cancers are centered on the use of DC.

Dendritic cells are often referred to as "the most potent APC." In order for a cell to be an efficient APC, it must take up soluble Ag, process and present Ag in a way that is stimulatory to T cells, ie. in the context of MHC molecules, express co-stimulatory molecules and produce immunostimulatory cytokines in order to engage and activate T-cells. Human DC reside in normal tissues, blood and lymphoid organs in trace populations. Tissue DC are termed immature due to their diminished capacity to stimulate T-cells, but are quite efficient at capturing Ag.[59] After Ag capture, DC then migrate to lymphoid tissue where they mature and upregulate their ability to present Ag and stimulate T-cells.[60] Our UCLA Kidney Cancer Program has performed in vitro studies characterizing DC obtained specifically from patients with RCC.[61] Using common cytokine based culture techniques (GM-CSF, IL-4 plus 10% autologous serum), DC can be consistently isolated and expanded from the PBL of patients with mRCC. Other studies confirm these findings of the ability to consistently generate functional DC from patients with RCC.[62] At UCLA, we have also demonstrated via a novel phase I dose escalation trial, that DC can be generated in vivo by administering GM-CSF plus IL-4 subcutaneously to patients with advanced cancers (including subjects with RCC).[63] These patients show minimally detectable DC at baseline, and have a marked increase in functional circulating DC after 7–14 days of combined cytokine administration.

Dendritic cells can be differentiated and expanded by ex-vivo or in-vivo cytokine exposure, loaded with TAA and used to induce a specific anti-tumor response. The various forms of antigens used to load DC include: peptide specific TAA,[64,65] tumor lysates[66,67] total RNA,[68] adenovirus transfected TAA[69] and apoptotic tumor cells.[70]

Dendritic Cell Based Clinical Trials In Renal Cell Carcinoma

At UCLA, we have completed a pilot trial of DC differentiated from PBL, loaded with TuLy obtained from the primary RCC.[67] We consistently cultured these DC for 3 consecutive weekly intradermal vaccine applications and did not observed any dose limiting toxicities. One subject showed in vitro evidence of enhanced anti-tumor immunity with upregulation of Th-1 cytokine production from PBL and enhanced cytotoxicity against autologous tumor. This subject sustained a short lived partial response, then developed brain metastases.

A similar study from Austria used cytokine generated DC loaded with TuLy plus Keyhole Limpet Hemacyanin (KLH) for intravenous application.[66] Again the vaccine was well tolerated with evidence of in vitro immune response to KLH and lysate. One of 5 subjects showed evidence of a partial clinical response.

Another novel approach to DC-based therapy is to fuse autologous tumor cells with either autologous or allogeneic DC. Allogeneic DC are used to recruit allo-reactive helper T-cells, possibly augmenting the immune response. Thus far, a tumor cell-DC hybrid vaccination has demonstrated remarkable clinical response in patients with RCC.[71] To prepare this vaccine, allogeneic cytokine derived DC plus autolo-gous tumor cells are hybridized using an "electrofusion" process. 17 subjects were vaccinated subcutaneously with a booster vaccine given after 6 weeks. All subjects without disease progression received further boosters every 3 months. Interestingly a different allogeneic DC donor was used to prepare each vaccine. There were 4 complete and 2 partial responses observed (mean follow up time of 13 months), with mild to moderate toxicity (fevers, tumor pain) and no evidence of auto-immune reaction. All subjects with objective response demonstrated a positive DTH reaction to autologous tumor. Importantly, confirmatory trials using fusions of allo-geneic DC with autologous tumor are now accruing.

The methods used to fuse DC to tumor cells include electrofusion as the above trial[71] and an alternative method uses polyethylene glycol (PEG) fusion. There is a trial accruing subjects with advanced RCC utilizing DC, PEG fused with tumor cells all in an autologous system.[72] Regardless of the fusion method, the theoretical advantage of tumor cell-DC hybrids as vaccines is the processing and presentation of tumor specific antigens along with MHC, co-stimulatory and other molecules provided by the DC and so important to inducing a CTL response against tumor antigens.

Tumor Associated Antigen Vaccines for RCC

The above mentioned clinical trials of DC based vaccines in mRCC rely on lysates or whole tumor cells. This is an important difference between vaccine development in RCC vs other cancers in which defined TAA have been elucidated. G250 has been identified and cloned and is the first widely expressed RCC TAA that con-tains both an HLA-A2 restricted CTL epitope and an HLA-DR restricted CD4+ T helper epitope.[73–75] Monoclonal Ab-G250 reacts with >75% of primary and mRCC while little to no cross reactivity exists with normal kidney.[76] These char-acteristics strongly suggest that G250 recognizes an RCC-TAA, and is potentially an attractive therapeutic target. This RCC-associated transmembrane protein, has been proven to be identical to MN/CA-IX, a cell adhesion molecule that was first identified in cervical cancer and that contains carbonic anhydrase activity.[77,78] In an attempt at improving DC vaccine potency in the treatment of RCC, investigators at UCLA recently constructed a chimeric protein consisting of G250 and GM-CSF.[79] The fusion protein maintains its GM-CSF biological activity and together with IL-4 is capable of differentiating potent DC capable of inducing CTL.

Identification of RCC-TAA will lead to important therapeutic advances in the treatment of RCC. Another method of circumventing the need for the identification of specific TAA are by using vaccines comprised of heat shock proteins (HSP). Heat shock proteins function as molecular chaperones, assisting the correct folding of polypepetides and assisting intracellular transport. They associate with a broad range of peptides derived from intracellular protein degradation including antigenic peptides produced in tumor cells. They interact with APC via a receptor leading to the secretion of pro-inflammatory cytokines and mediate maturation of DC.[80] Two clinical trials have demonstrated efficacy of a HSP vaccines in mRCC including objective responses, and prolonged disease stabilization.[81,82] A pivotal, 500 subject phase III trial of adjuvant HSP vaccine (Oncophage-Antigenic, inc.) in high risk RCC is underway.

GENE THERAPIES

Progress in the understanding of the genetic changes that are associated with the development of cancer, combined with a better understanding of the molecular basis of tumor immunity have lead to a new generation of genetic based therapies for RCC. Gene therapy usually involves the transfer of a functioning gene into a cell to correct an inborn genetic error, replace a defective/mutant gene, or to provide a new function to the cell. Commonly a gene is packaged into a vector that serves to transport the DNA of interest across the cell membrane. Most commonly, viruses such as adenovirus, vaccinia and retrovirus are used. Each has its own advantages and disadvantages that are exploited by the investigators needs. In fact, much research is centered on improving viral vectors including vectors that contain less viral genomic DNA, allowing for larger therapeutic DNA sequence insertions; and are less immunogenic, allowing for multiple vaccine administrations without the generation of neutralizing anti-viral antibodies. Other methods for incorporating genes into cells include physical methods such as the gene gun that produces high levels of gene expression without the use of a viral agent. Likewise, cationic lipsomes can also be used to "package" plasmid DNA for delivery into the cell via fusion with the membrane.

Currently the gene therapy of RCC has been in the form of transfer of genes into T lymphocytes to study their patterns of tumor localization "trafficking", or to increase their effectiveness as adoptive immunotherapy. The second category involves the introduction of genes into tumors to increase their immunogenicity and lastly preliminary attempts have been made at gene replacement therapy.

T-Lymphocyte Based Gene Therapy

Lymphocytes have attributes that make them attractive as a vehicle for delivery of a beneficial molecule to a targeted site. It is possible to expand them by many orders of magnitude in vitro in response to IL-2 or antigen or both. The use of IL-2 in vivo can lead to further proliferation of transfected cells and to prolonged cell survival. Cytokine gene transduced TIL can be theoretically used to deliver/produce high concentrations of cytokines locally at the tumor environment. This can serve to decrease systemic cytokine side effects and possibly increase efficacy. A phase I study of IL-2 transduced NK cells showed feasibility of this approach, lack of major toxicity, evidence of immune modulation and interesting clinical response.[83] These cells were able to proliferate in the absence of exogenous IL-2 and able to grow in an autocrine fashion. The responsiveness of RCC to adoptive immunotherapy makes it an ideal tumor type to utilize this cell based gene therapy.

Alternatively, gene therapy techniques can be used in the preparation of TIL for adoptive immunotherapy. Investigators at UCLA have propagated TIL in vitro in the presence of a tumor cell line infected with the IL-2 gene (RCC-Ad-IL-2).[84] Compared to standard TIL growth conditions in exogenous IL-2 alone, TIL grown in the presence of RCC-Ad-IL-2 were more immunologicaly potent. This work has implications for adoptive immunotherapy trials.

Labeling a cell with a marker gene allows for it's tracking in the body after infusion. Two clinical trials used genetically marked TIL to explore trafficking patterns after infusion.[85,86] Interestingly, neither study demonstrated selective homing/accumulation of TIL at the tumor site over other tissues tested. These labelling studies did however further demonstrate that a gene could be inserted and expressed in TIL, that went on to have long-term survival in the circulation.

Tumor Vaccines

Another category in the gene therapy of cancer is in the construction of tumor vaccines. This involves the transfection of tumor cell lines with genes that render the tumor more immunogenic. For example, an attempt can be made to convert the tumor cell into a better APC by restoring presentation of MHC molecules or co-stimulatory molecules. Alternatively, tumor cell transfection and subsequent expression of cytokine genes such as IL-2, IL-12, and GM-CSF can lead to attraction and stimulation of lymphocytes and APC. Successful cytokine gene transfer into RCC cell lines has been accomplished, resulting in potent antitumor activity when administered subcutaneously in murine models.[87] These studies clearly demonstrate that systemic tumor regression can result from a cytokine mediated local immune response.

Preclinical studies by investigators at Johns Hopkins have demonstrated that immunization with GM-CSF transduced tumors produced the greatest degree of systemic immunity likely due to induction of APC.[87] The phase I human gene therapy trial using cultured, irradiated autologous RCC cells either unmodified or genetically modified ex-vivo to secrete GM-CSF in patients with mRCC has been reported.[88] No significant toxicities were seen. Biopsies of the intradermal site of vaccine injection revealed APC and T-cell infiltrates in addition to eosinophils and neutrophils. One objective partial response was observed in a patient who also had the largest DTH conversion to unpassaged autologous tumor. Another group in Japan has made attempts to improve upon this vaccine strategy by using partially HLA matched allogeneic tumor cells, and/or varying the schedule of vaccinations.[89]

Investigators at Memorial Sloan Kettering Cancer Center have treated 12 patients with mRCC with a tumor vaccine consisting of an irradiated HLA A2+ allogeneic renal cell carcinoma cell line transfected with the IL-2 gene.[90] There were no toxicities greater than grade II, but there were also no objective responses seen. Pertaining to safety, there was no detection of the helper virus in any patient 1 week after vaccination.

Another strategy using B7-1 gene modified autologous tumor cells has been used in combination with systemic IL-2 in a phase I trial.[91] As anticipated, the toxicity was related to the IL-2. Interesting immunologic and clinical responses were observed, concluding that phase II trials are warranted.

Intratumoral Gene Therapy

Technology using liposomes to transfer genes into cells without the need for viral vectors has evolved into clinical trials in RCC. One trial involves the direct injection of a lipid formulated plasmid DNA encoding for the foreign class I MHC antigen, HLA B7 "Allovectin-7" (Genetic Therapy, Inc.) into accessible metastatic RCC lesions.[92] Fifteen HLA B7- patients were treated, without significant toxicity or objective responses. Detection of HLA-B7, mRNA and protein expression could be demonstrated in 8:14 tumor samples.

Similarly, trials using direct gene transfer of the IL-2/liposome complex "Leuvectin" (Vical, Inc.) into accessible metastatic RCC lesions indicate that Leuvectin is safe, is free of systemic toxicity, and has biologic activity.[93] Further phase II trials in RCC are planned.[94]

Corrective Gene Therapy

Since cancers represent an aberration in the regulation, transcription or translation of genes, attempts to treat resulting malignancy by correcting these derangements is appealing. Using a liposomal vehicle to deliver the VHL gene, Chen, et al transfected RCC cell lines that lacked expression of the normal VHL gene.[95] The expression of the wild type VHL gene resulted in growth suppression of the tumor cell line. This study implies that VHL protein is important in controlling the proliferation of kidney cells and that gene replacement therapy may have a role in the treatment of RCC.

Another potential target for gene replacement therapy is the p53 tumor suppressor gene which is commonly lost or mutated in RCC.[96] The in vitro liposomal delivery of wild type p53 into a RCC cell line resulted in decreased growth of tumor cells in culture. Using a mouse-xenograft model, the transfection of p53 resulted in a decrease in the number of pulmonary metastases.

CONCLUSION

Cell, vaccine and gene therapies for RCC are developing at an ever faster pace. Table 1 is a summary of current therapeutics that have been discussed in this chapter and have been applied in human clinical trials. Each of these treatment modalities has demonstrated that tumor regression can be achieved solely via manipulation of

Table 1. Classification of cell, gene and vaccine therapies of RCC.

Adoptive Immunotherapy

Lymphocyte Activated Killer Cells: non-MHC restricted cytotoxicity. Randomized trial evidence available.

Tumor Infiltrating Lymphocytes: MHC/non-MHC restricted cytotoxicity. Randomized trial evidence available.

Autolymphocyte Therapy: Activated memory cells. Randomized trial evidence available.

Vaccine Primed Lymph Node Cells   Phase I and II trial evidence.

T Cell Receptor Activated T Cells

Coactivated T Cells

Gene Therapy

Lymphocyte Based: TIL, NK cells transfected with cytokine genes. Phase I evidence.

Tumor Vaccines: Tumor cells transfected with cytokine genes, costimulatory molecules, MHC antigens. Phase I/II trial evidence.

Corrective Gene Therapy: Tumor cells transfected with tumor suppressor genes (VHL, p53). Clinical trials underway.

Vaccine Therapies

Dendritic Cell Based Therapies: DC loaded with tumor lysates, TAA. Fusions of tumor cells with DC. Phase I evidence.

Heat Shock Protein vaccine: Phase III trial acruing.

Table 2. Current clinical trials using tumor vaccines or adoptive immunotherapy for mRCC.

Adoptive Immunotherapy

Phase I/II Study of Interleukin-12-Primed Activated T Cells in Combination With Fluorouracil, Sargramostim (GM-CSF), and Pegylated Interferon alfa-2b in Patients With Metastatic Renal Cell or Colorectal Carcinoma. (St Lukes Medical Center, Milwaukee WI)

Phase II Study of Adjuvant Autologous Lymphocyte Therapy in Patients With Nonmetastatic Renal Cell Carcinoma. (St Lukes Medical Center, Milwaukee WI)

Tumor Vaccines/gene therapy

Phase III Randomized Study of Surgery and Adjuvant Autologous gp96 Heat Shock Protein-Peptide Complex Following Surgical Resection in Patients With Locally Advanced Renal Cell Carcinoma At High Risk For Recurrence. (Antigenics Inc. Wodburn MA)

Phase I/II Study of Immunization With In Vitro-Treated Autologous Tumor Cells and Dendritic Cells With Sargramostim (GM-CSF) in Patients With Stage III or IV or Recurrent Renal Cell Cancer (Hoag Memorial Hospital, Newport Beach CA)

Phase II Study of B7-1 Gene-Modified Autologous Tumor Cell Vaccine and Interleukin-2 in Patients With Stage IV Renal Cell Carcinoma. (H. Lee Moffitt Cancer Center, Tampa FL)

Phase II Study of Vaccine Therapy With Tumor-Specific Mutated von Hippel-Lindau Peptides in Patients With Renal Cell Carcinoma. (Warren Grant Magnusen Clinical Center, Bethesda MD)

Phase II Pilot Study of Cyclophosphamide and Active Intralymphatic Immunotherapy With a Vaccine Containing Interferon alfa or Interferon gamma-Treated Tumor Cells Followed by Sargramostim (GM-CSF) in Patients With Advanced Cancers. (St Vincents Medical Center, Los Angeles CA)

Source: National Cancer Institute—PDQ (Fall 2002).

the immune system or of the molecular pathways involved in tumor growth. Unfortunately, at present only a minority of patients have benefited from these treatment modalities. Progress continues to be made in the understanding of the genetic and cellular mechanisms that underlie tumorigenesis. This will feed improved translational applications of these therapies. Table 2 is a summary of current listings of cell, gene and vaccine based therapies for mRCC as found in the NCI-PDQ. This listing gives insight into the most recent directions of clinical investigations in the applications of these therapies. Continuing in vitro and clinical research in this area will no doubt yield effective treatments for mRCC.

REFERENCES

1. Boon T, Coulie P, Marchand M, Weynants P, Wolfel P, Brichard V. Genes coding for tumor rejection agents: perspectives for specific immunotherapy. In: DeVita VT, Hellman S, Rosenberg SA, eds. Biologic therapy of cancer updates. Philadelphia: JB Lippincott, 1994;14:2.
2. Morgan DA, Ruscetti FW, Gallo R. Selective in vitro growth of T lymphocytes from normal human bone marrows. Science 1976;193:1007.
3. Ruscetti FW, Morgan DA, Gallo RC. Functional and morphologic characterization of human T cells continuously grown in vitro. J Immunol 1977;119:131.
4. Linsley PS, Clark EA, Ledbetter JA. T-cell antigen CD28 mediates adhesion with B cells by interacting with activation antigen B7/BB-1. Proc Natl Acad Sci USA 1990;238:75.
5. Cheever MA, Greenberg PD, Fefer A, et al. Augmentation of the anti-tumor therapeutic efficacy of long-term cultured lymphocytes by in vivo administration of purified interleukin 2. J Exp Med 1982;155:968.
6. Donohue JH, Rosenstein M, Chang AE, et al. The systemic administration of purified interleukin 2 enhances the ability of sensitized murine lymphocytes to cure a disseminated syngeneic lymphoma. J Immunol 1984;132:2123.
7. Chever MA, Greenberg PD, Irle C, et al. Interleukin 2 administered in vivo induces the growth of cultured T cells in vivo. J Immunol 1984;132:2259.
8. Grimm EA, Mazumder A, Zhang HZ, et al. Lymphokine-activated killer cell phenomenon. Lysis of natural killer-resistant fresh solid tumor cells by interleukin-2 activated autologous human peripheral blood lymphocytes. J Exp Med 1982;155:1823.
9. Grimm EA, Robb J, Roth JA, et al. Lymphokine-activated killer cell phenomenon III. Evidence that IL-2 is sufficient for direct activation of peripheral blood lymphocytes into lymphokine-activated killer cells. J Exp Med 1983;158:1356.
10. Herberman RB, Hiserodt JC, Vujanovic NK, et al. Lymphokine-activated killer cell activity: characteristics of effector cells and progenitor cells in blood and spleen. Immunol Today 1987;8:178.
11. Lafreniere R, Rosenberg SA. Adoptive immunotherapy of murine hepatic metastases with lymphokine-activated killer cells and recombinant interleukin 2 can mediate the regression of both immunogenic and nonimmunogenic sarcomas and an adenocarcinoma. J Immunol 1985;135:4273.
12. Papa MZ, Mule JJ, Rosenberg SA. Antitumor efficacy of lymphokine-activated killer cells and recombinant interleukin 2 in vivo: successful immunotherapy of established pulmonary metastases from weakly immunogenic and nonimmunogenic tumors of three distinct histological types. Cancer Res 1986;46:4973.
13. Rosenberg SA. Immunotherapy of cancer by systemic administration of lymphoid cells plus interleukin 2. J Biol Response Mod 1984;3:501.
14. Mazumder A, Eberlein TJ, Grimm EA, et al. Phase I study of the adoptive immunotherapy of human cancer with lectin-activated autologous mononuclear cells. Cancer 1984;53:896.
15. Rosenberg SA, Lotze MT, Muul LM, et al. Observations on the systemic administration of autologous lymphokine-activated killer cells and recombinant interleukin 2 to patients with metastatic cancer. N Engl J Med 1985;313:1485.
16. Foon KA, Walther PJ, Bernstein ZP, et al. Renal cell carcinoma treated with continuous infusion interleukin-2 with ex vivo activated killer cells. J Immunother 1992;11:184.
17. Rosenberg SA. Karnofsky Memorial Lecture: the immunotherapy and gene therapy of cancer. J Clin Oncol 1992;10:180.
18. Thompson JA, Shulman KL, Benyunes MC, et al. Prolonged continuous intravenous infusion interleukin-2 and lymphokine-activated killer cell therapy for metastatic renal cell carcinoma. J Clin Oncol 1992;10:960.
19. Rosenberg SA, Lotze MT, Yang JC, et al. Prospective randomized trial of high dose interleukin 2 alone or in conjunction with lymphokine-activated killer cells for the treatment of patients with advanced cancers. J Natl Cancer Inst 1993;85:622.

20. McCabe M, Stablein D, Hawkins MJ. The modified Group C experience—phase III randomized trials of IL-2 versus IL-2/LAK in advanced renal cell cancer and advanced melanoma [abstract 714]. Proc Am Soc Oncol 1991;10:213.
21. Bajorin D, Sell KW, Richards JM, et al. A randomized trial of interleukin-2 plus lymphokine-activated killer cells versus interleukin-2 alone in renal cell carcinoma [abstract 1106]. Proc Am Assoc Cancer Res 1990;31:A1106.
22. Yron I, Wood TA, Speiss P, et al. In vitro growth of murine T cells V. The isolation and growth of lymphoid cells infiltrating syngeneic solid tumors. J Immunol 1980;125:238.
23. Yannelli JR, Hyatt C, McConnell S, et al. Growth of tumor-infiltrating lymphocytes from human solid cancers: Summary of a 5-year experience. Int J Cancer 1996;65:413–421.
24. Finke JH, Rayman P, Hart L, et al. Characterization of tumor infiltrating lymphocyte subsets from human renal cell carcinoma: specific reactivity defined by cytotoxicity, interferon gamma secretion, and proliferation. J Immunother 1994;15:91.
25. Rosenberg SA, Speiss PJ, Lafreniere R. A new approach to the adoptive immunotherapy of cancer with tumor-infiltrating lymphocytes. Science 1986;233:1318.
26. Belldegrun A, Pierce WC, Kaboo R, et al. Interferon alpha-primed tumor-infiltrating lymphocytes combined with interleukin 2 and interferon alpha as a therapy for metastatic renal cell carcinoma. J Urol 1993;150:1384.
27. Topalian SL, Solomon D, Frederick P, et al. Immunotherapy of patients with advanced cancer using tumor-infiltrating lymphocytes and recombinant interleukin 2: a pilot study. J Clin Oncol 1988; 6:839.
28. Dillman RO, Church C, Oldham RK, et al. A randomized phase II trial of continuous infusion interleukin 2 in 788 patients with cancer. The National Biotherapy Study Group Experience. Cancer 1993;71:2358.
29. Kradin RL, Lazarus DS, Dubinett SM, et al. Tumour-infiltrating lymphocytes and interleukin 2 in treatment of advanced cancer. Lancet 1989;1:577.
30. Bukowski RM, Sharfman W, Murthy S, et al. Clinical results and characterization of tumor-infiltrating lymphocytes with or without recombinant interleukin 2 in human metastatic renal cell carcinoma. Cancer Res 1991;51:4199.
31. Olencki T, Finke J, Lorenzi V, et al. Adoptive immunotherapy (AIT) for renal cell carcinoma (RCC) tumor infiltrating lymhocytes (TILs) cultured in vitro with rIL-2, rhIL-4, and autologous tumor: a phase II trial [Abstract 762]. Proc Am Soc Clin Oncol 1994;13:244.
32. Figlin RA, Pierce WC, Kaboo R, et al. Treatment of metastatic renal cell carcinoma with nephrectomy, interleukin-2 and cytokine-primed or CD8(+) selected tumor infiltrating lymphocytes from primary tumor. J Urol 1997;158:740–745.
33. Goedegebuure PS, Douville LM, Li H, et al. Adoptive Immunotherapy with tumor-infiltrating lymphoctes and interleukin-2 in patients with metastatic malignant melanoma and renal cell carcinoma: a pilot study. J Clin Oncol 1995;13:1939–1949.
34. Figlin RA, Thompson JA, Bukowski MD, et al. A multi-center, randomized, phase III trial of CD8+ tumor-infiltrating lymphocytes in combination with recombinant interleukin-2 in metastatic renal cell carcinoma. J Clin Oncol 1999;17(8):251–259.
35. Sawczuk IS. Autolymphocyte therapy in the treatment of metastatic renal cell carcinoma. Urol Clin North Am 1993;20:297–301.
36. Osband ME, Lavin PT, Babayan RK, et al. Effect of autolymphocyte therapy on survival and quality of life in patients with metastatic renal cell carcinoma. Lancet 1990;335:994–998.
37. Lavin PT, Maar R, Franklin M, et al. Autolymphocyte therapy for metastatic renal cell carcinoma: initial clinical results from 335 patients treated in a multisite clinical practice. Transplant Proc 1992;24:3057–3062.
38. Graham S, Babayan RK, Lamm DL, et al. The use of ex vivo activated memory T cells (autolymphocyte therapy) in the treatment of metastatic renal cell carcinoma: final results from a randomized controlled multisite study. Semin Urol 1993;11:27–34.
39. Sawczuk IS, Graham SD Jr, Miesowicz F and the ALT Adjuvant Study Group, Cellcor Inc, Newton MA, Emory Clinic, Atlanta GA, and Columbia University, NY, NY. Randomized, controlled trial of adjuvant therapy with ex vivo activated T cells (ALT) in $T_{1-3a,b,c}$ or $T_4N_+M_0$ renal cell carcinoma. Proc Am Soc Clin Oncol 1997;16:326a.
40. Chang AE, Shu S. Immunotherapy with sensitized lymphocytes. Cancer Invest 1992;10(5):357–369.
41. Aruga A, Aruga B, Cameron MJ, et al. Different cytokine profiles released by CD4 and CD8 tumor draining lymph node cells involved in mediating tumor regression. J Leuk Biol 1997;61:1–10.

42. Chang AE, Aruga A, Cameron MJ, et al. Adoptive immunotherapy with vaccine-primed lymph node cells secondarily activated with anti-CD3 and IL-2. J Clin Oncol 1997;15(2):796–807.
43. Chang 2002.
44. Tanigawa K, Takeshita S, Eickhoff GA, et al. Antitumor reactivity of lymph node cells primed in vivo with dendritic cell based vaccines. J Immunother 2001;24(6):493–501.
45. Li Q, Yu B, Grover AC, et al. Therapeutic effects of tumor reactive CD4+ cells generated from tumor-primed lymph nodes using anti-CD3/anti-CD28 monoclonal antibodies. J Immunother. 2002;25(4):304–313.
46. Sosman JA, Oettle KR, Hank JA, et al. Specific recognition of human leukemic cells by allogeneic T cell lines. Transplantation 1989;48:486–495.
47. Loeffler CM, Platt JL, Anderson PM, et al. Antitumor effects of interleukin-2, liposomes and anti-CD3-stimulated T-cells against murine MCA 38 hepatic metastasis. Cancer Res 1991;51:2127–2132.
48. Curti BC, Longo DJ, Ochoa AC, et al. Treatment of cancer patients with ex vivo anti-CD-3 activated killer cells and interleukin-2. J Clin Oncol 1993;11:653–660.
49. Curti BC, Ochoa AC, Powers CG, et al. Phase I trial of anti-CD-3 stimulated CD4+ T-cells, infusional interleukin-2 and cyclophosphamide inpatients with advanced cancer. J Clin Oncol 1998;16:2752–2760.
50. Thompson CB, Lindsten T, Ledbetter JA, et al. CD 28 activation pathway regulates the production of multiple T-cells derived lymphokines/cytokines. Proc Natl Acad Sci USA 1989;86:1333–1337.
51. Boise LH, Noel PJ, Thompson CS. CD28 and apoptosis. Curr Opin Immunol 1995;7:620–625.
52. Lum LG, LeFever AV, Treisman JS, et al. Immune modulation in cancer pts after adoptive transfer of anti-CD3/anti-CD28-costimulated T cells-phase I clinical trial. J Immunother 2001;5:408–419.
53. Finke JH, Rayman P, George R, et al. Tumor-induced sensitivity to apoptosis in T cells from patients with renal cell carcinoma: role of nuclear factor kappaB suppression. Clin Cancer Res. 2001;7(3 suppl):940s–946s.
54. Ng CS, Novick AC, Tannenbaum SC, et al. Mechanisms of immune evasion by renal cell carcinoma: tumor induced T-Lymphocyte apoptosis and NFκB suppression. Urology 2002;59(1):9–14.
55. Rayman P, Uzzo RG, Kolenko V, et al. Tumor-induced dysfunction in interleukin-2 production and interleukin-2 receptor signaling: a mechanism of immune escape. Cancer J Sci Am 2000;6(suppl 1):S81–S97.
56. Altman JD, et al. Phenotypic analysis of antigen-specific T-lymphocytes. Science 1996;274:94–95.
57. Romero P, et al. Ex-vivo stainng of metastatic lymph nodes by class I major histocompatability complex tetramers reveals high numbers of antigen experienced tumor-specific cytolytic T lymphocytes. J Exp Med 1998;188:1641–1650.
58. Becker C, Pohla H, Frankenberger B, et al. Adoptive tumor therapy with T lymphocytes enriched through an IFN-g capture assay. Nature Med 2001;7(4):1159–1162.
59. Steinman RM. The dendritic cell system and its role in immunogenicity. Ann Rev Immunol 1991;9:271–297.
60. Inaba k, Witmer-Pack M, Inaba M, et al. The tissue distribution of the B7–2 costimulator in mice: abundant expression on dendritic cells in situ and during maturation in vitro. J Exp Med 1994; 180:1849–1860.
61. Mulders P, Tso CL, Gitlitz B, et al. Presentation of renal tumor antigens by human dendritic cells activates tumor infiltrating lymphocytes against autologous tumor: Implications for live kidney cancer Vaccines. Clin Cancer Res 1999;5:445–454.
62. Radmayr C, Bock G, Hobisch A, et al. Dendritic antigen-presenting cells from the peripheral blood of renal-cell carcinoma patients. Int J Cancer 1995;63:627–632.
63. Roth MD, Gitlitz BJ, Kiertscher SM, et al. GM-CSF and interleukin-4 enhance the number and antigen presenting activity of circulating CD14+ and CD83+ cells in cancer patients. Cancer Res 2000;60(7):1934–1941.
64. Nestle FO, Alijagic S, Gilliet M, et al. Vaccination of Melanoma Patients with peptide- or Tumor Lysate-Pulsed Dendritic Cells, Nature Med 1998;4:328.
65. Murphy G, Tjoa B, Ragde H, et al. A Phase I Clinical Trial: T-Cell Therapy for Prostate Cancer Using Autologous Dendritic Cells Pulsed with HLA-A0201-Specific Peptides from Prostate-Specific Membrane Antigen. Prostate 1996;29:371.
66. Holtl L, Rieser C, Papesh C, et al. Cellular and Humoral Immune Responses in Patients with Metastatic Renal Cell Carcinoma After Vaccination with Antigen Pulsed Dendritic Cells. J of Urology 1999;161:777–782.
67. Gitlitz BJ, Belldegrun A, Zisman A, et al. A Pilot Trial of Tumor Lysate-Loaded Dendritic Cells for the Treatment of Metastatic Renal Cell Carcinoma. J. Immunother. In Press 2003.

68. Nair SK, Morse m, Boczkowski D, et al. Induction of tumor-specific cytotoxic T lymphocytes in cancer patients by autologous tumor RNA-transfected dendritic cells. Ann Surg 2002;235(4): 540–549.

69. Haluska F, Linette GP, Jonasch E, et al. Immunologic gene therapy of melanoma: Phase I study of therapy with autologous dendritic cells transduced with recombinant adenovirus encoding melanoma antigens. Proc AM Soc Clin Oncol (Abstr) #19, pg 1777, 2000.

70. Duclouet B, Lustgarten J, Shawler D, et al. Dendritic cells pulsed with apoptotic tumor cells induce potent antitumor immune response in vivo and in vivo. Proc AM Soc Clin Oncol (Abstr) # pg 1816, 2000.

71. Kugler A, Gernot S, Walden P, et al. Regression of human metastatic renal cell carcinoma after vaccination with tumor cell-dendritic cell hybrids. Nat Med 2000;6(3):332–336.

72. Avigan D, Atkins M, Gong J, et al. DC-tumor fusions as immunotherapy: A phase I clinical trial in patients with metastatic renal cancer. 16th Annual Meeting of Society for Biological Therapy, 2001.

73. Grabmaier K, Vissers JL, De Weijert MC, Oosterwijk-Wakka JC, Van Bokhoven A, Brakenhoff RH, Noessner E, Mulders PA, Merkx G, Figdor CG, Adema GJ, Oosterwijk E. Molecular cloning and immunogenicity of renal cell carcinoma-associated antigen G250. Int J Cancer 2000;85:865–870.

74. Vissers JL, De Vries IJ, Schreurs MW, Engelen LP, Oosterwijk E, Figdor CG, Adema GJ. The renal cell carcinoma-associated antigen G250 encodes a human leukocyte antigen (HLA)-A2.1-restricted epitope recognized by cytotoxic T lymphocytes. Cancer Res 1999;59:5554–5559.

75. Vissers JL, De Vries IJ, Engelen LP, et al. Renal cell carcinoma-associated antigen G250 encodes a naturally processed epitope presented by human leukocyte antigen-DR molecules to CD4+ lymphocytes. Int J Cancer 2002;100:441–444.

76. Steffens MG, Boerman OC, Oosterwijk-Wakka JC, et al. Targeting of renal cell carcinoma with iodine-131-labeled chimeric monoclonal antibody G250. J Clin Oncol 1997;15:1529–1537.

77. Opavsky R, Pastoreková S, Zelník V, Gibadulinová A, Stanbridge EJ, Závada J, Kettmann R, Pastorek J. Human MN/CA9 gene, a novel member of the carbonic anhydrase family: structure and exon to protein domain relationships. Genomics 1996;33:480–487.

78. Závada J, Závadová Z, Pastorek J, Biesová Z, Jezek J, Velek J. Human tumour-associated cell adhesion protein MN/CA IX: identification of M75 epitope and of the region mediating cell adhesion. Br J Cancer 2000;82:1808–1813.

79. Tso CL, Zisman A, Pantuck A, et al. Induction of G250-targeted and T-cell-mediated antitumor activity against renal cell carcinoma using a chimeric fusion protein consisting of G250 and granulocyte/monocyte-colony stimulating factor. Cancer Res 2001;61(21):7925–7933.

80. Srivastava PK, Amato RJ. Heat shock proteins: the 'Swiss Army Knife' vaccines against cancers and infectious agents Vaccine 2002;19(17–19):2590–2597.

81. Amato RJ, Murray L, Wood LA, Savary C, Tomasovic S, Srivastava PK, Reitsma D. Active specific immunotherapy in patients with renal cell carcinoma (RCC) using autologous tumor derived heat shock protein-peptide complex-96 (HSPPC-96) vaccine. Proc Am Soc Clin Oncol, 1999.

82. Amato R, Murray L, Wood L, Savary C, Tomasovic S, Reitsma D. Active specific immunotherapy in patients with renal cell carcinoma (RCC) using autologous tumor derived heat shock protein-peptide complex-96 (HSPP-96) vaccine. Proc Am Soc Clin Oncol, 2000.

83. Schmid-Wolf IG, Finke S, Trojaneck B, et al. Phase I clinical study applying autologous immunologicaly effector cells transfected with the Interleukin-2 gene in patients with metastatic renal cell cancer, colorectal cancer and lymphoma. Br J Cancer 1999;81:1009–1016.

84. Mulders P, Tso CL, Pang S, et al. Adenovirus-mediated interleukin-2 production by tumors induces growth of cytotoxic tumor-infiltrating lymphocytes against human renal cell carcinoma. J Immunother 1998;21:170–180.

85. Merrouche Y, Negrier S, Bain C, et al. Clinical application of retroviral gene transfer in oncology: Results of a French study with tumor-infiltrating lymphocytes transduced with the gene of resistance to neomycin. J Clin Oncol 1995;13:410–418.

86. Economou JS, Belldegrun AS, Glaspy J, et al. In vivo trafficking of adoptively transferred interleukin-2 expanded tumor-infiltrating lymphocytes and peripheral blood lymphocytes. Results of a double gene marking trial. J Clin Invest 1996;97:515–521.

87. Dranoff G, Jaffee EM, Lazenby A, et al. Vaccination with irradiated tumor cells engineered to secrete murine GM-CSF stimulates potent, specific and long lasting anti-tumor immunity. Proc Natl Acad Sci USA 1993;90:3539.

88. Simons JW, Jaffee EM, Weber C, et al. Bioactivity of autologous irradiated renal cell carcinoma vaccines generated by ex vivo granulocyte-macrophage colony stimulating factor gene transfer. Cancer Res 1997;57:1537–1546.

89. Kawai K, Tani K, Asano S, Akaza H. Ex-vivo gene therapy using granulocyte-macrophage colony stimulating factor transduced tumor vaccines. Mol Urol 2000;4(2):43–46.
90. Meyers ML, Minasian L, Motzer RJ, et al. Immunization with HLA-A2 matched allogeneic tumor cells that secrete Interleukin-2 in patients with metastatic melanoma or metastatic renal cell carcinoma. Proc AM Soc Clin Oncol 1997;16:441a.
91. Antonia SJ, Seigne J, Diaz J, et al. Phase I trial of B7.1 (CD80_ gnen modified autologous tumor cell vaccine in combination with systemic Interleukin-2 in patients with metastatic renal cell carcinoma. J Urol 2002;167(5):1995–2000.
92. Rini BJ, Selk LM, Vogelzang NJ. Phase I study of direct intralesional gene transfer of HLA-B7 into metastatic renal cell carcinoma lesions. Clin Cancer Res 1999;5(10):2766.
93. Hoffman DM, Figlin RA. Intratumoral Interleukin-2 for renal cell carcinoma by direct gene transfer of a plasmid DNA/DMRIE/DOPE lipid complex. World J Urol 2000;18(2):152–156.
94. Kaushik A. Leuvectin Vical Inc. Curr Opin Investig Drugs 2001;2(7):976–981.
95. Chen F, Kishida T, Duh FM, et al. Suppression of growth of renal carcinoma cells by the von Hippel-Lindau tumor suppressor gene. Cancer Res 1995;55(21):4804.
96. Zhang XH, Takenaka I, Sato C, Sakamoto. p53 and HER 2/neu alterations in Renal cell carcinoma. Urology 1997 oct 50(4):636–642.

12. MONOCLONAL ANTIBODY THERAPY OF KIDNEY CANCER

EGBERT OOSTERWIJK, PH.D.[1], ADRIENNE BROUWERS, M.D.[2],
OTTO C. BOERMAN, PH.D.[2], STEVEN M. LARSON, M.D.[3],
LLOYD J. OLD, M.D.[4], PETER MULDERS, M.D.[1], AND
CHAITANYA R. DIVGI, M.D.[3]

[1]Department of Urology, University Medical Center Nijmegen, Nijmegen, The Netherlands, [2]Department of Nuclear Medicine, University Medical Center Nijmegen, Nijmegen, The Netherlands, [3]Nuclear Medicine Service, Department of Radiology, Memorial Sloan Kettering Cancer Center, New York, U.S.A., [4]Ludwig Institute for Cancer Research, New York, U.S.A.

INTRODUCTION

There is a clear need for effective treatment of metastasized Renal Cell Carcinoma (RCC): despite intensive efforts to develop an effective treatment, once RCC has metastasized, treatment options are very limited. This tumor is not radiosensitive, resistant to chemotherapy, and treatment with biological response modifiers (IL-2, IFN) leads to low response rates.

One of the hallmarks of successful cancer therapy is the selective destruction of malignant cells over non-malignant cells. Much of the success of chemotherapy is based on the high proliferation rate of particular tumors whereby drugs without any selectivity can still provide selective kill of the proliferative fraction of tumor cells. Clearly, this approach has the disadvantage of serious side effects, because normal cells that proliferate, e.g., progenitor cells in the bone marrow, are also destroyed. Current cancer chemotherapeutic drugs are neither specific, i.e., they do not act exclusively on the metabolic pathway of cancer cells, nor do they target exclusively to cancer cells. Additionally, for various tumors, including Renal Cell Carcinoma (RCC), effective chemotherapeutics are not available[1] because they display resistance against the drugs, e.g. by expression of multidrug resistance genes [26,32]which act as ATP-dependant efflux pumps to reduce the intracellular accumulation of anthracyclines, vanca alkloids, taxanes, epipodophyllotoxins, dactinomycin, and other natural products.

The development of highly selective agents such as monoclonal antibodies (mAbs) might provide new treatment modalities for this disease. Here we discuss general

R.A. Figlin (ed.). KIDNEY CANCER. Copyright © 2003. Kluwer Academic Publishers. Boston. All rights reserved.

issues related to mAb treatment, and discuss our current knowledge of the effect of mAb G250 for the treatment of metastatic RCC patients. This mAb recognizes a target molecule expressed on virtually all cells of all clear cell RCC, and as such may provide a valuable highly selective agents able to specifically attack RCC cells.

MONOCLONAL ANTIBODIES: A QUANTUM LEAP

In 1975 Kohler and Milstein[23] described the monoclonal antibody technology, a feat for which they were awarded the Nobel price. Conceptually, monoclonal antibodies (mAb) were of great interest, because it was foreseen that specific tumor cell kill might become feasible. Already in the early 1900 Ehrlich discussed the possibility of antibody-guided therapy by suggesting the existence of tumor specific antigens that could serve as target molecules.[10] Thus, mAb were quickly called "magic bullets".

The hybridoma technique made it possible to produce large quantities of antibody with predefined specificity, directed against a single antigenic determinant. In fact, the description of mAbs represented a quantum leap in the field of tumor immunology. For the first time, B-lymphocytes from immunized hosts could be immortalized by means of fusion with drug-selected non-immunoglobulin secretor murine myeloma cells, allowing perpetual propagation and selection for mAbs recognizing antigens of interest.

Theoretically, appropriate screening methods could lead to the identification of mAbs recognizing tumor-associated (TAA) or tumor-specific antigens (TSA). Before the description and implementation of the hybridoma technology, many investigators tried to isolate and define tumor-specific or tumor-associated molecules, e.g. upregulated molecules, with polyvalent antisera. The presence of cross-reactive antibodies in these polyvalent sera severely hampered the identification of TAA/TSA that might be used as potential therapeutic targets. In general, even extensive absorption of polyclonal antisera failed to render these sera tissue or tumor specific. Because tumors express many normal (tissue-specific) differentiation antigens, the immune reaction of the challenged animal will be overwhelmingly tuned to those immunogenic moieties, and this was not an unexpected finding. Additionally, the sought after tumor-associated antigens might be poorly immunogenic. The description of mAb technology fuelled hopes that appropriate TAA/TSA could be identified. The scientific and pharmaceutical community expected fast implementation of these potentially very selective reagents.

Obviously, because selective tumor cell kill is desirable, one of the pivotal aspects of mAb-guided therapy is the tissue and tumor specificity of the chosen target molecule. As suggested by Ehrlich, and agreed upon by most investigators, mAb-guided therapeutics or mAb treatment alone could lead to selective tumor cell destruction, provided that appropriate fine specificity exists. Despite this scientific consensus, several mAbs with poor tumor or tissue specificity, i.e., with extensive cross-reactivity with normal tissues, have been investigated in clinical trials. Additionally, in the majority of clinical investigations cases mAbs were tested in patients with extensive tumor burden.

Since little was know about mAb dosing and effects, the majority of clinical trials, mostly aimed at therapeutic intervention, were negative, i.e. no clinical responses were seen. Indeed, the poor clinical results resulted in a declined interest in these highly specific agents. With the realization that many factors, including cross-reactive tissues, tumor heterogeneity, and tumor burden, are important, carefully designed clinical trials have been performed. Treatment with radiolabeled mAbs as well as unmodified mAb in combination with chemotherapy has shown significant anti-tumor effects, particularly in haematopoietic malignancies. This has lead to the acceptance of several mAbs as therapeutic drug by the FDA.

ISSUES RELATED TO THE USE OF MONOCLONAL ANTIBODIES

The potential application of mAbs in the management of human carcinomas can be divided grossly in three areas: diagnosis, prognosis and treatment. Depending on the chosen application, different requirements need to be met. Although specificity is seen as the most important factor in deciding whether or not a particular mAb can be successfully employed, this is not necessarily true. E.g., prognostic mAb can be cross-reactive with many normal organ tissues, as long as it can still prognosticate a particular patient population. Specificity is certainly an important issue when clinical implementation is wanted, but many other factors influence possible success.

Specificity can be defined as tumor-specificity, i.e., no cross-reactivity with non-malignant tissues, or tumor-type specificity. The latter is less important than tumor-specificity when a mAb is intended for therapeutic use. As a general rule, little or no cross-reactivity with normal tissues is desirable: this will diminish possible side effects. Additionally, cross-reactive tissues may necessitate administration of large amounts of mAb to saturate these tissues. In this situation unwanted side effects can occur when unconjugated mAb or conjugated mAb in the form of an immunotoxins or as radiolabeled material is administered. Conversely, overexpression of tissue differentiation antigens can provide sufficient difference in mAb targeting levels, and normal tissue damage may be acceptable in selected cases.

Secondly, preferably all tumors of a particular tumor type should express the antigen, including metastatic lesions, with as little heterogeneity as possible. Unfortunately very few antigens with true tumor-specificity have been detected. Ironically, the most prominent examples of TSA are the so-called cancer-testis genes, initially identified through the pioneering work of the group of Boon in Brussels[6] through expansion of cytotoxic T cells (CTL), isolated from cancer patients. These antigens are expressed in various tumors, albeit in only 30–40% of cases, and in normal testicular tissue. These antigens might serve as appropriate CTL targets and possibly be utilized in mAb-guided therapy. Unfortunately, cancer-testis antigen expression is quite heterogeneous[20,21,31], which would hamper complete tumor destruction.

While many see antigen expression as the main deciding factor for mAb guided tumor localization and therapy, several other parameters have been defined that may be equally important. Some of these are tumor cell related, whereas others are related to the mAb-antigen combination or tumor physiology. Size of the tumor mass, antigen density, fate of antigen/antibody complex, mAb dose, presence of circulating antigen, mAb format, mAb circulating time, administration route, have all been recognized as important parameters which can differ from one tumor type to the other. Additionally, many factors are interrelated, and it is likely that the importance of some variables differs between tumors and between patients. For example, for large tumor masses the protein dose may need to be adjusted.

Increased insight in tumor physiology, including metastatic lesions, especially through studies by Jain et al.,[4,18,19] has lead to the realization that parameters related to the tumor physiology may be extraordinary important besides antigen expression. The large, leaky blood vessels, impaired blood flow patterns, (neo) vascularization, high interstitial fluid pressures, and aberrant lymphoid vessels in tumors heavily influence the distribution of diffusion driven therapeutics, such as mAb. Some of these parameters are highly fluctuable in time, and accessibility of various parts of a tumor are influenced dramatically accordingly.

The different tumor physiology, particularly the vastly different vascular bed is worth mentioning. Large, leaky vessels realize tumor blood supply, and the presence of leaky vessels is in itself sufficient for selective uptake of mAb. Injection of control IgG can lead to positive tumor imaging, with tumor to background levels as high as $5:1$.[48] I.e., "specific" tumor uptake e.g., by an imaging modality, should always be viewed with caution, as this may be the result of the aberrant tumor vasculature. In fact, mAb uptake by tumor tissue is partly caused by the aberrant vasculature, and mAb tumor retention is dependant upon antigen expression.

The common view of RCC is that it is a highly vascular tumor, and thereby possibly a good target for mAb-guided therapy. However, one should keep in mind that high vascular density is not equivalent to high perfusion rates, which are required for optimal mAb delivery. Actually, the perfusion rate of RCC is lower than of e.g., normal kidney tissue, and thus adequate delivery of mAb may be hampered. The much lower perfusion rate in the vast majority, if not all, solid tumors, may explain some of the ineffectiveness of mAb-guided treatment of solid tumors.

MONOCLONAL ANTIBODY-GUIDED THERAPY

Monoclonal antibody-guided tumor therapy can be mediated via unmodified mAb through natural occurring effector mechanisms such as activation of effector cells, activation of complement, or through specific delivery of cytotoxic agents (toxins, drugs, radionuclides). The caveat for mAb therapies relying on effector cell mechanisms is the necessity of antigen expression by all tumor cells. Antigen negative tumor cells will escape and eventually lead to unwanted tumor recurrence and subsequent death of patients. Despite this disadvantage, many favor this form of passive immunotherapy, because administration of high doses of unconjugated, "naked" mAb is very well tolerated without any side effects.

For immunotoxins internalization of the mAb-antigen complex is absolutely required to mediate cell killing. Immunotoxins are extraordinary powerful, and internalization of as few as 50 immunotoxin molecules can kill a tumor cell. However, some cell-surface mAb-antigen complexes do not internalize at an appreciable rate, and differential internalization rates may occur between different tumor regions, hampering effectiveness. This internalization heterogeneity is almost certainly a reflection of clonal outgrowth or reflecting dissimilar tumor physiology. Although immunotoxins do have advantages, few studies have been performed, mainly because the toxins themselves are highly immunogenic, preventing multiple treatments.

Radionuclide conjugated mAbs have been studied extensively for therapy of solid tumors. Alpha or β emitters such as ^{131}I, ^{90}Y, [212]Bi, [211]At can kill at distances of up to 50 or more cell diameters. Thus, the antibody does not have to bind to every tumor cell for an efficient therapeutic effect, in contrast to unconjugated mAb or immunotoxins. Also, the radiolabeled mAb does not need to be internalized for cell killing. For reasons of convenience (easy handling, availability, easy of labeling techniques, costs) [131]I conjugated mAbs have been studied intensely, notwithstanding some major disadvantages. [131]I emits high-energy β emission and the γ emission is too strong for optimal imaging. The significant radiation dose to some normal organs, in particular bone marrow, limits the total amount of ^{131}I-mAb that can be given. Additionally, much of the γ radiation is delivered outside the body, requiring considerable safety measures.

The use of radiolabeled conjugates allows for in-situ tumor detection with a low scout dose followed by high dose therapy when adequate tumor targeting is demonstrated. This gives the opportunity to exclude patients with antigen negative tumors (poor mAb uptake), precluding unnecessary procedures, toxicity, and loss of quality of life. It may permit patient adjusted administration, although adequate dosimetry calculations are logistically demanding.

IMMUNOGENICITY OF RENAL CELL CARCINOMA: TUMOR-ASSOCIATED MOLECULES

Based on a number of independent observations Renal Cell Carcinoma, as melanoma, has long been considered an intrinsically immunogenic tumor:

- Spontaneous regression, mainly of pulmonary lesions, has frequently been described in metastasized RCC patients. The estimate of occurrence vary between 0.1–6%, and recent estimates have been as high as 2–6%.[11] While there is debate about the actual percentage, there is general consensus that spontaneous regressions do occur, suggestive for a role of the immune system. Whether the anti-tumor occurrences were mediated by cellular immune responses or by humoral immune responses has not been studied.
- Autologous typing studies by Ueda et al.[41] revealed tumor-specific humoral responses in (very few) RCC patients. These investigators were able to detect antibody specifically reactive with the autologous RCC cells without cross-reactivity to corresponding normal kidney tissue. True tumor-specificity was not demonstrated (complete immunohistochemical analysis was not performed), and the target molecule(s) was not defined molecularly. Recognition of upregulated kidney-associated molecules could not be ruled out.

- Several investigators have isolated RCC cytolytic CTL, able to kill autologous RCC cells while normal fibroblasts or peripheral blood mononuclear cells were not killed.[5,7,11–13,13,16,33] In one case (RAGE-1, Renal Antigen Gene-1) the gene was cloned.[16] Unfortunately, this gene was expressed by a very low percentage of RCC (2%), and was therefore discarded as appropriate immunotherapeutic target.
- Dramatic invasion of primary RCC by T cells and macrophages is quite common. This may be a non-specific response to the necrosis, which is certainly present in the larger tumors. However, the occurrence of these effector cells has been interpreted as an (abortive) active immune response.
- Finally, interleukine-2 and interferon-2α treatment can induce durable responses in patients with progressive metastatic RCC. Both cytokines induce non-specific activation of (parts of) the immune system, and the durable responses have been viewed as immune induced.

The collective evidence strongly suggests the presence of aberrantly expressed molecules in RCC. Yet, the studies only suggested the presence of molecules differentially expressed by RCC and normal kidney cells. The pivotal question: are molecules recognized that can serve as immunological targets, has not been answered. Nevertheless, these RCC-associated molecules not expressed by normal kidney tissue might serve as appropriate target molecules for mAb-guided therapy.

MONOCLONAL ANTIBODIES DEFINING RENAL CELL CARCINOMA ANTIGENS

In the wake of the description of the hybridoma technology, many investigators tried to isolate mAbs recognizing TAA or TSA. Several research groups have defined mAbs reactive with RCC-associated antigens.[2,3,14,15,22,28,29,40,46,49] Not surprisingly, most mAbs recognized kidney-differentiation antigens retained by (subsets of) RCC. For some mAbs strict kidney specificity was observed, whereas in isolated cases cross-reactivity with many non-kidney tissues. Unfortunately, in several cases the reactivity on tumor tissue has not been studied, despite a restricted tissue distribution that warranted further investigation. Little is known about the targeting ability and antitumor efficacy of these mAbs.[8,30,46]

In addition to mAbs recognizing kidney differentiation antigens, several mAbs recognizing RCC-associated antigens absent from normal kidney have been defined.[14,28,47] In general, antigen expression was quite heterogeneous and mostly only a proportion of the primary and metastatic RCC tested were positive for the respective antigen. Secondly, cross-reactivity with other tumors and few normal tissues was observed. A comparison between the fine-specificity analyses suggests that these mAbs recognize different RCC-tumor-associated antigens (RCC-TAA) because they display different cross-reactivity with normal tissues. Although all these mAbs are prime candidates for clinical investigations, proof of principle clinical studies with most RCC-TAA recognizing mAbs are rare, partly due to the difficulty to translate laboratory findings to clinical research without industrial interest.

Table 1. Immunohistochemical analysis of G250
expression: correlation with Renal Cell Carcinoma clear cell subtype.

Cell type	G250 expression		
	Positive	Negative	Percentage
Clear Cell type	171	2	99
Granular Cell type	19	10	66
Mixed Cell type	13	4	77
Spindle Cell type	0	2	0
TOTAL	203	18	88

MONOCLONAL ANTIBODY G250; GENERAL CHARACTERISTICS

The most extensively studied mAb in RCC is mAbG250. This mAb showed an exceptional tissue distribution in combination with very high expression in RCC, warranting clinical investigation. Immunohistochemical fine specificity analysis revealed cross-reactivity with gastric mucosal cells and large bile canals, whereas all other tissues tested, including normal kidney tissue, were antigen negative.[28] Subsequent in-depth analysis revealed slight reactivity of pancreas cells. More than 80% of primary RCC showed almost homogeneous G250 antigen expression as judged by immunohistochemistry. Cross-reactivity with non-RCC tumors was observed, but the percentage of a particular tumor type as well as the percentage of tumor cells stained was much lower than observed for RCC. Importantly, metastatic RCC investigated also showed quite high G250 expression.

In the initial analyses no clear-cut relation between G250 expression and morphological subtype was observed, but further studies showed that G250 is almost ubiquitously expressed in clear cell RCC (ccRCC), the most prominent RCC subtype, which comprises approximately 80% of cases[42] (Table 1).

After molecular definition of the G250 gene[17] it became clear that a direct link between mutational events intimately related to the development of ccRCC, mutation in the Von Hippel Lindau (VHL) gene product, and G250 expression existed: Expression of a non-functional VHL gene product leads to activation of the G250 promoter, resulting in G250 protein expression. This direct molecular link explained the ubiquitous G250 expression in ccRCC as well as the homogeneous expression in RCC clear cells. Provided that ccRCC metastases retain their VHL phenotype, all metastatic sites derived from G250-positive ccRCC are likely to be G250-positive. This would be an additional benefit for mAbG250-guided therapy, because the likelihood of antigen-negative tumor cells would be diminished. In fact, in clinical trials with mAbG250 patients with ccRCC only were included, and invariably excellent mAbG250 uptake has been observed.[9] In summary, this antibody met crucial requirements necessary for mAb-guided therapy: homogeneous expression in tumors and highly restricted normal tissue expression.

In RCC animal models as well as in ex vivo experiments on tumor-bearing kidneys selective uptake of mAbG250 in antigen positive tumors vs. antigen negative tumors or tissues was observed.[24,37,38,43-45] Several mAbG250 tumor targeting features were quite remarkable: extraordinary high uptake (up to more than 100% of the injected dose/ gram tumor tissue), paralleled by very high tumor: tissue ratios, and the requirement of a low protein dose to obtain tumor saturation. Based on these preclinical studies numerous clinical trials aimed at mAb-guided therapy in metastatic RCC patients have been performed.

CLINICAL STUDIES WITH MURINE MONOCLONAL ANTIBODY G250

The first clinical study with mAbG250 was a presurgical study of 131I labeled to escalating mass amounts of mG250, conducted to determine tumor uptake and mAb distribution.[27] Immediately after injection mAbG250 was evenly distributed in the blood pool, and no radioactivity in the tumor was visible. Tumor uptake was clearly evident 2–3 days after mAb administration. At the lowest protein dose (0.2 and 2 mg mAbG250), liver uptake was observed, but liver uptake decreased at higher protein dose levels, suggesting saturation of G250 antigen sites by the mAb. Because radical nephrectomy was part of the clinical management of these patients, extensively tumor tissue sampling was possible, and we were able to demonstrate that antibody targeting was not merely a function of the high vasculature nature of RCC. Additionally, gamma camera images of ^{99m}Tc-human serum albumin, administered immediately before surgery, and ^{131}I-mG250 were clearly disparate, demonstrating that the images were not a reflection of blood pool, but of true selective antibody accumulation.[27]

In tumor biopsy samples high levels of mG250 accumulation, with levels of up to 0.1% of the injected dose per gram of tumor (%ID/g) 7 days after infusion, were found, these levels being among the highest reported in studies of solid tumors. Additionally, normal tissue uptake, actually limited to the liver, was saturable, encouraging future development of mAbG250 in RCC.

Subsequently a phase I/II radioimmunotherapy trial with ^{131}I-mG250, to determine its safety and possible efficacy, was initiated at Memorial Sloan-Kettering Cancer Center, New York.[9] Escalating amounts of ^{131}I labeled to 10 mg of mG250 was administered as a single infusion. All patients had measurable, progressive, histology proven clear cell RCC. Targeting to all known disease 2 cm. or greater in diameter was excellent, highly suggestive that patient selection on the basis of clear cell RCC histology defined patients with G250-positive tumors. At dose levels ≥45 mCi ^{131}I hepatic toxicity was invariable, but the intensity otherwise unrelated to the amount of radioactivity administered or the radiation absorbed dose to the liver. More important, this toxicity was transient (symptoms usually resolved in 2 weeks) and not dose limiting. Dose-limiting toxicity, as in all radioimmunotherapy studies of radiolabeled antibodies, was haematopoietic, with the maximum tolerated dose of activity (MTDA) determined to be 90 mCi of ^{131}I per square meter. In the phase II arm of this trial, 15 patients were treated with 90 mCi 131I-mG250/m^2 to determine efficacy. No major responses were noted. However, the overall survival of patients treated with ^{131}I-mG250 seemed to be increased in comparison to historic control patients, and a few minor responses were observed.[9] The development of human anti-mouse antibody responses in all patients precluded re-treatment. The excellent targeting and the lack of significant nonhaematopoietic toxicity demonstrated the potential of (radiolabeled) mAbG250 in the treatment of renal cancer. This, in combination with the necessity for multiple injections, led to the development of chimeric mAbG250 (cG250).

CLINICAL STUDIES WITH CHIMERIC MONOCLONAL ANTIBODY G250

A chimeric version of the antibody was constructed (cG250) by molecular techniques (mouse heavy chain sequences were replaced by human heavy chain sequences) with the intention to diminish the immunogenicity of mG250. The design of the phase I clinical trial with cG250 was comparable with that of mG250.[35] All antigen-positive tumors (tested in retrospect by immunohistochemistry) showed excellent targeting of radioactivity, with uptake (measured at biopsy, 1 week after infusion), as high as 0.52% ID/g. As with mG250, hepatic uptake was saturable at doses of 5 mg cG250 and greater. Furthermore, and possibly more importantly, no evidence of human anti-chimeric antibody responses, as measured by enzyme-linked immunosorbent assay[35], were detectable. Thus, it appeared that chimerization had indeed lead to diminished immunogenicity, allowing multiple administrations.

In the subsequent phase I radioimmunotherapy trial, escalating doses of ^{131}I were labeled to 5 mg of cG250.[34] Although patients were screened for RCC with clear cell histology, patients received an imaging dose (6 mCi ^{131}I labeled to 5 mg cG250), to ensure that appropriate cG250-uptake was possible. Only patients showing targeting to tumor received the therapeutic infusion of ^{131}I-cG250 1 week later. Surprisingly, no hepatic toxicity was observed, in contrast to the mG250 radioimmunotherapy trial. This was most likely the consequence of saturation of the hepatic G250 antigen sites with the initial, imaging dose of cG250. Targeting of therapeutic ^{131}I-cG250 to disease was outstanding in those patients with positive "diagnostic" scans. As in all radiotherapy trials, dose-limiting toxicity was haematopoietic (approximately 60 mCi ^{131}I per meter square).

Despite excellent tumor targeting, uniform distribution of the radioactivity in tumors has been rare. To investigate mechanisms involved n these uneven distribution patterns a dual-labeling trial was performed. Patients received two independent administrations of cG250, labeled with ^{131}I or ^{25}I followed by surgery, allowing studies addressing the importance of variable factors.[36] Unexpectedly, cG250 distribution did not differ between different administrations, demonstrating that intrinsic tumor factors play a prominent role in mAb targeting. Thus, consistent "low uptake areas" may reflect intrinsically different tumor populations, e.g., consisting of fast internalizing subpopulations, resulting in apparent low uptake areas, because internalized iodinated proteins are quickly degraded and the iodine is lost. Possibly, avid mAb uptake may have occurred. Initially, this explanation was felt to be improbable, because ^{131}I-cG250 tumor retention in patients was in the order of weeks (see

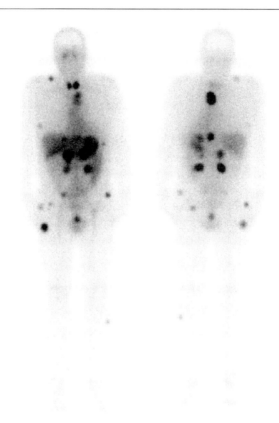

Figure 1. Immunoscintigram of metastatic RCC patient 2 weeks post-administration of 60mCi/m²
¹³¹I-cG250 (total dose 112mCi ¹³¹I)
Left: Anterior image, right, posterior image. Note the excellent cG250 uptake in all tumor lesions and
virtual absence of cG250 uptake in non-tumor tissues

also Figure 1), suggesting very low internalization rates. However, recent animal experiments have shown that internalization may play an important role in the cG250 distribution. The use of residualising radionuclides such as Yttrium or Lutetium may lead to a more noticeable homogeneous cG250 distribution, but more importantly, may deliver more potent radiation more evenly. Preliminary evidence in RCC patients treated with cG250 labeled with a residualising radionuclide (¹¹¹In) and ¹³¹I have indeed demonstrated increased uptake of the ¹¹¹In-labeled cG250 in comparison to ¹³¹I-cG250.

Currently we are performing a phase I/II trial where patients receive two high doses of ¹³¹I-cG250, separated by 3 months. An example of the excellent cG250 uptake is shown in figure 1. This image was obtained 2 weeks after cG250 administration and serves to show that 131I-cG250 uptake and retention can be exceptional. In this 131I–cG250 trial, toxicity is bone marrow related and toxicity appears to be more severe with the second administration, suggestive of moderate bone marrow damage by the first high dose. This trial is still open for recruitment and thus far no major responses have been observed.

As discussed earlier, administration of cold ("naked") antibody, can lead to effector cell recruitment or complement activation, both leading to target cell death. Although the intrinsic in vitro cG250 ADCC activity was low, a phase II study of cold cG250 was performed. Advanced, progressive RCC patients received 12 weekly intravenous infusions of 50 mg cG250/dose. Thirty-six patients were enrolled to detect a true response rate of 15%. Although this primary objective was not reached, a durable clinical benefit for at least six month or more was achieved in eight patients. This is certainly considered as clinically meaningful for this patient population, Six patients achieved a stabilization of their disease lasting more than 6 months. Beyond the observation period required by the clinical protocol, one patient achieved a CR more than 6 months after start of cG250 treatment and another patient experienced a minor response. Both patients were free of disease progression for more than 1 year. Based on the good tolerability of this treatment with cG250 together with the clinical benefit in 25% of this difficult treatment group warranted further investigation.

IL–2 has been known to enhance ADCC of mAbs. To investigate whether IL–2 or other cytokines might enhance cG250 ADCC, cG250 ADCC in combination with several cytokines was evaluated. IL–2 augmented and maintained cG250-mediated ADCC activity and K562 cytotoxicity when applied to PBMC in culture for seven days.[25,39] IFN-gamma also enhanced the ADCC of cG250 throughout the study period, but was not as effective as the IL–2 treatment. IFN-alpha 2a and 2b increased cG250-mediated ADCC and K562 cytotoxicity for only three days of the study period. The potent and sustained immune effector activity observed with cG250 and cytokines in these in vitro studies suggested that the combination immunotherapy of cG250 with cytokines such as IL–2 might be advantageous in the treatment of RCC. Indeed, subsequent trials with naked cG250 have focused on the combination of cG250 with biological response modifiers. In one trial the effects of cG250 (20 mg cG250/dose) and low dose IL–2 plus periodic IL–2 pulsing in advanced and metastatic RCC patient is studied, in another trial the effects of cG250 combined with IFN-α is being studied. In the cG250/IL2 clinical study objective responses have been observed, and this trial is currently being evaluated. The cG250/IFN-α trial has recently been initiated and is ongoing.

In summary, it appears that monoclonal antibody G250 treatment can play a role in the management of metastatic RCC. However, it may be important to delineate particular subgroups more prone to benefit from this treatment. Clearly, only patients with clear cell RCC should be eligible, but additional prognostic and predictive parameters are needed to improve definition of patients that can possibly benefit from this treatment. In particular high–risk patients may benefit from adjuvant treatment with this non-toxic treatment modality. Large cohort studies are needed to investigate this possibility.

ACKNOWLEDGEMENTS

The authors would like to acknowledge the many collaborators at Memorial Sloan Kettering Cancer Center, New York, U.S.A., and at the Ludwig Institute for Cancer Research, Melbourne Branch, Australia and New York Branch, New York, U.S.A., and at the University Medical Center Nijmegen, Nijmegen, The Netherlands, for their support and stimulating discussions. They also wish to acknowledge the patients participating in various clinical trials. Finally, Wilex GmbH, Munich, Germany is acknowledged for their support.

REFERENCES

1. Amato, RJ. Chemotherapy for renal cell carcinoma. Semin. Oncol., 27: 177–186, 2000.
2. Bander, NH, Cordon-Cardo, C, Finstad, CL, Whitmore, WF, Jr, Vaughan, ED, Jr, Oettgen, HF, Melamed, M, and Old, LJ. Immunohistologic dissection of the human kidney using monoclonal antibodies. J. Urol., 133: 502–505, 1985.
3. Bander, NH, Finstad, CL, Cordon-Cardo, C, Ramsawak, RD, Vaughan, ED, Jr, Whitmore, WF, Jr, Oettgen, HF, Melamed, MR, and Old, LJ. Analysis of a mouse monoclonal antibody that reacts with a specific region of the human proximal tubule and subsets renal cell carcinomas. Cancer Res., 49: 6774–6780, 1989.
4. Baxter, LT, and Jain, RK. Transport of fluid and macromolecules in tumors. I. Role of interstitial pressure and convection. Microvasc. Res., 37: 77–104, 1989.
5. Bernhard, H, Maeurer, MJ, Jager, E, Wolfel, T, Schneider, J, Karbach, J, Seliger, B, Huber, C, Storkus, WS, Lotze, MT, Meyer zum Buschenfelde, KH, and Knuth, A. Recognition of human renal cell carcinoma and melanoma by HLA-A2-restricted cytotoxic T lymphocytes is mediated by shared peptide epitopes and up-regulated by interferon-gamma. Scand. J. Immunol., 44: 285–292, 1996.
6. Boon, T, Coulie, PG, and Van den, EB. Tumor antigens recognized by T cells. Immunol. Today, 18: 267–268, 1997.
7. Brouwenstijn, N, Hoogstraten, C, Verdegaal, EM, Van der Spek, CW, Deckers, JG, Mulder, A, Osanto, S, and Schrier, PI. Definition of unique and shared T-cell defined tumor antigens in human renal cell carcinoma. J. Immunother., 21: 427–434, 1998.
8. Chiou, RK. Biodistribution and radioimmunoscintigraphy studies of renal cell carcinoma using tumor-preferential monoclonal antibodies and F(ab')2 fragments. J. Urol., 142: 1584–1588, 1989.
9. Divgi, CR, Bander, NH, Scott, AM, O'Donoghue, JA, Sgouros, G, Welt, S, Finn, RD, Morrissey, F, Capitelli, P, Williams, JM, Deland, D, Nakhre, A, Oosterwijk, E, Gulec, S, Graham, MC, Larson, SM, and Old, LJ. Phase I/II radioimmunotherapy trial with iodine-131-labeled monoclonal antibody G250 in metastatic renal cell carcinoma. Clin. Cancer Res, 4: 2729–2739, 1998.
10. Ehrlich, P. On immunity with special reference to cell life. In: the collected papers of Paul Ehrlich, volume II:Immunology and Cancer Research. Himmelweit F, Marquardt M, Dale H (Eds). Pergamon Press, London. 1957. Ref Type: Generic.
11. Elhilali, MM, Gleave, M, Fradet, Y, Davis, I, Venner, P, Saad, F, Klotz, L, Moore, R, Ernst, S, and Paton, V. Placebo-associated remissions in a multicentre, randomized, double-blind trial of interferon gamma-1b for the treatment of metastatic renal cell carcinoma. The Canadian Urologic Oncology Group. BJU. Int, 86: 613–618, 2000.
12. Finke, JH, Rayman, P, Alexander, J, Edinger, M, Tubbs, RR, Connelly, R, Pontes, E, and Bukowski, R. Characterization of the cytolytic activity of CD4+ and CD8+ tumor-infiltrating lymphocytes in human renal cell carcinoma. Cancer Res, 50: 2363–2370, 1990.
13. Finke, JH, Rayman, P, Edinger, M, Tubbs, RR, Stanley, J, Klein, E, and Bukowski, R. Characterization of a human renal cell carcinoma specific cytotoxic CD8+ T cell line. J. Immunother., 11: 1–11, 1992.
14. Finstad, CL, Cordon-Cardo, C, Bander, NH, Whitmore, WF, Melamed, MR, and Old, LJ. Specificity analysis of mouse monoclonal antibodies defining cell surface antigens of human renal cancer. Proc. Natl. Acad. Sci. U.S.A, 82: 2955–2959, 1985.
15. Fischer, P, Storkel, S, Haase, W, and Scherberich, JE. Differential diagnosis of histogenetically distinct human epithelial renal tumours with a monoclonal antibody against gamma-glutamyltransferase. Cancer Immunol. Immunother., 33: 382–388, 1991.

16. Gaugler, B, Brouwenstijn, N, Vantomme, V, Szikora, JP, Van der Spek, CW, Patard, JJ, Boon, T, Schrier, P, and Van den Eynde, BJ. A new gene coding for an antigen recognized by autologous cytolytic T lymphocytes on a human renal carcinoma. Immunogenetics, 44: 323–330, 1996.

17. Grabmaier, K, Vissers, JL, De Weijert, MC, Oosterwijk-Wakka, JC, Van Bokhoven, A, Brakenhoff, RH, Noessner, E, Mulders, PA, Merkx, G, Figdor, CG, Adema, GJ, and Oosterwijk, E. Molecular cloning and immunogenicity of renal cell carcinoma-associated antigen G250. Int. J. Cancer, 85: 865–870, 2000.

18. Jain, RK. Physiological barriers to delivery of monoclonal antibodies and other macromolecules in tumors. Cancer Res., 50: 814s–819s, 1990.

19. Jain, RK, and Baxter, LT. Mechanisms of heterogeneous distribution of monoclonal antibodies and other macromolecules in tumors: significance of elevated interstitial pressure. Cancer Res., 48: 7022–7032, 1988.

20. Jungbluth, AA, Busam, KJ, Kolb, D, Iversen, K, Coplan, K, Chen, YT, Spagnoli, GC, and Old, LJ. Expression of MAGE-antigens in normal tissues and cancer. Int. J. Cancer, 85: 460–465, 2000.

21. Jungbluth, AA, Stockert, E, Chen, YT, Kolb, D, Iversen, K, Coplan, K, Williamson, B, Altorki, N, Busam, KJ, and Old, LJ. Monoclonal antibody MA454 reveals a heterogeneous expression pattern of MAGE-1 antigen in formalin-fixed paraffin embedded lung tumours. Br. J. Cancer, 83: 493–497, 2000.

22. Kinouchi, T, Nakayama, E, Ueda, R, Ishiguro, S, Uenaka, A, Oda, H, and Kotake, T. Characterization of a kidney antigen defined by a mouse monoclonal antibody K2.7. J. Urol., 137: 151–154, 1987.

23. Kohler, G, and Milstein, C. Continuous cultures of fused cells secreting antibody of predefined specificity. Nature, 256: 495–497, 1975.

24. Kranenborg, MH, Boerman, OC, De Weijert, MC, Oosterwijk-Wakka, JC, Corstens, FH, and Oosterwijk, E. The effect of antibody protein dose of anti-renal cell carcinoma monoclonal antibodies in nude mice with renal cell carcinoma xenografts. Cancer, 80: 2390–2397, 1997.

25. Liu, Z, Smyth, FE, Renner, C, Lee, FT, Oosterwijk, E, and Scott, AM. Anti-renal cell carcinoma chimeric antibody G250: cytokine enhancement of in vitro antibody-dependent cellular cytotoxicity. Cancer Immunol. Immunother., 51: 171–177, 2002.

26. Nishiyama, K, Shirahama, T, Yoshimura, A, Sumizawa, T, Furukawa, T, Ichikawa-Haraguchi, M, Akiyama, S, and Ohi, Y. Expression of the multidrug transporter, P-glycoprotein, in renal and transitional cell carcinomas. Cancer, 71: 3611–3619, 1993.

27. Oosterwijk, E, Bander, NH, Divgi, CR, Welt, S, Wakka, JC, Finn, RD, Carswell, EA, Larson, SM, Warnaar, SO, Fleuren, GJ, Oettgen, HF, and Old, LJ. Antibody localization in human renal cell carcinoma: a phase I study of monoclonal antibody G250. J. Clin. Oncol., 11: 738–750, 1993.

28. Oosterwijk, E, Ruiter, DJ, Hoedemaeker, PJ, Pauwels, EK, Jonas, U, Zwartendijk, J, and Warnaar, SO. Monoclonal antibody G 250 recognizes a determinant present in renal-cell carcinoma and absent from normal kidney. Int. J. Cancer, 38: 489–494, 1986.

29. Oosterwijk, E, Ruiter, DJ, Wakka, JC, Huiskens-van der Meij JW, Jonas, U, Fleuren, GJ, Zwartendijk, J, Hoedemaeker, P, and Warnaar, SO. Immunohistochemical analysis of monoclonal antibodies to renal antigens. Application in the diagnosis of renal cell carcinoma. Am. J. Pathol., 123: 301–309, 1986.

30. Rachel, U, Baum, RP, Fischer, P, Jonas, D, and Scherberich, JE. Monoclonal antibody 138H11 in immunoscintigraphy of human kidney tumors—in vitro results. Investig. Urol. (Berl), 5:66–68, 66–68, 1994.

31. Scanlan, MJ, Altorki, NK, Gure, AO, Williamson, B, Jungbluth, A, Chen, YT, and Old, LJ. Expression of cancer-testis antigens in lung cancer: definition of bromodomain testis-specific gene (BRDT) as a new CT gene, CT9. Cancer Lett., 150: 155–164, 2000.

32. Schaub, TP, Kartenbeck, J, Konig, J, Spring, H, Dorsam, J, Staehler, G, Storkel, S, Thon, WF, and Keppler, D. Expression of the MRP2 gene-encoded conjugate export pump in human kidney proximal tubules and in renal cell carcinoma. J. Am. Soc. Nephrol., 10: 1159–1169, 1999.

33. Schendel, DJ, Gansbacher, B, Oberneder, R, Kriegmair, M, Hofstetter, A, Riethmuller, G, and Segurado, OG. Tumor-specific lysis of human renal cell carcinomas by tumor-infiltrating lymphocytes. I. HLA-A2-restricted recognition of autologous and allogeneic tumor lines. J. Immunol., 151: 4209–4220, 1993.

34. Steffens, MG, Boerman, OC, de Mulder, PH, Oyen, WJ, Buijs, WC, Witjes, JA, van den Broek, WJ, Oosterwijk-Wakka, JC, Debruyne, FM, Corstens, FH, and Oosterwijk, E. Phase I radioimmunotherapy of metastatic renal cell carcinoma with 131I-labeled chimeric monoclonal antibody G250. Clin. Cancer Res., 5: 3268s–3274s, 1999.

35. Steffens, MG, Boerman, OC, Oosterwijk-Wakka, JC, Oosterhof, GO, Witjes, JA, Koenders, EB, Oyen, WJ, Buijs, WC, Debruyne, FM, Corstens, FH, and Oosterwijk, E. Targeting of renal cell carcinoma with iodine-131-labeled chimeric monoclonal antibody G250. J. Clin. Oncol., 15: 1529–1537, 1997.

36. Steffens, MG, Boerman, OC, Oyen, WJ, Kniest, PH, Witjes, JA, Oosterhof, GO, van Leenders, GJ, Debruyne, FM, Corstens, FH, and Oosterwijk, E. Intratumoral distribution of two consecutive injections of chimeric antibody G250 in primary renal cell carcinoma: implications for fractionated dose radioimmunotherapy. Cancer Res., 59: 1615–1619, 1999.

37. Steffens, MG, Kranenborg, MH, Boerman, OC, Zegwaart-Hagemeier, NE, Debruyne, FM, Corstens, FH, and Oosterwijk, E. Tumor retention of 186Re-MAG3, 111In-DTPA and 125I labeled monoclonal antibody G250 in nude mice with renal cell carcinoma xenografts. Cancer Biother. Radiopharm., 13: 133–139, 1998.

38. Steffens, MG, Oosterwijk-Wakka, JC, Zegwaart-Hagemeier, NE, Boerman, OC, Debruyne, FM, Corstens, FH, and Oosterwijk, E. Immunohistochemical analysis of tumor antigen saturation following injection of monoclonal antibody G250. Anticancer Res., 19: 1197–1200, 1999.

39. Surfus, JE, Hank, JA, Oosterwijk, E, Welt, S, Lindstrom, MJ, Albertini, MR, Schiller, JH, and Sondel, PM. Anti-renal-cell carcinoma chimeric antibody G250 facilitates antibody-dependent cellular cytotoxicity with in vitro and in vivo interleukin-2-activated effectors. J. Immunother. Emphasis. Tumor Immunol., 19: 184–191, 1996.

40. Tokuyama, H, and Tokuyama, Y. Mouse monoclonal antibodies with restricted specificity for human renal cell carcinoma and ability to modulate the tumor cell growth in vitro. Hybridoma, 7: 155–165, 1988.

41. Ueda, R, Shiku, H, Pfreundschuh, M, Takahashi, T, Li, LT, Whitmore, WF, Oettgen, HF, and Old, LJ. Cell surface antigens of human renal cancer defined by autologous typing. J. Exp. Med., 150: 564–579, 1979.

42. Uemura, H, Nakagawa, Y, Yoshida, K, Saga, S, Yoshikawa, K, Hirao, Y, and Oosterwijk, E. MN/CA IX/G250 as a potential target for immunotherapy of renal cell carcinomas. Br. J. Cancer, 81: 741–746, 1999.

43. van Dijk, J, Oosterwijk, E, van Kroonenburgh, MJ, Jonas, U, Fleuren, GJ, Pauwels, EK, and Warnaar, SO. Perfusion of tumor-bearing kidneys as a model for scintigraphic screening of monoclonal antibodies. J. Nucl. Med., 29: 1078–1082, 1988.

44. van Dijk, J, Uemura, H, Beniers, AJ, Peelen, WP, Zegveld, ST, Fleuren, GJ, Warnaar, SO, and Oosterwijk, E. Therapeutic effects of monoclonal antibody G250, interferons and tumor necrosis factor, in mice with renal-cell carcinoma xenografts. Int. J. Cancer, 56: 262–268, 1994.

45. van Dijk, J, Zegveld, ST, Fleuren, GJ, and Warnaar, SO. Localization of monoclonal antibody G250 and bispecific monoclonal antibody CD3/G250 in human renal-cell carcinoma xenografts: relative effects of size and affinity. Int. J. Cancer, 48: 738–743, 1991.

46. Vessella, RL, Lange, PH, Palme, DF, Chiou, RK, Elson, MK, and Wessels, BW. Radioiodinated monoclonal antibodies in the imaging and treatment of human renal cell carcinoma xenografts in nude mice. Targeted Diagn. Ther., 1:245–282.: 245–282, 1988.

47. Vessella, RL, Moon, TD, Chiou, RK, Nowak, JA, Arfman, EW, Palme, DF, Peterson, GA, and Lange, PH. Monoclonal antibodies to human renal cell carcinoma: recognition of shared and restricted tissue antigens. Cancer Res., 45: 6131–6139, 1985.

48. Welt, S, Divgi, CR, Real, FX, Yeh, SD, Garin-Chesa, P, Finstad, CL, Sakamoto, J, Cohen, A, Sigurdson, ER, Kemeny, N, and . Quantitative analysis of antibody localization in human metastatic colon cancer: a phase I study of monoclonal antibody A33. J. Clin. Oncol., 8: 1894–1906, 1990.

49. Yoshida, SO, and Imam, A. Monoclonal antibody to a proximal nephrogenic renal antigen: immunohistochemical analysis of formalin-fixed, paraffin-embedded human renal cell carcinomas. Cancer Res., 49: 1802–1809, 1989.

13. ALLOGENEIC HEMATOPOETIC STEM CELL TRANSPLANTATION FOR CYTOKINE REFRACTORY RENAL CELL CARCINOMA

DARREL DRACHENBERG, M.D. AND RICHARD W. CHILDS, M.D.

E-mail Correspondence: Dr. Richard Childs, childsr@nih.gov and Dr. Darrel Drachenberg, DDrachenberg@sbgh.mb.ca

OVERVIEW

The treatment options for patients who develop metastatic renal cell carcinoma (RCC) are few. Conventional chemotherapeutics and radiotherapy rarely result in clinically beneficial responses. Fortunately, the past two decades has seen the development of promising immunotherapeutic approaches to treat metastatic RCC including the use of cytokines such as interleukin-2 and interferon-α, the adoptive infusion of lymphokine activated killer cells and tumor-infiltrating lymphocytes (TIL), and recently the development of dendritic cell based vaccination strategies. The promising results from these studies have forged the path for ongoing immunologically-based investigational approaches. Reduced intensity or nonmyeloablative allogeneic stem cell transplantation (NST) has recently been shown to produce potent immune-mediated anti-tumor responses in a variety of chemotherapy refractory hematologic malignancies while being associated with less morbidity and mortality compared to conventional "high dose" myeloablative regimens. Knowledge of RCC's proclivity to be regulated by the immune system recently led investigators to test this type of transplant strategy in this malignancy. Pilot trials were based on the hypothesis that graft versus tumor (GVT) effects, analogous to the graft-vs-leukemia (GVL) effect seen in hematological malignancies, might be generated against an immuno-sensitive solid tumor following the transplantation of allogeneic donor T lymphocytes. The recent observation of regression of metastatic RCC following NST has confirmed the susceptibility of RCC to a GVT effect. Disease responses have been seen in patients who have failed traditional cytokine regimens and have occasionally included complete responses. Here we review the development and outcome of pilot immunotherapy trials based on the use of an allogeneic immune system.

INTRODUCTION

Renal cell carcinoma [RCC] is the most common tumor affecting the kidney. It accounts for 2%–3% of all adult cancers and contributes 2% of all cancer deaths.[1] In the United States, approximately 30,000 new cases of RCC are diagnosed each year and the incidence is continuing to climb.[2] The increased utilization of diagnostic imaging modalities (ultrasound, computed tomography, magnetic resonance imaging) has led to 25 to 40% of new RCC's being diagnosed incidentally, with the majority presenting as localized disease. Unfortunately, however, the disease related mortality rate has not demonstrated a corresponding decrease, despite the apparent migration to detecting disease in an earlier stage.[3] Metastatic RCC is documented in approximately 25% of patients at the time of initial presentation and a further 25% will develop metastatic disease despite apparent localized disease at time of treatment.[4] The prognosis for patients with disseminated disease is poor with a median survival of less than 1 year with only a 1 to 2% survival at 5 years.[5] These mortality figures underscore the importance and necessity for the development of more efficacious systemic therapies for this disease.

Attempts to treat locally advanced and metastatic disease with conventional antitumor therapies such as chemotherapy have been largely unsuccessful. Agents with apparent *in vitro* activity such as vinblastine and floxuridine have response rates of only 2–4%, with none of the responses being durable and therefore rarely translating into a survival advantage for treated patients.[6] Hormonal manipulation, based on the observation of the production of RCC in Syrian hamsters exposed to estrogen, has also been largely ineffective.[7] Radiotherapy has its only role in the management of RCC relegated to the palliation of painful osseous metastasis or in emergent circumstances such as spinal cord compression or post-obstructive pneumonia.[8] The perceived failure of more conventional treatments to make an impact on long-term survival has led to the exploration of alternative therapeutic approaches, of which immunotherapy figures most prominently.

The highly variable and peculiar natural history of RCC with its occasionally protracted periods of stable disease and prolonged survival even in the face of disseminated disease has long fascinated and perplexed investigators. In 1928, the first documented case of spontaneous regression of pathologically confirmed metastatic RCC after nephrectomy was reported at the Mayo Clinic by Dr. HC Bumpus.[9] He surmised that "the body produces antibodies to render inert or destroy (tumor) cells . . . after removal of the primary focus by operation or through necrosis, the antibodies may be formed in sufficient quantity to overcome the invading cells and destroy the metastatic foci." Since then nearly 100 cases of spontaneous regression of metastatic RCC have been reported in the literature.[10] Evenson and Cole have observed that RCC appears to have the highest incidence of this phenomenon among all solid tumors.[11] The frequency of spontaneous regression is estimated at

0.3%,[12] but in a randomized study comparing recombinant INF-γ to placebo by Gleave et al. of the Canadian Urologic Oncology Group, a 6.6% objective response rate was noted in the placebo arm suggesting a higher rate of spontaneous regression than previously reported.[13] While not totally validated, the immune system is felt by many to be responsible for disease regression in the absence of systemic treatment. Therefore, the existence of spontaneous regression has been put forth as one of the rationales for the utilization of immunologic approaches in the treatment of RCC.

The presence of tumor-infiltrating lymphocytes, the isolation of tumor-specific autologous cytotoxic T lymphocytes, and the identification of tumor-associated antigens on renal cancer also support the notion that immune based therapies for RCC are worthy of exploration.[14,15] Furthermore, observations also suggest the presence of immune dysregulation and T-lymphocyte dysfunction in RCC patients. T-cell receptor abnormalities, abnormal NFκB activation, and enhanced apoptosis of T-lymphocytes both in peripheral blood and in the tumor have been noted.[16,17,18] Tumors may elude immuno-surveillance and become immuno-tolerant through the induction of T-lymphocyte apoptosis mediated through the Fas/Fas-ligand-receptor system. Indeed, Uzzo et al. reported that RCC tumor cells expressing Fas-L could induce apoptosis in activated T-cells from RCC patients.[18]

Based on the recognition of possible immunologic responsiveness, immunotherapy for RCC has undergone a metamorphosis since its inception over 2 decades ago. The first attempts were aimed at reinforcing the immune systems ability to recognize tumors as non-self through direct systemic administration of immunomodulatory cytokines such as interleukin-2 (IL-2), interferon-α (INF-α), interferon-γ (INF-γ), and combinations of cytokines with or without lymphokine-activated killer cells (LAK) or tumor-infiltrating lymphocytes (TIL). IL-2 treatment remains the only US Food and Drug Administration-approved treatment for metastatic RCC, however, controversy still exists as to its best route of administration (high vs low dose), method of infusion (bolus vs continuous), and synergy with other cytokines such as INF-α or LAK/TIL. Unfortunately, the excitement generated from *in vitro* and pre-clinical data supporting these cellular adjunctive immunotherapeutic strategies has not recapitulated into clinical responses. Nevertheless, IL-2 remains the most efficacious of all cytokine-based therapies with response rates between 15–25% and with occasional patients achieving complete and durable responses lasting over a decade. The recent observation of disease responses seen with dendritic cell vaccination strategies provides further impetus for the development of new immune based investigational approaches such as NST.[19,20]

BACKGROUND OF ALLOGENEIC IMMUNOTHERAPY

The first clinical applications of allogeneic stem cell transplantation (SCT) in cancer date back over 35 years. Despite many clinical advances, the complications following a fully myeloablative regimen remains high, with mortality rates of up to 40%. It was widely believed that to be effective, "mega-dose" conditioning would be required to eradicate all neoplastic disease. As a by-product of intensive chemo/radiotherapy, the recipient immune system is likewise eradicated. The resultant profound level of immuno-suppression that ensues prevents the host immune system form rejecting the donor allograft. An allogeneic stem cell allograft is then infused intravenously from a human leukocyte antigen (HLA) matched sibling donor consisting of hematopoietic stem cells (typically procured from donor blood by an apheresis procedure following granulocyte-colony stimulating factor (G-CSF)-mobilization). The allograft also serves to replace the patient's immune system, containing NK and T-cells that were eradicated in the patient by chemotherapy conditioning. It also serves to rescue the patient from ensuing marrow aplasia. Patients are usually placed on immunosuppressive agents such as cyclosporine (CSA) or tacrolimus for 6–12 months following the procedure to prevent donor immune cells from attacking normal host tissues such as the GI tract, liver, or skin, a process referred to as graft-vs-host disease (GVHD). This complication may be self-limiting to life threatening and occurs in 30%–50% of patients following the procedure. Besides toxicities directly related to "mega-dose" conditioning, acute GVHD remains one of the major contributors to transplant related morbidity and mortality (TRM). Despite these limitations, myeloablative SCT has been shown to exert powerful and curative immune mediated anti-tumor effects in chemotherapy resistant and refractory hematologic malignances that otherwise would be fatal.

The observation that even the most intensive of conditioning regimens commonly failed to eradicate all leukemic cells in patients that were ultimately cured by SCT, as well as the association of a decreased risk of leukemia relapse in patients with a history of graft-versus-host disease (GVHD) gave rise to the appreciation of the donor immune mediated anti-malignancy effect coined "graft-versus-leukemia" or the "graft-versus-tumor (GVT)" response. In the last two decades there has been increasing evidence that a graft-versus-leukemia (GVL) effect, mediated through an alloimmune response of donor lymphocytes against host leukemic cells, is likely the most important component that cures hematologic malignancies.[21] In fact, it has been demonstrated that donor lymphocyte infusions in the absence of any myeloablative chemotherapy can induce complete and durable remissions in patients with leukemia relapsing after allogeneic bone marrow transplantation.[22] These results support the notion that the GVT effect following allogeneic stem cell transplantation is a potent and effective form of immunotherapy that can be used to treat malignancies.[23-26] These observations have brought into question the need for frequently toxic myeloablative conditioning regimens. Reduced intensity conditioning regimens have therefore been proposed as a less toxic alternative to the traditional myeloablative SCT.[27,28] Such low-intensity or non-myeloablative stem cell transplants (NST) are designed to provide enough immunosuppression to allow engraftment of the HLA matched donor immune system while minimizing life-threatening toxicity associated with high dose chemotherapy/radiotherapy related conditioning. NST relies on the curative effect of GVT rather than the eradication of disease by dose intensive conditioning agents. Clinical results utilizing NST in the treatment of hematologic malignancies demonstrate that such regimens are generally well tolerated, have a decreased incidence of transplant related morbidity and mortality

Table 1. Principles of NST.

Conditioning regimen
Low intensity conditioning = Low toxicity profile
Immunosuppression to prevent rejection of donor allograft
Some degree of recipient hematologic recovery (mixed chimerism)
Immunosuppression given after the transplant
Prevents graft-vs-host disease (GVHD)
Mixed chimerism
Prevents GVHD
Prevents graft-vs-tumor (GVT) effects
Can transition from mixed to full donor chimerism by GVHD prophylaxis withdrawal or infusion of
    donor lymphocytes
Donor T-cells and donor lymphocyte infusions
Promotes transition from mixed to full donor chimerism
Can cause GVHD and/or a GVT effect

(TRM), and result in high levels of donor immune system engraftment sufficient to achieve sustained remissions in some diseases.[29-33] Some of the key principles of NST are summarized in Table 1.

ALLOGENEIC TRANSPLANTATION AS ALLOGENEIC IMMUNOTHERAPY FOR METASTATIC RENAL CELL CARCINOMA

The high mortality of traditional myeloablative SCT was largely prohibitive for the investigation of SCT as immunotherapy therapy in non-hematological malignancies. In light of the decreased toxicity profile and lower risk of TRM associated with low-intensity allotransplants, the potentially beneficial effects of GVT in incurable solid malignancies could now be safely investigated. Furthermore, the observation of a systemic immunosuppressed state in patients with metastatic RCC, the finding of increased apoptosis in circulating T-lymphocytes, abnormalities in T-cell receptors and NFκB activation, as well as tolerance to potential tumor-specific antigens makes complete immunologic replacement with a healthy donor immune system attractive.[34-36] Investigators hypothesized that a transplanted allogeneic system might be capable of overcoming tumor tolerance by providing non-tolerized T-cell populations which could recognize not only tumor-specific antigens but also minor histocompatibility allo-antigens, which if expressed on the tumor, might serve as targets for a GVT effect.

Recently a few groups have published the results of pilot trials investigating NST for the treatment of metastatic RCC (Table 2).[37-42] Although they vary according to conditioning regimens employed, post transplant GVHD prophylaxis, and post transplant complication rates, in general, they have all been reported to be well tolerated. The rate and degree of engraftment of the donor immune system is also variable depending on the patients pre-transplant immune status as well as the conditioning regimen agents and choice of post transplant immunosuppression. The common feature among the various transplant methodologies lies in the fact that they are all, by definition, nonmyeloablative and therefore allow a certain degree of

Table 2. Low intensity allogeneic regimens published in metastatic renal cell carcinoma.

Investigator	Conditioning regimens	GVHD prophylaxis	Other
Childs et al[38]	Cyclophosphamide 120 mg/Kg Fludarabine 125 mg/m^2	Cyclosporine	Regression of RCC in 10/19 patients. High incidence of GVHD. Addition of MMF to cyclosporine did not reduce incidence of GVHD. Decisions regarding tapering cyclosporine/DLI based on T-cell chimerism
Rini et al[39]	Cyclophosphamide 2 g/m^2 Fludarabine 90 mg/m^2	FK 506 and MMF	4/9 engrafted patients had a GVT effect
Bregni et al[40]	Thiotepa 10 mg/kg Fludarabine 60 mg/m^2 Cyclophosphamide 60 mg/kg	Cyclosporine and methotrexate	Delayed disease regression observed in 4/7 treated patients
Makimoto et al[41]	2-cladribine 0.1 mg/kg.day X6 days Busulfan 8/mg/kg Rabbit ATG 5 mg/kg	Cyclosporine	2/3 RCC patients observed to have disease regression

autologous (patient) lymphoid and hematopoietic recovery. This means that there will be, at least for some time, populations of donor and recipient hematopoetic and immune cells living in coexistence with donor immune cells, a state called "mixed chimerism". Mixed chimerism can have both a positive and negative impact on treatment sequellae. On one hand mixed chimerism promotes graft tolerance and therefore may decrease GVHD. On the other hand, mixed chimerism may produce undesirable graft versus tumor tolerance. The fact that the majority of metastatic RCC patients have undergone no pretransplant chemotherapy (given the chemo-resistance of RCC) appears to delay the engraftment process compared to that which is typically seen in patients with hematologic malignancies. Given the proclivity for metastatic RCC to be rapidly progressive, and because the conditioning regimen has no direct anti-tumor affect, it is most desirable to have rapid donor immune engraftment kinetics to minimize the potential of tumor escape through tolerance induction. Thus most NST protocols incorporate methodologies to convert patients from mixed to complete donor T cell chimerism (full engraftment) through early withdrawal of post-transplant immunosuppression or by the infusion of donor lymphocytes. Figure 1 shows the NST scheme utilized at the National Institutes of Health (NIH) to treat patients with cytokine refractory RCC. Patients with metastatic RCC receive a non-myeloablative conditioning regimen of cyclophosphamide (120 mg/kg) and fludarabine (125 mg/m^2) over a one-week period prior to transplant. Conditioning chemotherapy is followed by the infusion of an HLA identical or single antigen mismatched sibling donor G-CSF mobilized blood stem cell allograft on day 0. Cyclosporine (CSA) is started pre-transplant and low dose

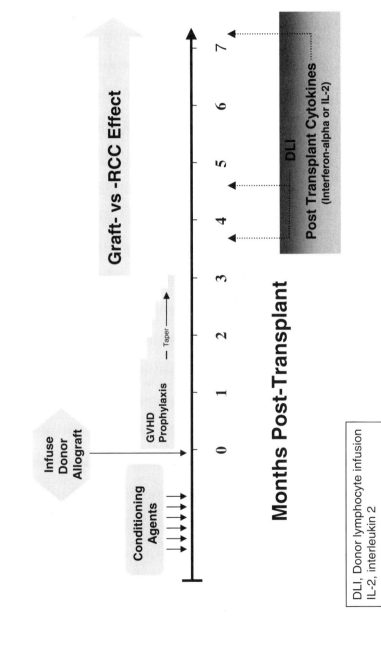

Figure 1. **Example of a typical non-myeloablative stem cell transplant strategy.** CSA, Cyclosporine; MTX, methotrexate

methotrexate is given IV on 3 separate occasions in the immediate post-transplant period as GVHD prophylaxis. Peripheral blood draws are performed at intervals after transplantation to assess T-lymphocyte and myeloid engraftment by polymerase chain reaction (PCR) based micro-satellite analysis. At day 30, patients with mixed chimerism are tapered off of immunosuppression and if needed, receive transfusions of donor lymphocytes (DLI) monthly until GVHD or disease regression occurs. Patients with full donor chimerism at day 30 receive a further 30 days of immuno-suppression until day 60, at which point a CSA taper begins.

RESULTS OF ALLOGENEIC TRANSPLANTS IN PATIENTS WITH METASTATIC RCC

NST remains an investigational approach for the treatment metastatic RCC, although definitive anti-tumor responses have been observed by several groups.[37–41] Bregni and associates recently reported the results of their nonmyeloablative-conditioning regimen that included thiotepa, fludarabine, and cyclophosphamide with CSA and methotrexate for GVHD prophylaxis. Four of 7 RCC patients treated with this regimen had a partial regression of metastatic disease. The regimen was reported to be extremely well tolerated with a low incidence of acute GVHD and with rapid and complete donor engraftment in the majority of treated patients. Rini and colleagues have also recently published their experience with NST in the treat-ment of metastatic RCC. Their initial nonmyeloablative-conditioning regimen was modified after an unacceptably high rejection rate associated with disease progres-sion in the setting of autologous hematopoiesis. Their original regimen of cyclophos-phamide $2 g/m^2$ and fludarabine $90 mg/m^2$ was increased to $4 g/m^2$ and $150 mg/m^2$ respectively, a modification that resulted in greater donor engraftment without addi-tional cases of graft rejection. Their overall response rate in 12 treated patients with greater than 180 days of follow-up was 33% in all patients and 44% in the nine patients who achieved sustained donor engraftment. Acute and chronic GVHD occurred in two and six patients respectively with a 30% incidence of transplant-related mortality. Pedrazzoli and associates also recently published their experience of reduced intensity transplantation in patients with cytokine refractory RCC.[42] They treated 7 patients with metastatic renal cell carcinoma refractory to immunotherapy/chemotherapy with a fludarabine and cytoxan based conditioning approach. Complete donor chimerism could only be achieved in patients who had a history of more intensive chemotherapy with mixed chimerism being observed in those who had received milder doses of previous chemotherapy or immunotherapy. Unfortunately, none the RCC patients achieved full donor chimerism, with 7 patients dying as a consequence of disease progression.

The preliminary results of our ongoing phase II trial at the NIH have been recently been published.[38] Ten of the first 19 patients treated with this approach had radiographic evidence of disease regression including 3 complete responders and 7 partial responses. More recently, a total of 47 patients have been treated with 21 patients (45%) having had radiographic evidence of disease regression consistent with a GVT effect. Two of the four patients who had a complete response survive in

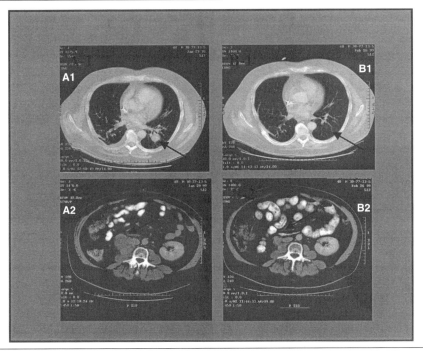

Figure 2. Graft-versus-tumor (GVT) effect following NST for metastatic RCC. a) Day 100 post-transplant CT images (**A1, A2**) of a patient with RCC with metastatic disease involving the lungs, pleura, and retroperitoneum. CT images from the same patient four weeks later, following the withdrawal of CSA showing regression of metastatic disease (**B1 and B2**)

remission 56 and 45 months after transplantation. Although pulmonary responses appear to occur most frequently, regression of metastasis in multiple sites has been observed (Figure 2 and 3). GVT effects were typically delayed by months with a median time to response of 6 months (range of 2–13 months). In most cases, disease regression did not occur until recipient T-cells were no longer detected and after CSA had been tapered. A prior history of acute GVHD was favorably associated with achieving a disease response although a few patients who had a disease response lacked evidence for GVHD and several others had resolved GVHD at the time of disease regression. The typical engraftment kinetics and their relation to clinical outcome are demonstrated in Figures 4 and 5.

TOXICITY AND LIMITATIONS OF ALLOGENEIC IMMUNOTHERAPY

Although NST may be associated with occasional dramatic regression of RCC in patients who have failed prior cytokine based immunotherapy, transplant associated toxicities appear to significantly limit this approach (Table 3). Despite the improved safety of lower intensity conditioning, the risk of TRM remains in the range of

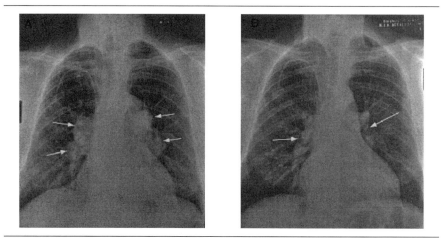

Figure 3. Pre-transplant chest x-ray of a patient with metastatic RCC with bulky bilateral hilar disease (**A**—white arrows). Regression of metastatic disease, which was markedly delayed by more than 8 months following transplantation is shown on a follow-up chest X-ray obtained 276 days post-transplant (**B**)

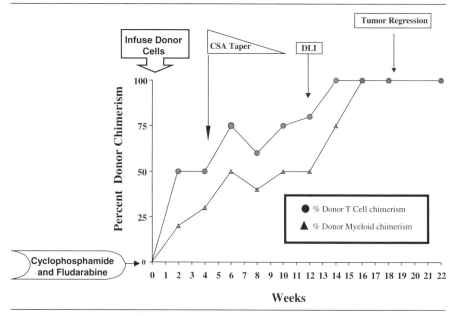

Figure 4. Engraftment profile and clinical outcome in a RCC patient undergoing non-myeloablative transplantation. T-cell engraftment (circles), and myeloid engraftment (triangles), shown as percentage donor, were initially mixed, although donor T-cell engraftment preceeded myeloid engraftment. Conversion from mixed to full donor myeloid chimerism is observed 16 weeks post-transplant Disease regression consistent with a GVT effect occurred shortly following the onset of acute GVHD

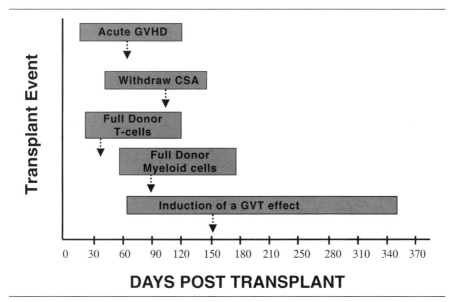

Figure 5. Time-line of events occurring after NST using cytoxan/fludarabine conditioning (Arrows represent median day of onset.)

Table 3. Limitations of allogeneic
stem cell transplantation in metastatic RCC.

Requirement for HLA matched donor (excludes approx. 2/3 of
  RCC pts.)
GVT effects delayed 4–6 months—patients with rapidly progressive
  disease less likely to survive to see benefit

Toxicity	Incidence (%)
GVHD	30–60%
CMV reactivation	20–40%
Graft rejection	5–10%
TRM	10–20%

TRM, Transplant Related Mortality

10–20%, mostly as a consequence of acute GVHD. Because of the significant risk of TRM associated with allogeneic stem cell transplantation, most investigational trials have required patients to have progressive metastatic disease and to have failed conventional cytokine based immunotherapy. Given the lag time between transplantation and a GVT effect, patients with rapid disease progression would be unlikely to gain clinical benefit from this form of therapy. Sound clinical judgment on tumor kinetics, clinical course, and expected survival must factor into the decision to treat patients with this form of therapy. Whether tumor debulking in poor prognosis patients can result in the prolongation of survival required for a GVT effect to occur is currently under investigation.

Table 4. Candidates for nonmyeloablative stem cell transplantation.

Progressive metastatic disease
Anticipated survival >6 months
Failed cytokine therapy
Absence of CNS involvement
HLA compatible sibling
No hypercalcemia

Because recent published data demonstrate a survival advantage among patients with pre-immunotherapy nephrectomy[43] and because cytokine-based immunotherapy does not typically cause regression of primary renal tumors[19] our patients routinely undergo nephrectomy prior to transplantation. This also permits accurate histological diagnosis as well as providing tissue for *in vitro* evaluation of the effector populations inducing disease regression in responding patients. At present, responses following NST have only been observed in patients presenting with the common clear cell variant of RCC. Finally, given the substantial risks of TRM associated with the use of unrelated HLA-matched donors, the majority of active NST trials in RCC require patients to have an HLA-matched sibling to serve as a stem cell donor. Unfortunately only 25–30% of patients with metastatic RCC will have such donors available to make NST a viable research option (Table 4).

CONCLUSION

Preliminary enthusiasm for NST as a novel investigational tool for metastatic RCC has been fueled to some extent by the lack of efficacious treatment provided by standard chemotherapeutics, radiotherapy, and cytokine-based immunotherapy. The observation that cytokine refractory metastatic RCC may regress following allogeneic transplantation attests to the powerful nature of the resultant GVT effect. These pilot trials provide the first clear evidence that a GVT effect can produce clinically meaningful regression of a metastatic solid tumor. With this new knowledge we have recently begun to expand the investigational use NST to other treatment refractory genitourinary tumors including metastatic bladder and prostate cancer. It is anticipated that the demonstration of GVT effects in solid malignancies will lay the groundwork for the development of future "tumor-targeted" adoptive immunotherapy approaches which might result in tumor specific GVT responses while decreasing the risk of acute GVHD. Advances in systemic and selective immunosuppressive agents that limit acute GVHD are needed to decrease the toxicity and mortality associated with allogeneic transplant approaches. Until that time, allogeneic NST should and must remain an investigational albeit promising methodology in the treatment of cytokine refractory RCC.

REFERENCES

1. Landis SH, Murray T, Bolden S, Wingo PA. Cancer statistics CA. Cancer J Clin 1999, 49:8–31.
2. Chow WH, Devesa SS, Warren JL, Fraumeni JFJ. Rising incidence of renal cell cancer in the United States. JAMA 1999, 281:1628–1631.

3. Motzer RJ, Bander NH, Nanus DM. Renal cell carcinoma. NEJM 1996, 335:856.
4. Lokich J, Harrison, JH. Renal cell carcinoma: natural history and chemotherapeutic experience. J Urol 1975:114–371.
5. Linehan WM, Shipley WU, Parkinson DR. Cancer of the kidney and ureter. In Devita VT Jr., ed. *Cancer: Principles and practice of oncology*, 4th edition. Philadelphia: JB Lippincott, 1993.
6. Yagoda A, Petrylak D, Thompson S. Cytotoxic chemotherapy for advanced renal cell carcinoma. Urol Clin North Am 1993, 20:303–314.
7. Bloom HJG. Medroxyprogesterone acetate (Provera) in the treatment of metastatic renal cell cancer. Br J Cancer 1971, 25:250.
8. Smith EM, Kursh ED, Makley J, Resnick MI. Treatment of osseous metastasis secondary to renal cell carcinoma. J Urol 1992, 148:784.
9. Bumpus HC. The apparent disappearance of pulmonary metastasis in a case of hypernephroma following nephrectomy. J Urol 1928, 20:185.
10. Fairlamb DJ. Spontaneous regression of metastatic renal cell cancer. Cancer 1981, 47:2102.
11. Evanson TC, Cole WH. Spontaneous regression of cancer. WB Saunders, Philadelphia, 1996, 11–87.
12. Bloom HJG. Renal Cancer. In *Endocrine therapy of Malignant disease*. WB Saunders, Philadelphia, 1972, 339–367.
13. Gleave ME, Elhilali M, Fredet Y, et al. Interferon Gamma-1b compared with placebo in metastatic renal cell carcinoma. NEJM 1998, 338:1265.
14. Finke JH, Rayman P, Hart L, et al. Characterization of TIL subsets from human renal cell carcinoma: specific reactivity defined by cytotoxicity, INF-γ secretion and proliferation. J Immunother 1994, 15:91.
15. Gaugler B, Brownvenstijn N, Vantomme V, et al. A new gene coding for an antigen recognized by autologous cytolytic T-Lymphocytes on human renal cell carcinoma. Immunogenetics 1996, 44: 323.
16. Finke JH, Zea AH, Stanley J, et al. Loss of T-cell receptor Zeta chain and p56lck in T-cells infiltrating human renal cell carcinoma. Cancer Res 1993, 53:5613.
17. Li X, Liu J, Park JK, et al. T cells from renal cell carcinoma patients exhibit an abnormal pattern of Kappa B-specific DNA binding activity: a preliminary report. Cancer Res 1994, 54:5424.
18. Uzzo RG, Rayman P, Bloom T. Mechanisms of apoptosis in T-cells from patients with renal cell carcinoma. Clin Cancer Res 1999, 5:1219–1229.
19. Bukowski RM. Natural history and therapy of metastatic renal cell carcinoma: the role of Interleukin-2. Cancer 1997, 80:1198–1220.
20. Kugler A, Stuhler G, Walden P, et al. Regression of human metastatic renal cell carcinoma after vaccination with tumor cell-dendritic cell hybrids. Nat Med 2000, 6:332–336.
21. Horowitz M, Gale RP, Sondel P, et al. Graft-versus-leukemia reactions after bone marrow transplantation. Blood 1991, 78:2120–2130.
22. Kolb HJ, Mittermueller J, Clemm C, et al. Donor leukocyte transfusions for treatment of recurrent chronic myelogenous leukemia in marrow transplant patients. Blood 1990, 76:2462–2465.
23. van Besien KW, de Lima M, Giralt SA, et al. Management of lymphoma recurrence after allogeneic transplantation: the relevance of graft-versus-lymphoma effect. Bone Marrow Transplant 1997, 19:977–982.
24. Verdonck L, Lokhorst H, Dekker A, et al. Graft-versus-myeloma effect in 2 cases. Lancet 1996, 347: 800–801.
25. Eibl B, Schwaighofer H, Nachbaur D, et al. Evidence of a graft-versus-tumor effect in a patient treated with marrow ablative chemotherapy and allogeneic bone marrow transplantation for breast cancer. Blood 1996, 88:1501–1508.
26. Ueno NT, Rondon G, Mirza NQ, et al. Allogeneic peripheral-blood progenitor-cell transplantation for poor-risk patients with metastatic breast cancer. J Clin Oncol 1998, 16:986–993.
27. Giralt S, Estey E, Albitar M, et al. Engraftment of allogeneic hematopoietic progenitor cells with purine analog-containing chemotherapy: harnessing graft-versus-leukemia without myeloablative therapy. Blood 1997, 89:4531–4536.
28. Slavin S, Nagler A, Naparastak E, et al. Nonmyeloablative stem cell transplantation and cell therapy as an alternative to conventional bone marrow transplantation with lethal cytoreduction for the treatment of malignant and non malignant hematologic diseases. Blood 1998, 91:756–763.
29. Khouri J, Keating MJ, Korbling M, et al. Transplant lite: induction of graft vs malignancy using fludarabine based nonablative chemotherapy and allogeneic progenitor-cell transplantation as treatment for lymphoid malignancies. J Clin Oncol 1998, 16:2817–2824.

30. Sykes M, Preffer F, McAfee S, et al. Mixed lymphohaemopoietic chimerism and graft-versus-lymphoma effects after non-myeloablative therapy and HLA mismatched bone-marrow transplantation. Lancet 1999, 353:1755–1759.

31. Childs R, Clave E, Contentin N, et al. Engraftment kinetics after nonmyeloablative allogeneic peripheral blood stem cell transplantation: full donor T-cell chimerism preceded alloimmune responses. Blood 1999, 94:3234–3241.

32. Sandmaier BM, McSweeney P, Yu C, Storb R. Nonmyeloablative transplants: preclinical and clinical results. Semin Oncol 2000, 27(suppl 5):78–81.

33. Bornhauser M, Thiede C, Schuler U, et al. Dose-reduced conditioning for allogeneic blood stem cell transplantation: durable engraftment without antithymocyte globulin. Bone Marrow Transplant 2000, 26:119–125.

34. Finke JH, Zea AH, Stanley J, et al. Loss of T-cell receptor zeta chain and p56lck in T-cells infiltrating human renal cell carcinoma. Cancer Res 1993, 53:5613–5616.

35. Li X, Liu J, Park JK, et al. T cells from renal cell carcinoma patients exhibit an abnormal pattern of kappa B-specific DNA binding activity: a preliminary report. Cancer Res 1994, 54:5424–5429.

36. Uzzo RG, Rayman P, Bloom T. Mechanisms of apoptosis in T-cells from patients with renal cell carcinoma. Clin Cancer Res 1999, 5:1219–1229.

37. Childs R, Clave E, Tisdale J, et al. Successful treatment of metastatic renal cell carcinoma with a nonmyeloablative allogeneic peripheral blood progenitor cell transplant: evidence for a graft-versus-tumor effect. J Clin Oncol 1999, 17:2044–2051.

38. Childs R, Chernoff A, Contentin N, et al. Regression of metastatic renal-cell carcinoma after nonmyeloablative allogeneic peripheral-blood stem-cell transplantation. N Engl J Med 2000, 343: 750–758.

39. Rini B, Zimmerman TM, Stadler W, et al. Allogeneic stem-cell transplantation of Renal Cell Cancer after nonmyeloablative chemotherapy: Feasibility, engraftment, and clinical results. J Clin Onc 2002, 20(8):2017–2024.

40. Bregni M, Dodero A, Peccatori J, et al. Nonmyeloablative conditioning followed by hematopoietic cell allografting and donor lymphocyte infusions for patients with metastatic renal and breast cancer. Blood 2002, 99(11):4234–4236.

41. Makimoto A, Mineishi S, Tanosaki R, et al. Nonmyeloablative stem cell transplantation (NST) for refractory solid tumors [abstract]. Proc Am Soc Clin Oncol 2001, 20:44.

42. Pedrazzoli P, Da Prada G, Giorgiani G, et al. Allogeneic blood stem cell transplantation after reduced intensity, preparative regimen—a pilot study in patients with refractory malignancies. Cancer 2002, 94(9):2409–2416.

43. Flanigan RC, Salmon SE, Blummenstein EA, et al. Nephrectomy followed by interferon alpha-2b compared with interferon alpha-2b alone for metastatic renal cancer. NEJM 2001, 345:1655–1659.

14. NOVEL THERAPIES FOR RENAL CELL CARCINOMA

SAMIRA SYED M.D.

Division of Medical Oncology, University of Texas Health Science Center at San Antonio

ANTHONY W. TOLCHER M.D., FRCP(C)

Associate Director Clinical Research, Institute for Drug Development, Cancer Therapy and Research Center and Associate Clinical Professor of Medicine, University of Texas Health Science Center at San Antonio.

INTRODUCTION

The treatment of advanced renal cell carcinoma presents a daunting challenge to medical, surgical and radiation oncologists. Although patients with localized renal cell carcinoma can be effectively treated by surgery with a 5 year survival of up to 88%, the treatment options are limited for patients with advanced disease with the 5 year survival rate under 10%.[1,2] Furthermore, systemic chemotherapeutic agents have had little impact on the natural history of this disease. A comprehensive review by Yagoda *et al*[3] encompassed 4542 patients enrolled in 83 clinical trials published from 1983 through 1993. Among the 4093 evaluable patients, a 6% overall response rate was determined which was comprised of 53 (1.3%) complete responses and 192 (4.7%) partial responses. This dismal level of antitumor activity is comparable to the reported rate of spontaneous objective responses observed for placebo treated patients entered in a randomized study.[4]

The failure of conventional chemotherapy to have a significant impact on the long-term survival of those individuals with metastatic renal cell carcinoma has prompted the exploration of alternative treatment strategies. In recent years cytokine-based immunotherapy has emerged as the primary option for the systemic treatment of advanced renal cell carcinoma. The quality and durability of the responses with interleukin-2 (IL-2) based immunotherapy, while superior to those

Address for Correspondence: Anthony W. Tolcher, 7979 Wurzbach Suite 414, San Antonio, TX 78229.
E-mail: atolcher@saci.org

R.A. Figlin (ed.). KIDNEY CANCER. Copyright © 2003. Kluwer Academic Publishers. Boston. All rights reserved.

seen with chemotherapy, remain modest. In addition, due to associated toxicity of this treatment, only a minority of patients with advanced disease are appropriate candidates for therapy. As a result, there is a tremendous impetus to examine novel therapies for patients with renal cell carcinoma. In the following chapter several novel investigational approaches for the treatment of advanced renal cell carcinoma that are currently in clinical trials are described.

ANTIANGIOGENESIS STRATEGIES IN RENAL CELL CARCINOMA

The critical role of tumor-associated angiogenesis in promoting maximal growth, invasion and metastasis has been demonstrated in the pioneering studies of Folkman and his colleagues.[5,6] They demonstrated that tumor growth beyond a minimal volume requires the formation of new capillary blood vessels from pre-existing microvessels by endothelial cell outgrowth. This process involves appropriate changes in the extracellular matrix that allows proliferating endothelial cells to migrate and form new vessels within the surrounding tissue. The process of angiogenesis is regulated by a dynamic equilibrium of positive and negative regulators. Under normal circumstances, the net outcome of this equilibrium is a nearly static vasculature. In advanced cancer, the balance is shifted in favor of angiogenesis. There are two main classes of angiogenic factors, the first includes specific factors released by numerous cell types that bind specifically to receptors on endothelial cells and stimulate their growth, migration and differentiation. Vascular endothelial growth factor (VEGF) is among the specific factors that stimulate angiogenesis. The second class consists of non-specific angiogenic factors that either indirectly or directly promote angiogenesis. These factors include the fibroblast growth factors, transforming growth factor–α, epidermal growth factor, platelet derived growth factor, and integrins.[7–11] Agents that target many of these factors represent rational drug development strategies for patients with renal cell and other advanced solid malignancies.

The vascular nature of renal cell carcinoma (RCC) has led to a rapid expansion of research elucidating the role of angiogenesis in the growth of this tumor and its metastases. Clear-cell carcinoma is characterized by both a high degree of vascularity and a high prevalence (75–80%) of mutations and hypermethylation in the von-Hippel-Lindau (VHL) gene.[12] Wild-type VHL protein is a ubiquitin ligase which ubiquinates and thereby causes the degradation of hypoxia-inducible factor-alpha (HIF-1α), a transcription factor that regulates a number of genes involved in angiogenesis including VEGF and PDGF.[13] Mutations in the VHL gene inhibit the function of the VHL protein thereby resulting in an overproduction of HIF-1α and overexpression of angiogenic factors, including VEGF, downstream.[13]

Increased VEGF expression has also been found in the majority of hypervascular renal cell carcinoma, whereas hypovascular tumors express low levels of this factor.[14] Increased serum levels of VEGF have been correlated with tumor burden.[15,16] and shortened progression free survival and overall survival.[17] Furthermore, decreases in serum VEGF levels have been correlated with successful therapy.[16] Similar evidence of a worse prognosis has been described with other pro-angiogenic factors. Pathologic evidence indicates that basic fibroblast growth factor (bFGF) is expressed immunohistochemically in the extracellular matrix of 87% of renal cell carcinoma pathologic specimens and also predicts a worse disease specific survival in patients with localized disease following nephrectomy (p = 0.008).[18]

Based on these findings, therapeutic approaches that target angiogenesis are particularly attractive in renal cell carcinoma.

VEGF TARGETED THERAPIES

VEGF is a potent mitogen that induces endothelial cell migration, invasion, and *in vitro*, the formation of endothelial tube-like structures at picomolar concentrations.[16,19] VEGF receptors (VEGFR) are expressed almost exclusively on endothelial cells and following VEGF ligand binding the receptors undergo dimerization and activation of the intracellular tyrosine kinase with downstream signaling. Activation of VEGFR2 increases vascular permeability, leads to the formation of a lattice network of endothelial cells that acts as a substrate for tumor cell growth.[20] In addition, VEGF acts as an endothelial cell survival factor[7,8,9] with experimental evidence that inhibition of VEGF activity will induce endothelial cell apoptosis. Based on the multiplicity of available targets available with receptor tyrosine kinase pathways, various strategies are currently in clinical evaluation to inhibit VEGF pathway including antibodies to VEGF or its receptors, use of hammerhead ribozymes to inhibit receptor expression, and tyrosine kinase inhibitors that block receptor activation and downstream signaling.[7,21]

An anti-VEGF neutralizing antibody (Bevacizumab) is currently being studied in several phase III trials. This recombinant humanized monoclonal antibody to VEGF contains the human immunoglobulin G_1 framework (93%) with a murine VEGF-binding region (7%). The antibody blocks the binding of all VEGF isoforms to the receptors and inhibits the biologic activities of VEGF as measured by assays for endothelial mitogenesis, vascular permeability and *in vivo* angiogenesis.[22]

In the phase I study of rhuMab VEGF, 30 patients with advanced solid tumors were evaluated. The serum half life of rhuMab VEGF was found to be approximately 13 days and at doses ≥0.3 mg/kg rhuMab VEGF provided complete suppression of circulating VEGF. The toxicities encountered occurred during the first several hours after antibody infusion and were limited to grade 1 or 2 headache, nausea, asthenia and low grade fever in fewer than 20% of patients treated. Intratumoral hemorrhage was reported in two patients who received treatment with rhuMab VEGF at the 3 mg/kg dose level.[23]

The synergistic anti-tumor activity of antibodies to VEGF and cytotoxic chemotherapy has been demonstrated in at least two human cell lines in animal models. In the Calu-6 human lung cancer cell line, this synergy was demonstrated with cis-platinum, whereas in the MCF-7 breast cancer cell line the enhanced anti-tumor effect was seen with doxorubicin.[24,25] Based on preclinical and phase I studies, the safety of combining rhu Mab VEGF with chemotherapy was tested. One recently completed phase I study, combined rhuMab VEGF (3 mg/kg weekly) with three standard chemotherapy regimens: doxorubicin 50 mg/m2 every 4 weeks, carboplatin AUC 6 plus paclitaxel 175 mg/m2 every 4 weeks and 5-FU 500 mg/m2 with leucovorin 20 mg/m2 weekly.[22] This study demonstrated that the drug could be delivered safely in combination with chemotherapy at doses associated with VEGF blockade without synergistic toxicity.

A recently completed double blind placebo controlled phase III trial assessed the activity of rhuMAb in metastatic RCC.[26] In this study, 110 patients were randomized to receive placebo or rhu Mab VEGF at either a low dose (3 mg/kg) or a high dose (10 mg/kg). The primary endpoints of this study were time to disease progression and response rate. Interim analysis showed a highly significant prolongation of time to progression in patients receiving high dose rhuMab VEGF compared to placebo (p = 0.001). The difference between the low dose rhuMab VEGF and placebo was of borderline significance. Furthermore, four objective responses were observed in the high dose arm (10 mg/kg). Toxicity at both doses of the antibody was minimal, however hypertension and asymptomatic proteinuria were most prominent in the high dose arm. This study provides important "proof of concept" for angiogenesis strategies in renal cell carcinoma and supports the further investigation of this agent alone or in combination with other therapies for patients with advanced RCC.

An alternate strategy for inhibiting VEGF activity is the use of selective inhibitors of membrane receptor tyrosine kinases. These competitive inhibitors of tyrosine kinase activation localize at the ATP binding site and inhibit phosphorylation and activation of downstream signaling following VEGF receptor binding. The prototypic VEGFR tyrosine kinase inhibitor is SU5416 (semaxanib). This small, lipophilic, highly protein bound synthetic molecule selectively inhibits the autophosphorylation of flk-1 induced by the interaction of VEGF with its receptor.[27] In preclinical studies SU5416 was shown to be a potent inhibitor of VEGF-mediated signaling, inhibited VEGF dependent mitogenesis of human endothelial cells, and following systemic administration of SU5416 to mice, inhibited a broad spectrum of subcutaneously implanted tumor cell lines.[28] The maximum tolerated dose (MTD) for SU5416 in 63 patients with advanced malignancies enrolled onto a phase I study was determined to be 145 mg/m^2.[29] This dose resulted in systemic exposure comparable to what was required in animals to produce effective growth inhibition.[29] Phase I studies have suggested that this agent is generally well tolerated, the dose limiting toxicities (DLT) being projectile vomiting, nausea and severe headache. Other adverse effects included superficial and deep phlebitis, dry and raspy voice and fatigue.[29-31] This agent however possessed an unfavorable pharmacokinetic profile with rapid elimination, poor oral bio-availability requiring intravenous administration, and a brief plasma half-life that required twice-weekly intravenous dosing. These features may ultimately have limited the efficacy of this agent in randomized studies.

Several orally bio-available VEGFR 2 tyrosine kinase inhibitors are currently being evaluated in phase I studies.[32-34] *In vitro*, these agents inhibit VEGF stimulated VEGFR-2 autophosphorylation and the proliferation in endothelial cells. In human tumor cell line xenografts these agents elicit substantial tumor growth delay in a broad spectrum of tumors. Toxicities encountered in phase I studies include hypertension and proteinuria that may represent a "class effect" for toxicities associated with VEGF targeting strategies.[32-34] Favorable pharmacokinetic profiles, and the oral route of administration may permit clinical studies that will ultimately test these agents' proof of concept.

In summary, therapies targeting VEGF and the VEGFR pathway appear to be promising investigational strategies for patients with renal cell carcinoma with preliminary evidence of proof of concept.

OTHER INHIBITORS OF ANGIOGENESIS

Anti-angiogenic properties have been identified in agents used initially for different effects. Thalidomide, which was withdrawn from the market because of its severe teratogenic effects, has potent anti-angiogenic activity *in vitro* and *in vivo*. Thalidomide is thought to inhibit angiogenesis through the non-specific inhibition of multiple cytokines and components of the angiogenic process including TNF-alpha, bFGF, VEGF, interleukin 6 and interleukin 8.[7,35-37] The anti-angiogenic potential of thalidomide has precipitated a number of clinical trials either alone or in combination with other agents.

In renal cell carcinoma the results have been mixed and conflicting. In one study of 25 patients the objective response rate was 9% with 32% percent of patients experiencing stable disease for more than 6 months.[38] In contrast, in 26 patients treated with escalating doses of thalidomide there were no objective responses. In this latter study, because the natural history of renal cell carcinoma includes persistent stable disease in some patients, the authors concluded that routine use in renal cell patients should not be considered.[39] Further studies are underway to evaluate the role of thalidomide alone or in combination with other agents in the treatment of RCC.

Interferon-α has been evaluated significantly in patients with advanced renal cell carcinoma with an overall response rate of up to 16%.[1] Interferon alpha has known anti-angiogenic effects mediated, at least in part, by suppression of b-FGF expression.[40] However, the dose and schedule of interferon alpha that maximizes the anti-angiogenic potential of this drug is not known. Based on a presumption that continuous exposure to anti-angiogenetic agents will be required to achieve tumor growth inhibition, modified formulations of interferon alpha that sustain plasma concentrations over prolonged periods of time, such as pegylated interferon, may allow the angiogenesis inhibitory properties of interferon alpha to be further explored.[41]

Compounds that inhibit the function of proliferating endothelial cells are also under evaluation. TNP-470 is a synthetic analogue of fumagillin, a naturally occurring secreted product of the fungus Aspergillus fumigates fresenius. Accidental contamination of an endothelial cell culture led to the identification of fumagillin as an inhibitor of angiogenesis.[42] TNP-470 *in vitro* inhibits endothelial cell proliferation including growth stimulated by basic fibroblast growth factor (b-FGF) and also inhibits tumor growth and metastases *in vivo* in a number of rodent tumor model systems including a rodent renal cell carcinoma.[42-46] A phase II study using this compound has recently been completed in patients with refractory renal cell carcinoma.[43] Of the thirty-three patients treated, one had an objective response and prolonged stable disease was observed in six patients. Since the trial was not specifically designed to assess disease stabilization the clinical significance of the proportion of patients experiencing stable disease is not known.

Carboxyamidotriazol (CAI) is an oral agent in phase II trials for the treatment of renal cell carcinoma. CAI is an inhibitor of phospholipase C-□ and phospholipase A2 phosphorylation.[16,47,48] Blockade of this pathway prevents the release of arachadonic acid, which inhibits malignant proliferation and metastasis.[49] CAI also has anti-angiogenic effects mediated by bFGF inhibition.[16,49] In phase I studies this agent has been well tolerated with asthenia and reversible ataxia the dose limiting toxicity.[16] In these trials, minor responses and disease stabilization was observed in a number of patients with metastatic renal cell carcinoma which has resulted in the evaluation of this agent in phase II studies for RCC.[16]

EPIDERMAL GROWTH FACTOR RECEPTOR TARGETING AGENTS

The epidermal growth factor receptor (EGFR) represents a potentially attractive therapeutic target for the treatment of renal cell carcinoma. The epidermal growth factor receptor is a type I receptor tyrosine kinase involved in cellular differentiation and proliferation of both normal and malignant cells. The receptor is composed of three major domains: the extracellular ligand binding domain, a transmembrane lipohilic component, and the cytoplasmic tyrosine kinase domain. Following binding by ligand (EGF, transforming growth factor α, and others) EGFR undergoes hetero and homodimerization that induces tyrosine kinase autophosphorylation. Expression and overexpression of EGFR occurs in the majority of patients with clear cell carcinoma, and therefore, inhibition of EGFR represent a logical experimental therapeutic strategy in the management of this malignancy.[41] A number of inhibitors of the epidermal growth factor receptor (EGFR) are currently under development including monoclonal antibodies directed to the extracellular domain of EGF receptor and small molecule inhibitors of the internal tyrosine kinase domain.

C225 (cetuximab) is an investigational chimeric monoclonal antibody directed against the extracellular domain of the erbB1 receptor. This antibody binds with an affinity 10 fold greater than those of the natural ligands (epidermal growth factor and transforming growth factor alpha).[50–55] C225 inhibits EGF-induced activation, auto-phosphorylation and internalization of EGFR.[52,54,55] Cetuximab and other monoclonal antibodies directed to EGFR inhibit the growth of erbB1 expressing cancers in vitro.[52,53,55,56] and inhibit tumor growth in vivo and increase survival of a wide range of EGFR expressing subcutaneously implanted human tumor xenograft models including pancreas, breast, colon, head and neck and prostate cancers.[54,55] C225 has been shown to enhance radio-sensitivity in vitro and in vivo.[55,56] There is also evidence that the growth inhibitory effects are additive and synergistic when combined with various chemotherapeutic agents including cisplatin and doxorubicin.[55,57] In phase I studies C225 had a half-life of approximately seven days with saturation of EGFR binding sites at 200 mg/m2 IV.[55,58] The most common toxicity of this agent is an acneiform rash and folliculitis. The skin reaction usually involves the face, upper chest, and back, and is likely related to the prominent role of EGFR and EGF-like ligands in epidermal tissues. C225 is currently being evaluated in several phase II studies both alone and in combination with other chemotherapeutic agents for a variety of advanced solid tumors known to over-express EGFR. A recently completed phase II study evaluated C225 in 54 patients with advanced renal cell carcinoma. There was one partial response (PR) and two minimal responses (MR) reported with this therapy however, more than 25% of the patients treated achieved stable disease for at least six months.[59]

ABX-EGF (Abgenix) is a fully humanized IgG2k monoclonal antibody specific to EGFR with nearly a 10-fold higher binding affinity for EGFR than C225. This monoclonal antibody exhibits marked tumor growth inhibition including tumor regressions in a broad spectrum of human tumor xenograft models.[60,61] The degree of cellular EGFR expression appears to be relevant for antitumor activity. Tumors that express greater number of EGFR molecules per cell demonstrated marked growth inhibition when treated with ABX-EGF whereas tumors that did not express EGFR did not.[54] Preliminary results of a phase I study of ABX-EGF in solid tumors that express EGFR indicate that this agent is well tolerated at doses predicted to induce anti-tumor activity.[61] As with C225, transient acneiform rashes have been reported with ABX-EGF. In the preliminary report of a phase II evaluation of the ABX-EGF antibody in metastatic renal cell carcinoma patients, objective responses have been observed in approximately 10% of patients. Furthermore, some patients experienced prolonged stable disease exceeding 40 weeks.[62]

Inhibition of EGFR may also be mediated by small molecule inhibitors of the tyrosine kinase domain. These molecules that contain common quinazoline backbone structures, including ZD 1839 (Iressa) and OSI 774 (Tarceva), demonstrate competitive inhibition of ATP binding of the tyrosine kinase domain.[54] Inhibition of the receptor tyrosine kinase function inhibits autophosphorylation associated with ligand binding, induces cell cycle arrest and reduces cell proliferation in EGFR expressing cells.[54] In some experimental models that are dependent upon EGFR activation for growth, tumor regressions are observed following exposure to EGFR tyrosine kinase inhibitors.[63] Inhibition of EGFR tyrosine kinase activity may also demonstrate tumor growth properties mediated by mechanisms independent of the antiproliferative mechanism of action. Inhibition of EGFR tyrosine kinase activity also inhibits malignant angiogenesis through downstream inhibition of VEGF expression.[64]

The preliminary results of phase 1 studies of ZD1839 and OSI 774 in patients with advanced malignancies known to overexpress erbB demonstrate that these agents are generally well tolerated.[65–70] The most common toxicity is an acneiform rash, nausea, vomiting, hyperbilirubinemia, and diarrhea. Both intermittent and continuous schedules have been evaluated. The pharmacokinetic profile of ZD1839 and OSI 774 indicate that these agents are suitable for once daily dosing.[64–66,70]

Preliminary evidence of antitumor activity in patients with metastatic renal cell carcinoma was observed during the phase I study of OSI 774.[70] A complete response in pulmonary, retroperitoneal and peritoneal lymph node metastases was observed in one patient who subsequently underwent resection of the primary tumor. This observation provided the impetus for further development of this agent in renal cell carcinoma. However, since these agents will likely have a low objective response rate and may represent cytostatic rather than cytotoxic agents, careful clinical trial design accompanied by the identification of predictive biomarkers of response will be critical to determine the utility of these agents and the optimal patient population that will most benefit from EGFR-inhibiting therapy.

OTHER INVESTIGATIONAL STRATEGIES FOR RENAL CELL CARCINOMA

A novel chemotherapeutic agent under investigation for patients with renal cell carcinoma is BMS-247550. This compound is a semi-synthetic epothilone B analogue. Epothilone B agents bind to tubulin at distinct sites from those of the taxane molecules and induce tubulin polymerization. Similar to paclitaxel, this agent blocks the cell cycle at G_2-M transition stage and induces cellular apoptosis.[71] In vitro, it is twice as potent as paclitaxel in inducing tubulin polymerization and is a highly potent cytotoxic agent capable of killing cancer cells at low nanomolar concentrations. Significant anti-tumor activity has also been demonstrated in both paclitaxel-sensitive and -refractory cell lines.[72] This drug is currently in broad phase II testing including trials for patients with advanced renal cell carcinoma.

CCI-779, an ester of the immunosupressive agent sirolimus (rapamune), has also demonstrated some anti-tumor activity in patients with advanced renal cell carcinoma in phase I clinical studies.[73] This compound has potent immunosuppressant and anti-proliferative properties. This stems from the drug's ability to modulate the Akt/phosphoinosital-3-kinase (PI3 kinase) signal transduction pathways linking growth stimuli from receptor tyrosine kinases to the synthesis of specific proteins required for cell cycle progression from G1 to S phase. In addition, CCI-779 inhibits proliferation of endothelial cells and therefore, may also have an anti-angiogenesis effect independent of direct tumor cytostasis and apoptosis.[74] CCI-779 demonstrated single agent activity in patients with renal cell carcinoma during the phase I clinical development, and has modest rate of antitumor activity in a phase II evaluation.[75]

Modified formulations of immunotherapy agents are being developed to improve efficacy and reduce toxicity. One such agent in phase I trials is albuleukin, a genetic-engineered fusion protein consisting of the mature form of recombinant human albumin attached to the C-terminal end of the mature form of recombinant IL2. The fusion protein is designed to have the favorable pharmacological properties, particularly the sustained half-life of human albumin, combined with the lymphocyte activation properties of IL2. This agent, while still in the earliest stages of clinical evaluation, may hold promise for patients with advanced renal cell carcinoma.

A similar strategy utilizes the addition of polyethylene glycol moieties to Interferon-α which is has also been evaluated in renal cell carcinoma. The metabolism of this formulation, through the sequential elimination of PEG molecules, allows for sustained drug levels and therefore may provide a more continuous exposure to the immunostimulatory properties of Interferon-α[41].

In conclusion, conventional chemotherapy is largely ineffective for advanced renal cell carcinoma and immunobiologic approaches to this disease have some valid utility but can be applied but only a minority of patients. There exists a tremendous impetus for the development of novel treatment for this disease. Newer targeted based therapies have demonstrated encouraging, albeit preliminary, evidence of anti-tumor activity and provide some optimism that effective treatments may be on the horizon.

REFERENCES

1. DeVita VT, Hellman S, Rosenberg SA (2001) Cancer Principles and Practice of Oncology, 6th Edition. pp 1362–1394.
2. Cancer Facts and Figures 2002: Surveillance, Epidemiology and End Results Program (1973–1998). Division of Cancer Control and Population Sciences, National Cancer Institute, Bethesda.
3. Yagoda A, Abi-Bached B, Petrylak D (1995) Chemotherapy for advanced renal cell carcinoma: 1983–1993. Semin Oncol 22: 42.
4. Gleave ME, Elhilali M, Fradet Y, et al (1998) Interferon Gamma-1b compared with placebo in metastatic renal cell carcinoma. N Engl J Med 338: 1265–1271.
5. Folkman J (1971) Tumor angiogenesis: therapeutic implications. N Engl J Med 285: 1182–1186.
6. Folkman J (1990) What is the evidence that tumors are angiogenesis dependent? J Nat Cancer Inst 82: 4–6.
7. Ellis LM (2002) Angiogenesis. Horizons in cancer therapeutics. 3: 4–22.
8. Gerber HP, Dixit V, Ferrara N (1998) Vascular endothelial growth factor induces expression of the antiapoptotic proteins Bcl-2 and A1 in vascular endothelial cells. J Biol Chem 273: 13313–13316.
9. Gerber HP, McMurtrey A, Kowalski J, et al (1998) Vascular endothelial growth factor regulates endothelial cell survival through the phosphatidylinositol 3'-kinase/Akt signal transduction pathway. J Biol Chem 273: 30336–30343.
10. Eliceiri BP, Cheresh DA (1999) The role of alpha v integrins during angiogenesis: insights into potential mechanisms of action and clinical development. J Clin Invest 103: 1227–1230.
11. Scatena M, Almeida M, Chaisson ML, et al (1998) NF-Kappa B mediates alpha v beta 3 integrin-induced endothelial cell survival. J Cell Biol 141: 1083–1093.
12. Zbar B (1995) Von Hippel-Lindau disease and sporadic renal cell carcinoma. Cancer Surveys 25: 219–232.
13. Clifford SC, Astuti D, Hooper L, et al (2001) The pVHL-associated SCF ubiquitin ligase complex: molecular genetic analysis of elongin B and C, Rbx 1 and HIF-1 alpha in renal cell carcinoma. Oncogene 20: 5067–5074.
14. Takahashi A, Sasaki H, Kim SJ, et al (1994) Markedly increased amounts of messenger RNAs for vascular endothelial growth factor and placenta growth factor in renal cell carcinoma associated with angiogenesis. Cancer Res 54: 4233–4237.
15. Baccala AA, Zhong H, Clift SM, et al (1998) Serum vascular endothelial growth factor is a candidate biomarker of metastatic tumor response to ex vivo gene therapy of renal cell cancer. Urology 51: 327–332.
16. Bigelow KR, Spiotto MT, Stadler WM (2001) Anti-angiogenic Agents and Strategies in Renal Cell Carcinoma. Current Clin Oncol pg 381–395.
17. Blay JY, Pallardy M, Ravaud A, et al (1999) Serum VEGF is an independent prognostic factor in patients with metastatic renal carcinoma treated with IL-2 and/or interferon: Analysis of the CRECY trial. Proc Am Soc Clin Oncol. 18: 433a; A 1669.
18. Nanus DM, Schmitz-Drager BJ, Motzer RJ, et al (1993) Expression of basic fibroblast growth factor in primary human renal tumors: Correlation with poor survival. J Natl Cancer Inst 85: 1597–1599.
19. Asano M, Yukita A, Matsumoto T, et al (1995) Inhibition of tumor growth and metastatses by an immuno-neutralizing monoclonal antibody to human vascular endothelial growth factor/vascular permeability factor 121, Cancer Res. 55: 5296–5301.
20. Ferrara N, Houck K, Jakeman L, et al (1992) Molecular and biological properties of the vascular endothelial cell growth factor family of proteins. Endocrine Rev 13: 18–32.
21. Basche M, Sandler AB, Eckhardt SG, et al (2002) Angiozyme, an anti-VEGFR1 ribozyme, carboplatin and paclitaxel: results of a phase I study. Proc Am Soc Clin Oncol 21: 112a abst 445.

22. Margolin K, Gordon MS, Holmgren E, et al (2001) Phase 1b Trial for Intravenous Recombinant Humanized Monoclonal Antibody to Vascular Endothelial Growth Factor in Combination with Chemotherapy in Patients with Advanced Cancer: Pharmacologic and Long-Term Safety Data. J Clin Oncol 19: 851–856.

23. Gordon MS, Margolin K, Talpaz M, et al (2001) Phase I safety and pharmacokinetic study of recombinant human anti-vascular endothelial growth factor in patients with advanced cancer. J Clin Oncol 19: 843–850.

24. Kabbinavar FF, Wong JT, Ayala RE, et al (1995) The effect of antibody to vascular endothelial growth factor and cisplatin on the growth of lung tumors in nude mice. Proc Am Assoc Cancer Res 36: 488; abst 2906.

25. Borgström P, Gold DP, Hilan KJ, et al (1999) Importance of VEGF for breast cancer angiogenesis in vivo: Implications from intravital microscopy of combination treatments with an anti-VEGF neutralizing monoclonal antibody and doxorubicin. Anticancer Res 19: 4203–4214.

26. Yang JC, Haworth L, Steinberg SM, et al (2002) A randomized double-blind placebo-controlled trial of bevacizmab (anti-VEGF antibody) demonstrating a prolongation in time to progression in patients with metastatic renal cancer. Proc Am Soc Clin Oncol 21: 5a; A15.

27. Strawn LM, Mc Maho G, App H, et al (1996) Flk-1 as a target for tumor growth inhibition. Cancer Res 56: 3540–3545.

28. Fong TA, Shawver LK, Sun L, et al (1999) SU5416 is a potent and selective inhibitor of the vascular endothelial growth factor receptor (Flk-1/KDR) that inhibits tyrosine kinase catalysis, tumor vascularization and growth of multiple tumor types, Cancer Res 59: 99–106.

29. Rosen L, Mulay M, Mayers A, et al (1999) Phase I dose-escalating trial of SU5416, a novel angiogenesis inhibitor in patients with advanced malignancies. Proc Am Soc Clin Oncol. 18: 161a; A618

30. Cropp G, Rosen L, Mulay M, et al (1999) Pharmacokinetics and pharmacodynamics of SU5416 in a phase I, dose escalating trial in patients with advanced malignancies. Proc Am Soc Cliin Oncol 18: 161a; A619.

31. Stopeck A. (2000) Results of a phase I dose-escalating study of the anti-angiogenic agent, SU5416, in patients with advanced malignancies. Proc Am Soc Clin Oncol 19: 206a; A802.

32. Tolcher A, Karp DD, O'leary DD, et al (2002) A phase I and biologic correlative study of an oral vascular endothelial growth factor receptor-2 (VEGF-2) tyrosine kinase inhibitor, CP 547,632 in patients with advanced malignancies. Proc Am Soc Clin Oncol 21: 84a; A334.

33. Hurwitz H, Holden SN, Eckhardt SG, et al (2002) Clinical evaluation of ZD6474, an orally active inhibitor of VEGF signaling in patients with solid tumors. Proc Am Soc Clin Oncol 21: 82a; A325.

34. Drevs J, Schmidt-Gersbach IM Mross K, et al (2002) Surrogate markers for the assessment of biologic activity of the VEGF-receptor inhibitor PTK787/ZK 222584 (PTK/ZK) in two clinical trials. Proc Am Soc Clin Oncol 21: 85a; A337.

35. D'Amato RJ, Loughnan MS, Flynn E, et al (1994) Thalidomide is an inhibitor of angiogenesis. Proc Natl Acad Sci USA. 91: 4082–4085.

36. Rowland TL, McHugh SM, Deighton J, et al (1998) Differential regulation by thalidomide and dexamethasone of cytokine expression in human peripheral blood mononuclear cells. Immunopharmacology. 40: 11–20.

37. Koch HP (1985) Thalidomide and congeners as anti-inflammatory agents. Prog Med Chem. 22: 165–242.

38. Stebbing J, Benson C, Eisen T, et al (2001) The treatment of advanced renal cell cancer with high-dose oral thalidomide Br J Cancer 85: 953–958.

39. Motzer RJ, Berg W, Ginsberg M, et al (2002) Phase II trial of thalidomide for patients with advanced renal cell carcinoma. J Clin Oncol 20: 302–306.

40. Singh RK, Gutman M, Bucvana CD, et al (1995) Interferons alpha and beta down-regulate the expression of basic fibroblast growth factor in human carcinomas. Proc Natl Acad Sci USA 92: 4562–4566.

41. Berg WJ, Divgi CR, Nanus DM, et al (2000) Novel Investigative Approaches for Advanced Renal Cell Carcinoma. Semin Oncol 27: 234–239.

42. Ingber D, Fujita T, Kishimoto S, Sudo K, et al (1990) Synthetic analogues of fumagillin that inhibit angiogenesis and suppress tumor growth. Nature 348: 555–557.

43. Stadler WM, Kuzel T, Shapiro C, et al (1999) Multi-Institutional Study of the Angiogenesis Inhibitor TNP-470 in Metastatic Renal Carcinoma. J Clin Oncol 17: 2541–2545.

44. Yanase T, Tamura M, Fujita K, et al (1993) Inhibitory effect of angiogenesis inhibitor TNP-470 On tumor growth and metastases of human cell lines in vitro and in vivo. Cancer Res 53: 2566–2570.

45. Fujioka T, Hasegawa M, Ogiu K, et al (1996) Anti-tumor effects of angiogenesis inhibitor 0-(chloroacetyl-carbamoyl) fumagillol (TNP-470) against murine renal cell carcinoma. J Urol 155: 1775–1778.
46. Morita T, Shinohara N, Tokue A. (1994) Anti-tumor effect of a synthetic analogue of fumagillin on murine renal carcinoma. Br J Urol 74: 416–421.
47. Kohn EC, Reed E, Sarosy G, et al (1996) Clinical investigation of a cytostatic calcium influx inhibitor in patients with refractory cancers, Cancer Res 56: 569–573.
48. Kohn EC, Felder CC, Jacobs W, et al (1994) Structure-function analysts of signal and growth inhibition by carboxyamido-triazole, CAI Cancer Res 54: 935–942.
49. Kohn EC, Liotta LA. (1995) Molecular insights into cancer invasion: strategies for prevention and intervention, Cancer Res 55: 1856–1862.
50. Fan Z, Baselga J, Masui H, et al (1993) Antitumor effect of anti-epidermal growth factor receptor monoclonal antibodies plus cis-diamminedichloroplatinum on well established A431 cell xenografts. Cancer Res 53: 4637–4642.
51. Masui H, kawamoto T, Sato JD, et al (1984) Growth inhibition of human tumor cells in athymic mice by anti-epidermal growth factor receptor monoclonal antibodies. Cancer Res 44: 1002–1007.
52. Prewett M, Rockwell P, Rockwell RF, et al (1996) The biologic effects of C225, a chimeric monoclonal antibody to the EGFR on human prostate carcinoma. J Immunother 19: 419–427.
53. Kawamoto T, Sato JD, Le A, et al (1983) Growth stimulation of A431 cells by epidermal growth factor: identification of high-affinity receptors for epidermal growth factor by an anti-receptor monoclonal antibody. Proc Natl Acad Sci USA 80: 1337–1341.
54. Rowinsky EK (2001) Signal transduction inhibitors. Horizons in cancer therapeutics. 2: 3–35.
55. Mendelsohn J, (2000) Blockade of receptors for growth factors: an anticancer therapy: the fourth annual Joseph H. Burchenal American Association for Cancer Research Clinical Research Clinical Award Lecture. Clin Cancer Res 6: 747–752.
56. Huang SM, Bock JM, Harari PM. (1999) Epidermal growth factor receptor blockade with C225 modulates proliferation, apoptosis, and radio-sensitivity in squamous cell carcinoma of the head and neck. Cancer Res 59: 1935–1940.
57. Shin DM, Donato NJ, Perez-Soler R, et al (2001) Epidermal growth factor receptor-targeted therapy with C225 and cisplatin in patients with head and neck cancer. Clin Cancer Res 7: 1204–1213.
58. Baselga J, Pfister D, Cooper MR, et al (2000) Phase I studies of anti-epidermal growth factor receptor chimeric antibody C225 alone and in combination with cisplatin. J Clin Oncol 18: 904–914.
59. Gunnett K, Motzer R, Amato R, et al (1999) Phase II study of anti-epidermal growth factor receptor antibody C225 alone in patients with metastatic renal cell carcinoma. Proc Am Soc Clin Oncol 18: 340a; A1309.
60. Yang XD, Jia XC, Corvalan JR, et al (1999) Eradication of established tumors by a fully human monoclonal antibody to the epidermal growth factor receptor without concomitant chemotherapy. Cancer Res 59: 1236–1243.
61. Figlin RA, Belldegun A, Lohner ME (2001) ABX-EGF: A fully humanized anti-EGF receptor antibody in patients with advanced cancer. Proc Am Soc Clin Oncol 20: 276a; A1102.
62. Schwartz G, Dutcher JP, Vogelzang NJ, et al (2002) Phase 2 clinical trial evaluating the safety and effectiveness of ABX-EGF in renal cell cancer (RCC) Proc Am Soc Clin Oncol 21: 24a; A91.
63. Woodburn J, Kendrew J, Fennel M (2000) ZD1839 ("Iressa") a selective epidermal growth factor receptor tyrosine kinase inhibitor (EGFR-TKI): inhibitor of c-fos mRNA, an intermediate marker of EGFR activation, correlates with tumor growth inhibition. Proc Am Assoc Cancer Res 41: 402; A2552.
64. Ciardiello F, Caputo R, Bianco R, et al (2001) Inhibition of growth factor production and angiogenesis in human cancer cells by ZD1839 (Iressa), a selective epidermal growth factor receptor tyrosine kinase inhibitor. Clin Cancer Res 7: 1459–1465.
65. Ranson M, Hammond L, Ferry D, et al (2002) ZD1839 a selective oral epidermal growth factor receptor—tyrosine kinase inhibitor, is well tolerated and active in patients with solid malignant tumors: results of a phase I trial. J Clin Oncol 20: 2240–2250.
66. Baselga J, Herbst R, LoRusso P, et al (2000) Continuous administration of ZD1839 (Iressa), a novel oral epidermal growth factor receptor tyrosine kinase inhibitor, in patients with five selected tumor types; evidence of activity and good tolerability. Proc Am Soc Clin Oncol 19: 177a; A 686.
67. Goss GD, Hirte H, Lorimer I, et al (2001) Final results of the dose escalation phase of a phase I pharmacokinetics, pharmacodynamic and biological activity study of ZD1839: NCIC CTG IND, 122. Proc Am Soc Clin Oncol. 20: 85a; A 335.

68. Hammond LA, Figueroa J, Schwartzberg L, et al (2001) Feasibility and pharmacokinetic trial of ZD1839 (Iressa), an epidermal growth factor receptor tyrosine kinase inhibitor, in combination with 5-fluorouracil and leucovorin in patients with advanced colorectal cancer. Proc Am Soc Clin Oncol. 20: 137a; A 544.

69. Miller VA, Johnson D, Heelan RT, et al (2001) A pilot trial demonstrates the safety of ZD1839 (Iressa), an oral epidermal growth factor receptor tyrosine kinase inhibitor, in combination with carboplatin and paclitaxel in previously untreated advanced non-small cell lung cancer. Proc Am Soc Clin Oncol 20: 326a; A1301.

70. Hidalgo M, Siu LL, Nemunaitis J, et al (2001) Phase I and pharmacologic study of OSI-774, an epidermal growth factor receptor tyrosine kinase inhibitor in patients with advanced solid malignancies. J Clin Oncol 19: 3267–3279.

71. Yamaguchi H, Paranawithana SR, Lee MW, et al (2002) Epothilone B Analogue (BMS-247550)-Mediated Cytotoxicity through Induction of Bax Conformational Change in Human Breast Cancer Cells. Cancer Res 62: 466–471.

72. Lee FYF, Borzilleri R, Fairchild CR, et. Al. (2001) BMS-247550: A Novel Epothilone Analog with a Mode of Action Similar to Paclitaxel but Possessing Superior Anti-tumor Efficacy Clin Cancer Res 7: 1429–1437.

73. Hidalgo M, Rowinsky EK. (2000) The rapamycin-sensitive signal transduction pathway as a target for cancer therapy. Oncogene. 19: 6680–6686.

74. Mills GB, Lu Y, Kohn EC (2001) Linking molecular therapeutics to molecular diagnostics: Inhibition of the FRAP/RAFT/TOR component of the P13K pathway preferentially blocks PTEN mutant cells in vitro and in vivo. Proc Natl Acad Sci 98: 10031–10033.

75. Atkins MB, Hidalgo M, Stadler W, et al (2002) A randomized double-blind phase 2 study of intravenous CCI-779 administered weekly to patients with advanced renal cell carcinoma. Proc Am Soc Clin Oncol. 21: 10a; A36.

INDEX